Cancer-Associated Thrombosis

New Findings in Translational Science, Prevention, and Treatment

Edited by

Alok A. Khorana

University of Rochester
Rochester, New York, USA

Charles W. Francis

University of Rochester
Rochester, New York, USA

informa
healthcare

New York London

Informa Healthcare USA, Inc.
52 Vanderbilt Avenue
New York, NY 10017

Printed in the United States of America on acid-free paper
10 9 8 7 6 5 4 3 2 1

International Standard Book Number-10: 1-4200-4799-X (Hardcover)
International Standard Book Number-13: 978-1-4200-4799-8 (Hardcover)

Library of Congress Cataloging-in-Publication Data

Cancer-associated thrombosis : new findings in translational science, prevention, and treatment / edited by Alok A. Khorana, Charles W. Francis.
p. ; cm.
Includes bibliographical references and index.
ISBN-13: 978-1-4200-4799-8 (hardcover : alk. paper)
ISBN-10: 1-4200-4799-X (hardcover : alk. paper)
1. Thrombosis. 2. Cancer--Complications. I. Khorana, Alok A. II. Francis, Charles W.
[DNLM: 1. Venous Thrombosis--etiology. 2. Venous Thrombosis--prevention & control. 3. Anticoagulants--therapeutic use. 4. Heparin--therapeutic use. 5. Neoplasms--complications. 6. Risk Factors. WG 610 C215 2007]

RC394.T5C36 2007
616.99'4--dc22 2007020502

Visit the Informa Web site at
www.informa.com

and the Informa Healthcare Web site at
www.informahealthcare.com

To my parents:
Anand B. Khorana and Suman A. Khorana
from whom I first learned medicine, and scholarship.
A. A. K.

To my wife, Anne, for her support and advice.
C.W.F.

Foreword

As we achieved senior professorial status, we have both been referred to by some of our esteemed colleagues as the "grandfathers" of the modern field of cancer and thrombosis—perhaps a dubious distinction indicative more of our collective ages than our collective wisdom—but at least we now get the privilege of being asked by the editors of this impressive volume to look back and provide perspective.

When we got together in 1971, to plan the first randomized controlled trial of an anticoagulant for the adjuvant treatment of cancer (VA Cooperative Study #75), we had no idea how this crossover area of research would grow over the next 36 years. However, we also could not have predicted that in spite of a positive result in that first trial (the patients with small cell lung cancer, who received warfarin in addition to traditional chemotherapy, lived significantly longer than the control group, who received chemotherapy alone), it would take another 26 years for the concept to truly enter the consciousness of the clinical oncology community. Indeed, most oncologists would probably say that thrombosis is still far from being a mainstream issue in the clinical practice of oncology, and most tumor biologists have yet to embrace the notion that the activation of clotting is intrinsic to the process of tumorigenesis. Nevertheless, with the publication over the past several years of the results of several randomized controlled trials to test the hypothesis that low-molecular-weight heparin (LMWH) can prolong survival in patients with cancer, it would certainly appear that a tacit understanding now exists regarding the importance to the biology of neoplasia of heparin-sensitive reactions.

While the efficacy of various preparations of LMWH in cancer survival may or may not be related to the anticoagulant properties of these compounds, the results of these clinical trials have reawakened interest in the basic concept that hemostasis plays an important role in cancer, perhaps beyond thrombogenesis. In the current volume dedicated to this topic, Khorana and Francis have assembled an "all-star" cast to address the various aspects of this intriguing relationship, from basic epidemiology and the molecular biology of oncogenesis, to an up-to-date assessment of clinical trials of anticoagulant drugs.

It was the great diagnostician from Paris, Professor Armand Trousseau, who in his lecture to the New Syndeham Society of London in 1865 first drew our attention to the phenomenon of *phlegmasia alba dolens* (migratory thrombophlebitis) as a harbinger of an occult cancer. His observation that "There appears in the cachexiae …a particular condition of the blood that predisposes it to spontaneous coagulation…" made it clear that cancer patients are hypercoagulable. Ever since that remarkable lecture we, the disciples of Trousseau, have been trying to refine his observations and use them to understand better the pathophysiology of thrombosis in cancer. We now understand that activation of clotting occurs in response to the genetic program(s) that govern the process of neoplastic transformation, at least in experimental tumor systems such as those described in this volume by Boccaccio and colleagues. Furthermore, we have discovered that key signaling reactions are shared by growing tumor cells and hemostatic pathways, further refining the picture of an intimate association between the development of cancer and the use of clotting as a host defense mechanism. As our knowledge of the importance of one or more of these oncogene-driven signaling pathways of individual tumors expands, it seems likely that drugs will be designed to target for inhibition of both thrombus formation and tumor growth. In the meantime, the various aspects of the overlap between cancer biology and clotting biology reviewed in this text may explain in part how systemic anticoagulation appears to inhibit tumor growth and should stimulate the design and implementation of new clinical trials to test this paradigm in individual tumor types. We share the enthusiasm of the editors of this volume, who have done us all a service by pushing this important field forward.

Frederick R. Rickles, MD, FACP
Noblis, Falls Church, Virginia, and the George Washington University, Washington, D.C., U.S.A.

Leo R. Zacharski, MD
VA Medical Center, White River Jct, Vermont, and the Dartmouth Medical School, Hanover, New Hampshire, U.S.A.

Preface

The study of hemostasis in cancer is an exciting area of research that involves investigators from disparate fields including molecular biology, hematology, oncology, and epidemiology. The results of investigations in this area have direct implications for cancer patients and their providers, including medical and surgical oncologists, hematologists, internists, and hospitalists.

The field has seen an explosion of research in recent years. Five developments are particularly noteworthy. First, we understand more fully that the coagulation cascade is inextricably linked with tumor biologic processes, in particular tumor angiogenesis, and that the hypercoagulable state is under oncogene regulation. Tissue factor is an excellent example of this linkage, and its importance in both thrombosis and angiogenesis in cancer is being increasingly recognized. Second, the burden of cancer-associated thrombosis has been increasing since the late 1990s and likely will continue to rise with the advent of anti-angiogenic therapy. Oncologists in particular have become more aware of this problem because of the vascular toxicity of regimens containing anti-angiogenic drugs. Third, we are able to identify risk factors predictive of cancer-associated thrombosis; this enhances the clinician's ability to stratify patients and develop effective prophylaxis strategies. Fourth, low-molecular-weight heparins are playing an increasingly important role in both prevention and treatment of this illness. These drugs appear to be more effective than older anticoagulants and may also impact tumor outcomes and survival in cancer patients. Other new anti-thrombotics are in development as well. Finally, two major United States cancer panels—the American Society of Clinical Oncology (ASCO) VTE Guidelines Panel and the National Comprehensive Cancer Network Practice Guidelines on Venous Thromboembolic Disease—are in the midst of releasing guidelines on this subject. These represent the first guidelines on this topic issued by the US oncology community and reflect the increasing need for guidance in treating this difficult illness.

In this book we present a synthesis of this new literature and place it in its proper context. We are pleased that all of the chapters are written by internationally renowned experts in their respective fields, including the co-chairs and many other members of the ASCO VTE Guidelines Panel. Together, these authors have collaborated to provide a comprehensive, balanced, and thought-provoking perspective on state-of-the-art research in this area. In addition, the authors have provided executive summaries highlighted in a box at the beginning of each chapter. We hope these will provide a useful reference tool for practitioners and that this book will be of interest not only to hematologists and oncologists but also to internists, surgeons, hospitalists and midlevel providers, all of whom provide care to the many cancer patients with thromboembolism.

Alok A. Khorana
Charles W. Francis

Contents

Contributors

Giancarlo Agnelli Division of Internal and Cardiovascular Medicine—Stroke Unit, Department of Internal Medicine, University of Perugia, Perugia, Italy

M. E. Belderbos Department of Medical Oncology, Johns Hopkins Medical Institutions, Baltimore, Maryland, U.S.A.

J. W. Blom Department of Public Health and Primary Care, Leiden University Medical Center, Leiden, The Netherlands

Carla Boccaccio Institute for Cancer Research and Treatment (IRCC), University of Turin Medical School, Torino, Italy

Lubor Borsig University of Zürich, Zürich, Switzerland

Paolo M. Comoglio Institute for Cancer Research and Treatment (IRCC), University of Turin Medical School, Torino, Italy

Jay L. Degen Division of Developmental Biology, Cincinnati Children's Hospital Research Foundation, and University of Cincinnati College of Medicine, Cincinnati, Ohio, U.S.A.

C. J. M. Doggen Department of Clinical Epidemiology, Leiden University Medical Center, Leiden, The Netherlands

Anna Falanga Hematology Division, Ospedali Riuniti di Bergamo, Bergamo, Italy

Charles W. Francis James P. Wilmot Cancer Center and the Department of Medicine, University of Rochester, Rochester, New York, U.S.A.

Sylvia Haas Institut für Experimentelle Onkologie und Therapieforschung, Technische Universität München, Munich, Germany

Ajay Kakkar Centre for Surgical Sciences, Institute of Cancer, Barts and the London Queen Mary's School of Medicine and Dentistry, and Thrombosis Research Institute, London, U.K.

Alok A. Khorana James P. Wilmot Cancer Center and the Department of Medicine, University of Rochester, Rochester, New York, U.S.A.

Nicole M. Kuderer Department of Medicine, Duke University and the Duke Comprehensive Cancer Center, Durham, North Carolina, U.S.A.

Agnes Y. Y. Lee Department of Medicine, McMaster University, Hamilton, Ontario, Canada

Howard A. Liebman Division of Hematology, Department of Medicine, University of Southern California Keck School of Medicine and the Kenneth J. Norris, Jr. Comprehensive Cancer Center, Los Angeles, California, U.S.A.

Gary H. Lyman Department of Medicine, Duke University and the Duke Comprehensive Cancer Center, Durham, North Carolina, U.S.A.

Marina Marchetti Hematology Division, Ospedali Riuniti di Bergamo, Bergamo, Italy

Aidan McManus Thrombosis Research Institute, London, U.K.

Eric S. Mullins Divisions of Hematology/Oncology, Cincinnati Children's Hospital Research Foundation, and University of Cincinnati College of Medicine, Cincinnati, Ohio, U.S.A.

Joseph S. Palumbo Divisions of Hematology/Oncology, Cincinnati Children's Hospital Research Foundation, and University of Cincinnati College of Medicine, Cincinnati, Ohio, U.S.A.

Gloria Petralia Centre for Surgical Sciences, Institute of Cancer, Barts, and the London Queen Mary's School of Medicine and Dentistry, and Thrombosis Research Institute, London, U.K.

A. Piccioli Department of Medical and Surgical Sciences, University of Padua, Padua, Italy

R. Pili Department of Medical Oncology, Johns Hopkins Medical Institutions, Baltimore, Maryland, U.S.A.

H. M. Pinedo Department of Medical Oncology, VU Medical Center, Amsterdam, The Netherlands

P. Prandoni Department of Medical and Surgical Sciences, University of Padua, Padua, Italy

Maithili V. Rao James P. Wilmot Cancer Center and the Department of Medicine, University of Rochester, Rochester, New York, U.S.A.

F. R. Rosendaal Department of Clinical Epidemiology, Hemostasis and Thrombosis Research Center, Leiden University Medical Center, Leiden, The Netherlands

Wolfram Ruf Department of Immunology, The Scripps Research Institute, La Jolla, California, U.S.A.

Jennifer L. Stevenson University of California, San Diego, California, U.S.A.

Mark B. Taubman Department of Medicine and Cardiovascular Research Institute, University of Rochester, Rochester, New York, U.S.A.

Ajit Varki University of California, San Diego, California, U.S.A.

H. M. W. Verheul Department of Medical Oncology, University Medical Center Utrecht, Utrecht, The Netherlands, and Department of Medical Oncology, Johns Hopkins Medical Institutions, Baltimore, Maryland, U.S.A.

Melina Verso Division of Internal and Cardiovascular Medicine—Stroke Unit, Department of Internal Medicine, University of Perugia, Perugia, Italy

Ilene Weitz Division of Hematology, Department of Medicine, University of Southern California Keck School of Medicine and the Kenneth J. Norris, Jr. Comprehensive Cancer Center, Los Angeles, California, U.S.A.

Richard H. White Department of Internal Medicine, Division of General Medicine, University of California, Davis, Sacramento, California, U.S.A.

Ted Wun Department of Internal Medicine, Division of Hematology and Oncology, University of California, Davis, Sacramento, California, U.S.A.

1

Oncogenes, Cancer, and Hemostasis

Carla Boccaccio and Paolo M. Comoglio
Institute for Cancer Research and Treatment (IRCC),
University of Turin Medical School, Torino, Italy

- Hemostatic activation is controlled at a genetic level, likely as an adaptive response, and provides a growth advantage to tumors.
- Three different experimental models provide complementary evidence that genetic lesions commonly associated with human tumors modulate the expression of genes controlling hemostasis.
- Activation of the *MET* oncogene leads to a thrombohemorrhagic syndrome in a model of hepatocellular carcinoma, in association with upregulation of plasminogen activator inhibitor-1 and cyclooxygenase-2.
- Mutations in *EGFR*, *RAS* oncogenes, and tumor-suppressor genes *P53* and *PTEN* are associated with upregulation of tissue factor, which in turn is associated with hemostatic activation as well as angiogenesis.
- Hemostasis proteins expressed as a result of specific genetic mutations may cause protumorigenic effects independent of hemostatic activation.
- Hemostasis proteins may serve as novel targets for therapeutic intervention in malignancy.

CANCER GENES, CELLS, AND THEIR MICROENVIRONMENT

The prevailing molecular theory of tumors postulates that cancer is a genetic disease caused by mutations in genes belonging to three main families: oncogenes, tumor-suppressor genes, and stability genes. Oncogenes and tumor-suppressor genes encode proteins that regulate cell number in tissues; that is, the balance between cell increase (proliferation) and loss (apoptosis). Stability genes (often referred to as "caretaker" genes) encode proteins that maintain the integrity of the genome through the monitoring and repair of lesions (1). Each family includes an ample (tens) but defined number of genes. A tumor derived from a single patient usually contains alterations in multiple genes, combining members of the three families. It is believed that no single gene alteration is capable, alone, to drive the entire process of transformation of a normal cell into a fully malignant cancer cell (1). Cancer malignancy is indeed a complex phenotype characterized by multiple traits, which can be summarized as the ability (*i*) to autonomously increase in cell number, independently of extracellular signaling, (*ii*) to proliferate for an unrestricted number of cell cycles (so-called "replicative immortality"), (*iii*) to induce the formation of new vessels, and (*iv*) to trespass normal tissue boundaries. Tissue invasion is a prerequisite for the formation of secondary tumors in distant organs (metastasis) (2). In the last 10 years, experimental proof has been provided to support the old notion that, in the tumor mass, not all the cells are equal, and only a small cell subset is necessary and sufficient for the generation of the primary tumor and its metastases. These are called "tumor-initiating cells" or "cancer stem cells," by analogy with normal stem cells that are responsible for regeneration of tissues, either by default (such as in the bone marrow or epidermis) or on demand (such as in the nervous tissue) (3). Cancer stem cells divide, giving rise to two kinds of progeny: cells that replenish the cancer stem cell pool (that is, they self-renew and are endowed with replicative immortality), and cells destined to aberrantly differentiate into the heterogenous and nontumorigenic cell types of the tumor bulk. If unaffected by therapies, cancer stem cells cause tumor relapse, while their "differentiated" progeny, although numerically predominant, should be relatively innocent. The cancer stem cell paradigm predicts that this is the cell that accumulates genetic lesions responsible for cancer, and that this cell must be targeted by therapies in order to cure the patient (4,5).

In most cases, cancer patients do not inherit the genetic lesions responsible for the cancer phenotype from their parents. Instead, genetic alterations occur in their somatic cells as a result of chemical, physical, and biological agents, defined as carcinogens, which are endowed with the ability to mutate genes. Simplistically, the mutagenic property of carcinogens can be considered as the only direct cause of cancer onset and progression. In fact, carcinogens cause activating mutations of oncogenes (resulting in increased proliferation ability), and loss of function in tumor-suppressor genes and stability genes, resulting in insensitivity to antiproliferative stimuli, resistance to apoptosis, and predisposition to accumulate mutations. However, as it is well accepted that the cancer cell populations undergo a process of "Darwinian evolution" (6–8), we must take into account that genetic lesions responsible for cancer oncogenes are first "induced" by mutagens and then "selected" by environmental conditions (9). Some carcinogens act in a straightforward manner, because they provide both induction and selection of mutations. For instance, a mutagen such as ultraviolet light hitting the epidermis first causes extensive DNA mutation, which is followed by a blockage of cell proliferation (to allow DNA repair) and apoptosis of irreparably damaged cells. This fosters the process of tissue regeneration, favoring the emergence of clones where, by chance, mutations provide the ability to escape apoptosis and to circumvent growth arrest. In other cases, the action of the carcinogen is more subtle, and the development of neoplastic clones must rely on selection by environmental conditions independent of the carcinogen itself. Inflammation, associated with tissue damage and regeneration, is a well-known environmental condition that favors selection of cancer clones (10). The "tumor stroma," that is, the extracellular matrix and its associated cells provided by the host, and the "tumor parenchyma", formed by cancer cells, appear to share the responsibility for the outcome of the disease (11,12). The extracellular environment provides clonal selection, and modulates angiogenesis, cell invasion, and metastasis, thus controlling tumor growth and spread independently of the genetics of the cancer clone. In turn, cancer cells influence the structure and function of the stroma, by secreting signaling and structural molecules. As we discuss below, activation of the hemostasis process is one of the events that cancer cells cause to take place in their microenvironment, and it is likely an adaptive response controlled at a genetic level (Fig. 1). As such, it provides a growth advantage to tumors and emerges as a property that can be targeted in the frame of a multifaceted therapeutic approach to cancer (13).

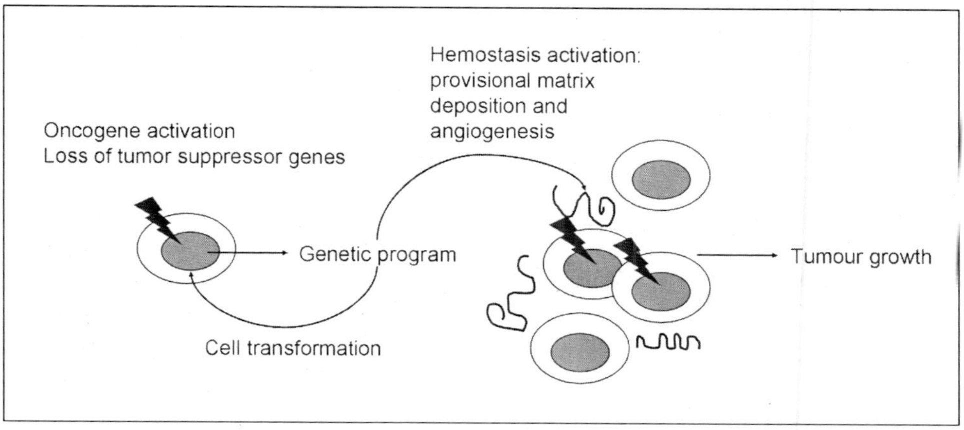

Figure 1 Cell transformation causes activation of hemostasis. Genetic lesions (such as oncogene activation and loss of tumor-suppressor genes) drive genetic programs responsible for cell transformation and for modification of the extracellular matrix, including hemostasis activation. In turn, hemostasis favors tumor growth.

CANCER AND BLOOD COAGULATION: TROUSSEAU'S SYNDROME

In 1865, the French clinician Armand Trousseau described the association between *thrombophlebitis migrans* ("a condition of the blood that predisposes it to spontaneous coagulation") and the presence of an occult malignancy (14). Since then, the term "Trousseau's syndrome" has been used to indicate the association of a blood coagulation disorder, mostly venous thromboembolism (VTE), with a cancer at any stage. Interestingly, the clinical correlation between cancer and VTE is two-way. On one hand, it has been demonstrated that cancer patients have a higher risk of developing a thrombotic event when compared to noncancer patients. On the other, idiopathic VTE can be the harbinger of an otherwise asymptomatic cancer, offering the chance for early diagnosis. Epidemiological studies indicate that the risk of developing a tumor is three to nine times higher in patients with idiopathic VTE than in patients with secondary VTE (15–17). Unfortunately, evidence suggests that when it is heralded by VTE, a tumor has a more severe prognosis than when it is not accompanied by coagulation disorders (18). However, although in some cases we might still be incapable of exploiting the anticipated diagnosis to cure or better treat the patient, it is clear that extensive cancer screening after VTE can uncover tumors in very early and completely attachable stages.

From a biological perspective, the association of VTE with incipient cancer is intriguing. It suggests that the ability to interfere with blood coagulation is an inherent property of cancer cells and/or their microenvironment, a property that can be functionally related to the onset of neoplastic transformation. Moreover, this early correlation suggests that the interference of cancer cells with blood coagulation could be progressive, and lead to overt hemostasis disturbances only in a subset of patients, possibly depending on host-derived predisposing factors. Therefore, even in the absence of overt coagulation disorders, there might be abnormalities in laboratory coagulation tests specifically associated with tumor onset. It might be possible to exploit these abnormalities for screening of early cancer. Thus it is important to identify the molecular pathways through which cancer cells affect the process of hemostasis. This could allow for the identification of specific markers for cancer diagnosis. Moreover, as discussed below, increasing evidence indicates that the procoagulant activity of tumors is not a mere epiphenomenon, but it is likely to be instrumental in tumor growth. Hence, understanding the mechanisms that support the procoagulant activity of cancer cells could uncover targets to fight both the secondary (VTE) and the primary (cancer) disease.

Investigation of the pathogenesis of Trousseau's syndrome has revealed a complex picture. It is likely that VTE results from the interaction between cancer cells and host factors. All the elements of the so-called "Virchow's triad" can simultaneously account for the prothrombotic state in the same cancer patient (19,20). These elements include: (*i*) *stasis of the blood*, due to extrinsic compression of blood vessels by the tumor or patient immobilization; (*ii*) *vascular injury*, which follows invasions of vessels by cancer cells, but also therapeutic interventions, such as insertion of a central venous catheter or administration of chemotherapy toxic to endothelial cells; (*iii*) *blood hypercoagulability*, mostly due to release of procoagulant molecules by cancer cells, to increased platelet aggregation and to adhesive interactions among tumor cells, endothelium, and blood cells (Fig. 2). In the following sections, within this ample spectrum of pathogenetic mechanisms, we will discuss in detail the direct effect of cancer cells on blood hypercoagulability. In particular, we will describe recent studies showing that oncogene activation upregulates genes controlling hemostasis in cancer cells.

In order to understand how cancer cells can interfere with hemostasis, it may be useful to briefly recall the key regulatory mechanisms of this process. The endothelium plays a central role in hemostasis regulation (21). In normal conditions, it actively inhibits hemostasis, while when damaged, it unleashes the process in order to stop bleeding. The endothelium modulates platelet adhesion and aggregation through the expression of several membrane-bound and soluble molecules. Among these, an important role is played by prostacyclin and

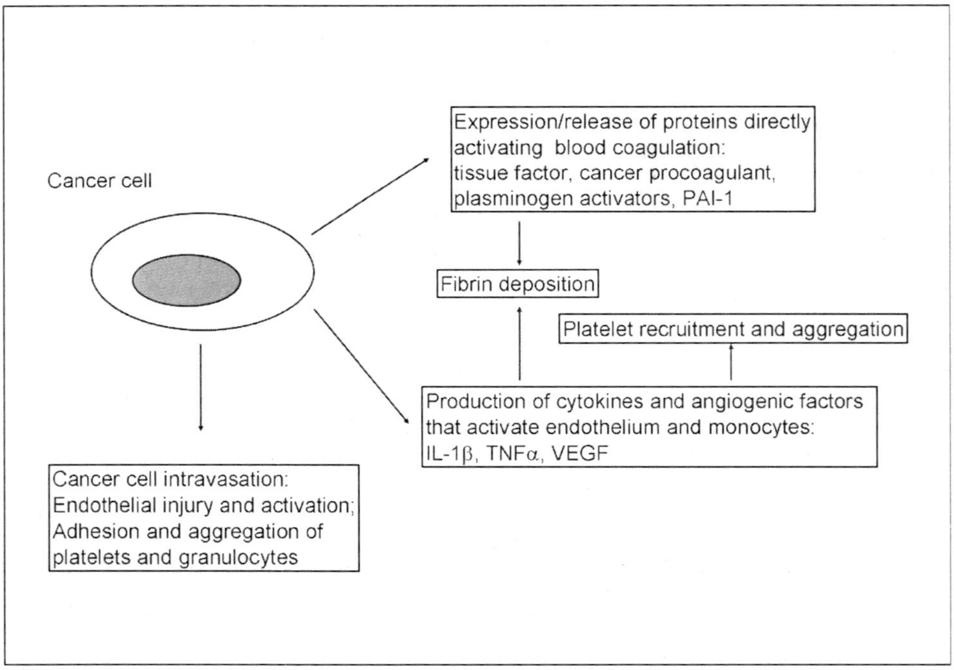

Figure 2 The procoagulant activities of cancer cells in the pathogenesis of Trousseau's syndrome. Cancer cells can interfere with blood clotting in three main ways, including: release of proteins directly involved in blood coagulation, release of cytokines modulating the activities of endothelial cells and monocytes, intravasation and mechanical endothelial injury.

thromboxane, which are derivatives of prostaglandins (PGs). These are synthesized from arachidonic acid through a multistep process that involves cyclo-oxygenases 1 and 2 (Cox-1 and Cox-2) (22). Injured endothelial cells express tissue factor (TF) on their membrane. TF is a receptor and a cofactor for the activation of coagulation factor VII, a circulating zymogen (precursor of a serine protease) that commonly initiates the blood coagulation cascade. The ensuing recruitment and sequential activation of other serine proteases (coagulation factors X, IX, VIII, and V) leads to the generation of thrombin. The latter catalyzes the conversion of circulating fibrinogen into insoluble fibrin, which is then further modified to form the fibrin–gel matrix. This matrix acts as a net, trapping platelets and blood cells, which results in the production of a blood clot. This clot seals the wound in the vessel wall and provides a scaffold for tissue repair (23,24). Blood clotting is counteracted by specific inhibitors at many steps in the coagulation process. Finally, when the injured vessel is repaired, the clot is removed by fibrinolytic enzymes, mostly plasmin. The latter derives from plasminogen, through the intervention of urokinase-type plasminogen activators (uPAs) or tissue-type plasminogen activators (tPAs). Generation of plasmin, and thus removal of the blood clot, is inhibited by plasminogen-activator inhibitors-1 and -2 (PAI-1 and PAI-2) (25).

ONCOGENES AND TUMOR-SUPPRESSOR GENES MODULATE THE EXPRESSION OF GENES CONTROLLING HEMOSTASIS

At least three different experimental models have provided complementary evidence that genetic lesions commonly associated with human tumors modulate the expression of genes that control hemostasis, such as *TF*, *PAI-1*, and *COX-2* (Fig. 3) (26–28). Most importantly,

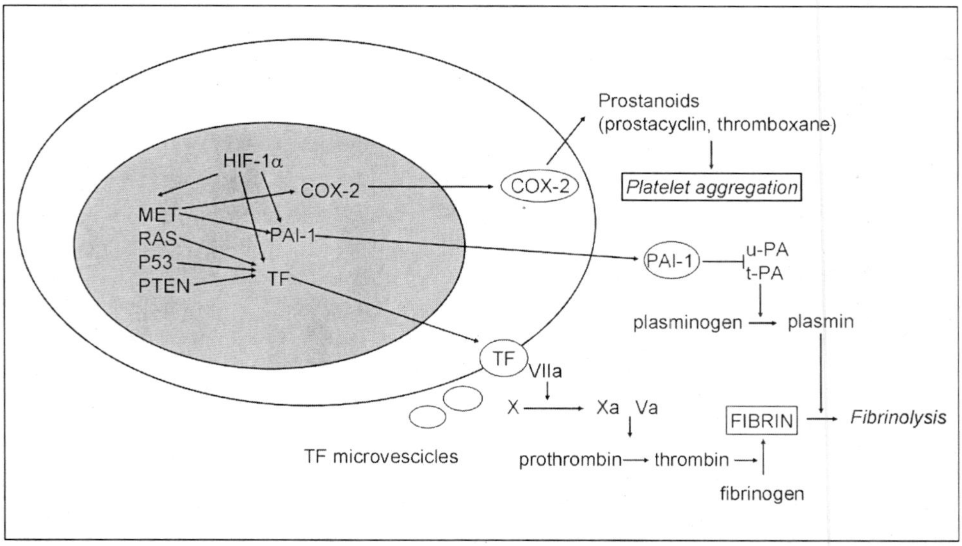

Figure 3 Oncogenes and tumor suppressors modulate the expression of genes controlling hemostasis. Oncogenic activation of *MET*, *RAS*, *p53*, or *PTEN* leads to transcriptional induction of genes involved in hemostasis regulation, including *PAI-1*, *COX-2*, and *TF*. HIF-1α is a transcriptional factor activated by low oxygen concentration (hypoxia), which frequently occurs in tumors. HIF-1α controls the expression of hemostasis genes directly, or through *MET*. The scheme illustrates the steps of hemostasis in which *TF*, *PAI-1*, and *COX-2* products are involved (for detailed explanation, see text). *Abbreviation*: HIF, hypoxia-inducible factor.

these studies show that hemostasis genes controlled by cancer genes play a functional role in tumor development, thus suggesting potential targets for tumor therapy.

MET Activation Upregulates PAI-1 and COX-2

The *MET* oncogene encodes the tyrosine kinase receptor for hepatocyte growth factor/scatter factor (HGF/SF). This receptor elicits a genetic program known as "invasive growth," which is physiologically activated in embryonic cells during gastrulation, and later during the development of striated muscle, and epithelial and nervous tissues. In adult tissues, *MET* is expressed by stem/progenitor cells, and the invasive growth program is activated so as to attain tissue regeneration and repair (29). During this process, stem/progenitor cells can be mobilized throughout the organisms by MET signaling. Pathological activation of MET and of the invasive growth program in tumors is likely to support invasion and metastasis of cancer stem cells (30). Interestingly, the ligand of *MET*, HGF/SF, shares several properties with the proteins of the coagulation system. In fact, HGF/SF contains structural motifs named "kringles" and a serine protease-like domain that are highly homologous to those found in plasminogen (see above). Moreover, like clotting factors, HGF/SF is released as an inactive molecule (pro-HGF) that must undergo a proteolytic cleavage to become biologically competent; this cleavage is performed by enzymes belonging to the coagulation system, including uPA, factor XII, and a factor XII-like (31). This means that the blood coagulation process results in the activation of HGF and thus of *MET*.

Oncogenic activation of *MET* is found in several types of human tumors. Point mutations, which can be sporadic or inheritable, as in the case of papillary kidney cancer, are relatively rare. In contrast, *MET* gene amplification or overexpression in the absence of structural alteration is quite common and is mostly associated with an invasive phenotype and poor prognosis (32). Interestingly, *MET* expression is upregulated by hypoxia-inducible factor-1 (HIF-1), a transcription factor activated by decreased oxygenation, a frequent occurrence in the inner tumor mass. Moreover, hypoxia and MET synergize in inducing the invasive growth program (33). As hypoxia upregulates a set of genes involved in tissue repair, angiogenesis, and blood coagulation (including the procoagulant proteins TF and PAI-1, see above) (34), it is likely that *MET* can amplify the biological response to hypoxia, sustaining the expression of the same genes.

Recently, we have developed a model of hepatocarcinoma by targeting an activated form of *MET* to the mouse liver (26). The oncogene was directly inserted into the genome of adult hepatocytes by means of a lentiviral vector driving expression through a hepato-specific promoter. This technology allowed the transformation of cells scattered through the liver parenchyma and development of dysplastic foci slowly progressing into overt hepatocarcinoma. Interestingly, the neoplastic process was preceded and accompanied by a biphasic thrombohemorrhagic syndrome. In the first phase, which started before the onset of detectable hepatocellular alterations and was highly reminiscent of Trousseau's syndrome, venous thrombosis and hyperactivation of the coagulation system occurred. In the second phase, the thrombotic disorder evolved into a disseminated intravascular coagulopathy, leading to exhaustion of the hemostatic system and lethal hemorrhages. In this phase, the mice displayed elevated blood levels of the fibrin degradation product d-dimer, a prolonged prothrombin time, and a significant reduction in the platelet count. The occurrence of a phenotype comprising a neoplastic process and a hemostatic disorder in association with a single, specific genetic lesion (the *MET* oncogene) offered the opportunity to investigate the genetic link between neoplastic transformation and the procoagulant activity of cancer cells. Genome-wide transcriptional profiling of hepatocytes expressing the activated *MET* oncogene showed a prominent induction of *PAI-1* and *COX-2*, together with an overall weak modulation of about 70 genes involved in hemostasis regulation. Interestingly, *PAI-1* and *COX-2* were the two most heavily induced genes within the entire gene set analyzed by the microarray. Consistently, both proteins were overexpressed in vivo in hepatocytes transformed by *MET*, and increased levels of PAI-1 and COX-2 products were released in the mouse blood.

Although the transcriptional profile offers an incomplete picture of the cellular events occurring after oncogene activation, overexpression of *PAI-1* and *COX-2* can provide an explanation for the *MET*-dependent thrombohemorrhagic phenotype. Interestingly, both enzymes have been implicated in both control of hemostasis and cancer progression. As mentioned, PAI-1 is a circulating protein with antifibrinolytic activity that can exert a systemic prothrombotic effect (25). This property is supported by the phenotype of PAI-1 transgenic mice, featuring venous occlusions (35), and by the finding that patients with high levels of plasma PAI-1 display increased risk of venous and artery occlusion (36). Interestingly, in cancer patients, elevated levels of PAI-1 have been correlated with tumor aggressiveness and poor prognosis (37). PAI-1 is supposed to foster cancer onset and progression mostly favoring angiogenesis (see below) (38,39). As mentioned, COX-2 catalyzes an intermediate step in the synthesis of lipid-derived signaling molecules such as prostacyclins and thromboxane, which are released in the blood and modulate platelet functions, and thus hemostasis (22). *COX-2* is well known as a critical gene in cancer development. Indeed, administration of COX-2 inhibitors (such as the nonsteroid anti-inflammatory drug Rofecoxib®) can prevent onset and progression of colorectal cancer (CRC), both in human patients and mouse models (40). As in the case of *PAI-1*, the involvement of *COX-2* in cancer has been associated with regulation of angiogenesis (41), cell invasion, and metastasis (see below). Studies in mice developing the *MET*-associated Trousseau's syndrome suggest that genes such as *PAI-1* and *COX-2*, directly controlled by *MET*, can be responsible for both the thrombohemorrhagic disturbance and the neoplastic process. In fact, administration of specific inhibitors of PAI-1 (XR5118) or COX-2 (Rofecoxib) prevented both laboratory and clinical signs of coagulopathy and, in the case of Rofecoxib, the drug also caused liver dysplastic nodules to regress by necrosis (26).

Mutant Epidermal Growth Factor Receptor, RAS, *p53*, and *PTEN* Loss Upregulate TF

Epidermal growth factor receptor (EGFR), also known as ERB-B1, is a tyrosine kinase receptor broadly involved in the control of cell proliferation (42). EGFR overexpression has been found in several types of cancers, especially from breast, lung, pancreas, and head and neck, often in association with aggressive behavior and poor prognosis (43). RAS proteins (encoded by *N-RAS*, *K-RAS*, or *H-RAS* oncogenes) are small GTPases that play a key role in the transduction of proliferative, motile, and antiapoptotic signaling generated by growth factor receptors, including EGFR, MET, and many others. RAS proteins control a complex network of downstream effectors, among which the RAF-mitogen-activated protein kinase (MAPK) cascade and the phosphatidylinositol 3-kinase (PI3K)-AKT pathway (see below) play a pivotal role in carcinogenesis. *RAS* genes are affected by activating point mutations in about 20% of human tumors, with the highest frequencies in pancreatic, thyroid, colorectal, and lung cancer (44). *p53* and *PTEN* are tumor-suppressor genes, critically involved in the control of apoptosis. p53 is a transcription factor that activates genetic programs leading to cell-cycle arrest, DNA repair, and apoptosis in the case of genetic and cellular damage, or aberrant proliferation (45). Loss of *p53*, which results in increased cell survival and accumulation of mutations, is found in about 50% of human tumors of any kind (46). PTEN is a lipid and protein phosphatase that negatively regulates the PI3K signaling pathway. PI3K is activated by growth factor receptors and stimulates cell proliferation and survival, through the protein kinase AKT. Thus, in the absence of *PTEN*, the antiapoptotic pathway regulated by PI3K is hyperactivated (47). *PTEN* is considered the second most commonly mutated tumor-suppressor gene after *p53*. Mutations of *PTEN* (as well as of other members of the PI3K pathways) are found in many cancer types, most frequently in glioblastoma, and breast, ovarian, and colon carcinoma (48).

Recent evidence shows that mutation of *EGFR*, *RAS*, *p53*, or *PTEN* can support the expression of TF, the main initiator of the blood-clotting cascade (see above), again providing a direct link between transformation and the procoagulant activity of cancer cells (27,28). As in the case of *PAI-1* and *COX-2* (the genes upregulated by the *MET* oncogene), TF expression correlates both with hemostatic disturbance in patients and with enhanced tumor angiogenesis and aggressiveness (49–51). As this correlation is present in CRC patients, Yu et al. investigated the connection between *TF* expression and the genetic status of CRC cell lines. Further, they studied the requirement of TF for the tumorigenic and angiogenic potential of CRC cell lines (28). The reported experimental model included (*i*) CRC cell lines DLD-1 and HCT116 (indicated hereafter as CRC cells), both bearing one mutant *K-RAS* allele and normal *p53* alleles; (*ii*) genetically modified CRC cells, engineered through homologous recombination so as to obtain inactivation of the mutated *K-RAS* allele (referred to hereafter as CRC-RAS$^-$ cells), or inactivation of both *p53* alleles (referred to hereafter as CRC-p53$^{-/-}$ cells). Thus CRC-RAS$^-$ are representative of an early stage of CRC progression, where *RAS* or *p53* are normal; CRC cells correspond to a more advanced stage of malignancy, characterized by *RAS* activation, and CRC-p53$^{-/-}$ represents an even more malignant stage, characterized by *p53* loss in addition to *RAS* activation. It was found that TF expression increases as cells accumulate lesions in *RAS* and *p53* genes, that is, as they progress toward a higher degree of malignancy. Interestingly, it was shown that although TF is an integral protein of the plasma membrane, CRC and CRC-p53$^{-/-}$ cells transplanted in mice generated levels of circulating TF proportional to TF expression on the cell membrane (which is higher in CRC-p53$^{-/-}$ than in CRC cells). The presence of TF in the blood was correlated to the shedding of TF-containing microvesicles from the cancer cell surface. It was then shown that, although CRC-RAS$^-$, expressing low levels of TF, were poorly tumorigenic in vivo, after transplantation in mice, these cells occasionally gave rise to tumors, which arose from genetically unstable cells. Interestingly, these tumorigenic cells had usually reacquired an activating mutation in a *RAS* allele and, concomitantly, reestablished high levels of TF expression. The functional role of TF in tumorigenesis was explored in HCT116 cell lines, expressing high levels of TF. These cells were engineered to express a small interfering RNA (siRNA) to silence TF expression. It was found that TF silencing, although not affecting the in vitro growth properties, prevented neoangiogenesis and tumor vascularization in vivo, thus inhibiting tumor formation by HCT116 cells. These findings imply that activation of TF, and possibly of the downstream blood clotting cascade, are required for efficient vascularization of tumors bearing activated *RAS*. The same study mentions that inhibitors of EGFR markedly decrease the expression of TF in the A431 cell line, bearing amplification of the *EGFR* gene, again supporting a direct correlation between oncogene and hemostasis activation (28).

In another recent work, Rong et al. studied the procoagulant activity of glioblastoma, a high-grade astrocytoma frequently causing a severe Trousseau's syndrome. Glioblastoma is characterized by the presence of hypoxic zones, including a central focus of intravascular thrombosis and necrosis, surrounded by a dense collection of neoplastic cells (pseudopalisading cells). Interestingly, these have been interpreted as a "wave of cells actively migrating away from a central hypoxic zone" (27). This aspect is suggestive of cells executing the invasive growth program elicited by the *MET* oncogene, which is upregulated by hypoxia and is indeed overexpressed in pseudopalisading cells (52). Another genetic lesion frequently found in glioblastoma is inactivation of *PTEN*. This lesion is considered a specific marker of high-grade malignancy, as it is absent in lower-grade astrocytoma. Therefore, the correlation between *PTEN* loss and the ability of cancer cells to cause a procoagulant activity (specific to glioblastoma patients) was investigated (27). In human glioblastoma cell lines with biallelic inactivation of *PTEN*, it was found that hypoxia increased the expression of transmembrane TF, as well as the release of TF in the culture medium. Consistently, in human histological samples of glioblastoma, hypoxic areas (pseudopalisading cells) were found positive for TF expression. The culture medium of hypoxic glioblastoma cells could promote plasma clotting in vitro, an ability that was strictly dependent on the presence of TF, as shown by inhibition of TF through neutralizing antibodies. Conversely, restoration of the *PTEN* gene in glioblastoma cells led to a significant decrease in TF transcription. Among the pathways negatively regulated by PTEN (see above), it was found that both PI3K-AKT and, although to a lesser extent, RAS-MAPK were responsible for TF induction (27). Thus, this study also supports a direct correlation between a genetic lesion (*PTEN* inactivation) associated with high malignancy on one hand, and activation of signaling pathways that upregulate transcription of TF on the other hand.

Although the studies by the groups of Yu and Rong do not provide conclusive proof that TF released by tumor cells is responsible for the hemostatic disturbance associated with Trousseau's syndrome, they convincingly show that TF is a transcriptional target of pathways (RAS and AKT) commonly activated in cancer. Moreover, Yu et al. provide strong evidence that TF is instrumental to tumorigenesis by supporting angiogenesis. This is an essential contribution to establishing the functional significance of hemostasis activation by cancer cells, and to elucidate molecules and mechanisms that can be targeted for tumor therapy.

A FUNCTIONAL ROLE FOR HEMOSTASIS GENES IN CANCER DEVELOPMENT

Tumors have been defined as wounds that never heal and therefore keep the mechanisms of tissue regeneration constantly activated (53). This observation likely reflects the fact that oncogenic events cause aberrant activation of genetic programs responsible for tissue regeneration. In this respect, *MET* is a paradigmatic gene as it is physiologically involved in epithelial morphogenesis during development, postnatal tissue regeneration, wound healing, and angiogenesis (29). Thus, it is conceivable that oncogenic activation of *MET* leads to constitutive activation of the above biological processes and development of "never healing wounds." Increasing evidence indicates that hemostasis is a crucial player in normal tissue regeneration, and thus of its pathological counterpart, tumor onset and progression. In the above section, we analyzed how cancer cells can affect blood coagulation. Here we will summarize the processes and molecular mechanisms through which hemostasis can favor tumor growth and progression (Fig. 4) (for a more detailed discussion, see the following chapters).

It is now well established that the hemostatic system regulates angiogenesis, which is the process of sprouting and organization of new blood vessels from preexisting vessels (54). In the case of common tissue injury, damaged vessels must be occluded rapidly in order to prevent hemorrhage. Thus, platelets are activated to adhere to the wound margins, and to form a provisional barrier that is quickly stabilized by deposition of a fibrin mesh. This clot rapidly reconstitutes the vessel wall and provides a scaffold for invasion by endothelial cells and for the rebuilding of the normal tissue. It has been suggested that

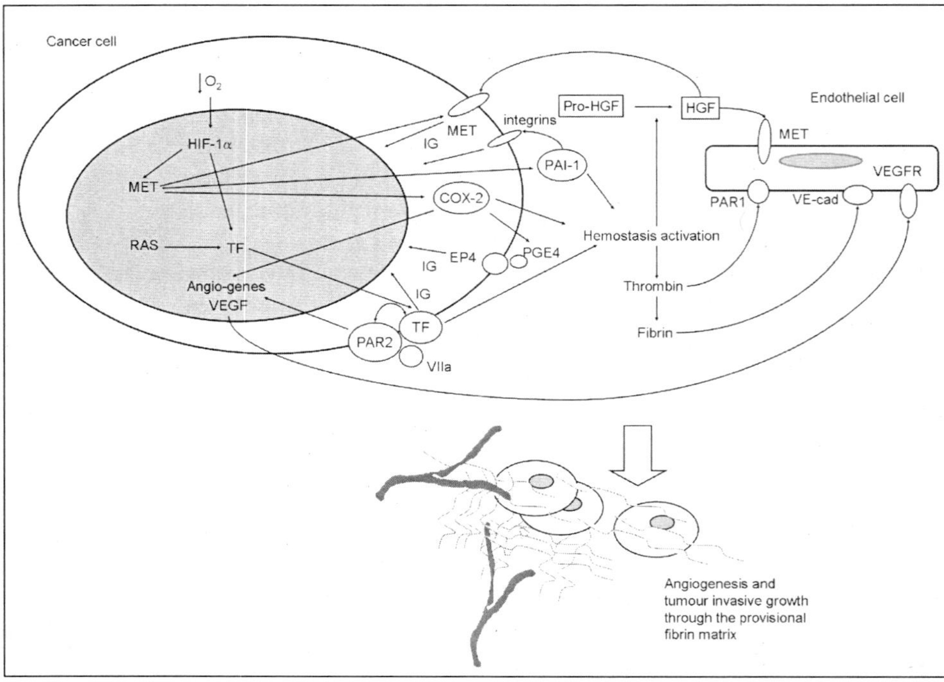

Figure 4 Hemostasis genes play a functional role in cancer development. *TF*, *COX-2*, and *PAI-1*, induced by oncogenes such as *MET* and *RAS*, and by hypoxia, stimulate hemostasis activation and fibrin deposition in the pericellular environment. Fibrin forms a provisional matrix that favors angiogenesis and supports cell adhesion and migration. Proteases activated during hemostasis activate HGF, the ligand of MET, which is expressed by endothelial and cancer cells. *MET* activation by HGF results in angiogenesis and cancer IG. TF and thrombin activate cell surface receptors (PAR), which transduce an invasive signal and upregulate the expression of genes involved in angiogenesis (angio-genes, including VEGF). COX-2 catalyzes the synthesis of prostaglandins that modulate platelet aggregation and of PGE_4. The latter binds cell surface receptors (EP4) that control cell invasion. PAI-1 modulates cancer cell adhesion through the stimulation of integrin recycling at the cell surface (for detailed explanation, see text). *Abbreviations*: HGF, hepatocyte growth factor; TF, tissue factor; PAR, protease activated receptor; IG, invasive growth; VEGF, vascular endothelial growth factor; PGE_4, prostaglandin E4; PAI, plasminogen-activator inhibitor.

proteins generated by hemostasis activation "coordinate the spatial localization and temporal sequence of clot/endothelial cell stabilization followed by endothelial cell growth and repair of a damaged blood vessel," therefore implying a direct role for hemostasis proteins in the control of angiogenesis (54). We can speculate that cancer cells that are able to unleash the hemostatic process (independently of vessel injury, or concomitantly with it during cancer cell intravasation) have a selective advantage, as they are more efficient in inducing the new vessels required to oxygenate and nourish the tumor mass. Consistently, hypoxia controls a set of genes, including *VEGF*, hemostasis genes, and *MET*, which enable cells to restore the vehicle of oxygen, i.e., blood vasculature.

Fibrin, the end product of the blood coagulation cascade, plays a prominent role in orchestrating vascular repair and angiogenesis. In fact, fibrin serves as a reservoir of growth factors, such as fibroblast growth factor, HGF, vascular endothelial growth factor (VEGF), and others, which bind fibrin directly or through the fibrin-associated heparin. Moreover, fibrin contains sequences that bind E-cadherins and integrins, thereby providing anchorage to endothelial cells and, possibly, to a wide variety of cell types (55). Interestingly, when angiogenesis is induced by cancer cells through aberrant activation of hemostasis and growth factor signaling, the resulting blood vessels are frequently abnormal in structure and permeability. These leaky vessels allow extravasation of fibrinogen and clotting factors, resulting in the activation of the coagulation cascade. This is followed by formation of fibrin deposits directly around the tumor cells (49,56). These deposits provide a quick-setting extracellular matrix offering anchorage and a support for migration to tumor cells. Interestingly, it has been shown that fibrinogen-deficient mice can permit growth and vascularization of implanted tumors, but not tumor metastasis (57). This suggests that the fibrin matrix is required for building an invasive trail and/or a "metastatic niche" in secondary sites. Moreover, fibrin can protect cancer cells from attack by the immune system (58).

As we have discussed in the previous paragraphs, blood clotting and production of fibrin can be unleashed or supported by cancer cells through different mechanisms. Interestingly, hemostasis proteins expressed as a result of specific genetic lesions (TF, PAI-1, COX-2) cause also protumorigenic effects that are independent of fibrin deposition and, in some instances, also of blood clotting activation.

TF plays a crucial role in angiogenesis during the development of the embryonic vasculature, as shown in *TF* gene knockout mice, which die around mid-gestation by impaired vascular integrity and abnormal development of the yolk sac (59,60). Interestingly, this phenotype largely overlaps that of embryos deficient for VEGF. Recent evidence indicates that TF, which is a transmembrane protein, behaves as a cellular receptor, capable of initiating transducing events ending in upregulation of genes that mediate angiogenesis, cell survival, adhesion, and migration (50,51). Signal transduction is elicited by binding of coagulation factor VII to the extracellular domain of TF, which is followed by activation of the short TF cytoplasmic domain. In this domain, a couple of serine residues become phosphorylated, possibly upon recruitment of membrane-associated kinases. Signaling downstream of TF is only partially known. Among classical pathways activated in cancer cells, TF induces p38, MAPK, and Rac-1, which appear to be responsible for TF-dependent cell migration (61). A peculiar mechanism of signal transduction elicited by TF involves protease-activated receptors (PARs). As a result of the activation process initiated by the TF/factor VIIa complex, coagulation proteases including factor VIIIa, FXa, and thrombin (see above) are recruited in the proximity of the cell surface and of PAR receptors. Cleavage of the PAR extracellular domain by coagulation proteases generates a tethered ligand that binds intramolecularly to the receptor and elicits cytoplasmic signaling. Factor VIIa appears to specifically cleave PAR2, while thrombin cleaves and activates PAR1, 3, and 4 (62). These receptors play a complex role in tumors, being expressed by cancer cells, but also by endothelial, inflammatory, and stromal cells, and by platelets (63). It has been shown that TF and PAR2 cross-talk in cancer cells, again playing the role of pivotal regulator of angiogenesis. In the resting condition, the cytoplasmic domain of TF inhibits PAR2. This inhibition is removed as a result of TF phosphorylation by protein kinase C, which, in turn, is activated downstream of PAR2. This allows full activation of PAR2 signaling, which leads to upregulation of genes involved in angiogenesis (64). TF/PAR2 signaling has been implicated also in protection from apoptosis induced by serum deprivation and loss of adhesion (65). We can conclude that TF fosters tumor growth by both environmental and cell-autonomous effects. The environmental effects include induction of the coagulation cascade ending in fibrin deposition, which is proangiogenic and proadhesive for tumor cells. The cell-autonomous effects elicited by TF are partly mediated by PAR2, which is expressed on the surface of cancer cells and activated by factor VIIa. These effects include the induction of genes that modulate angiogenesis, and two activities leading to invasive growth, such as cell motility and protection from apoptosis. Although TF is the orchestrator of the coagulation cascade and of PAR signaling, thrombin is also thought to play a predominant role in cancer, invasive growth, and angiogenesis. Much evidence suggests that through the activation of PARs, thrombin can modulate the properties of multiple cell types, including cancer, endothelial and inflammatory cells, and platelets. This results in the stimulation of cancer cell invasion and in the organization of a metastatic niche (63). Interestingly, it has been shown that treatment with the thrombin inhibitor hirudin does not suppress the growth of established tumors, but prevents metastasis and primary tumor implantation, which are critically dependent on the cell's ability to engraft in a new extracellular environment (66).

PAI-1 also seems to play a central role in cell invasion and metastasis (67,68). PAI-1 acts as part of an enzymatic system, which includes plasmin, plasminogen activators (uPA and tPA), and uPA receptor. The latter, expressed on the surface of epithelial and other types of cells, localizes plasminogen activation at specific pericellular sites. The resulting plasmin provides not only fibrin degradation but also activation of other proteases and direct digestion of several components of the extracellular matrices, thus favoring cell migration (67,68). The role of PAI-1 in cancer invasion is counterintuitive, as PAI-1 inhibits plasminogen activation, and thus extracellular matrix degradation. However, as discussed above, PAI-1, promotes persistence and expansion of the blood clot, which provides the proangiogenic and proadhesive provisional matrix. Moreover, it has been shown that PAI-1 binds vitronectin, a structural component of the extracellular matrix, thereby blocking the binding of cell surface integrins to vitronectin and promoting the detachment of several cell types from their substratum (69). It has been also found that PAI-1 promotes endocytosis of cell surface multimolecular complexes, which include uPA receptor, uPA, PAI-1, and several types of integrins. The endocytosed integrins can then recycle to the plasma membrane, where they can reengage their substratum (70). It has been proposed that, by this mechanism, PAI-1 stimulates dynamic cell adhesion and multiple cycles of attachment–detachment–reattachment, resulting in the promotion of cell migration, invasion, and metastasis (71). Finally, PAI-1 activity has been associated with the modulation of angiogenesis. In fact, growth and vascularization of tumor xenografts are compromised in *PAI-1* knockout mice, while they are increased in mice overexpressing *PAI-1* (38,39). However, the molecular mechanism(s) through which *PAI-1* regulates angiogenesis, and to what extent these mechanisms rely on the procoagulant effect of *PAI-1* or on its ability to modulate cell adhesion are still unclear.

COX-2 participates in the synthesis of prostanoids [PGE_2, $PGF_{2\alpha}$, PGD_2, thromboxane A_2 (TxA_2), and PGI_2], lipid-derived signaling molecules that are released in the extracellular environment and modulate the functions of several cell types, including platelets, endothelial cells, and cancer cells (21,22). In particular, COX-2 catalyzes the synthesis of intermediate prostanoids (PGG_2 and PGH_2) that are then transformed into final prostanoids by tissue-specific synthases (22). Although it is known that in endothelial cells, the activity of COX-2 mostly supports the synthesis of PGI_2 (also known as prostacyclins), which prevent platelet aggregation, the final outcome of COX-2 activation in cancer cells is largely unpredictable. In fact, besides PGI_2, TxA_2 can be produced, which promotes platelet aggregation. In any case, increased production of either PGI_2 or TxA_2 or both can cause the hemostasis disturbances associated with tumors having a high COX-2 expression. Recently, the prostanoid PGE_2 has received much attention as a prominent player in the protumorigenic activity of COX-2. Cellular effects of PGE_2 are mediated through the (EP) Prostaglandin E receptor family of G-protein–coupled receptors, including four members (EP 1–4), each characterized by the ability to activate a distinct intracellular signaling pathway. Interestingly, EP4, which is coupled to adenyl cyclase and cAMP production, signals also through MAPK and PI3K pathways, which are commonly activated by oncogenic signals and are known to support cell proliferation and invasion (72). Taking advantage of mice defective for EP receptor expression, and of specific inhibitors of EP receptor subtypes, it has been shown that these receptors, and in particular EP4, are involved in tumor invasion and metastasis, as they affect the motile behavior of cancer cells, their resistance to apoptosis, and, possibly, their sensitivity to killing by natural killer cells (73,74).

REFERENCES

1. Vogelstein B, Kinzler KW. Cancer genes and the pathways they control. Nat Med 2004; 10(8):789–799.
2. Hanahan D, Weinberg RA. The hallmarks of cancer. Cell 2000; 100(1):57–70.
3. Huntly BJ, Gilliland DG. Leukaemia stem cells and the evolution of cancer-stem-cell research. Nat Rev Cancer 2005; 5(4):311–321.
4. Clarke MF, Fuller M. Stem cells and cancer: two faces of eve. Cell 2006; 124(6):1111–1115.
5. Wicha MS, Liu S, Dontu G. Cancer stem cells: an old idea—a paradigm shift. Cancer Res 2006; 66(4):1883–1890.
6. Nowell PC. The clonal evolution of tumor cell populations. Science 1976; 194(4260):23–28.
7. Cahill DP, Kinzler KW, Vogelstein B, Lengauer C. Genetic instability and darwinian selection in tumours. Trends Cell Biol 1999; 9(12):M57–M60.
8. Merlo LM, Pepper JW, Reid BJ, Maley CC. Cancer as an evolutionary and ecological process. Nat Rev Cancer 2006; 6(12):924–935.
9. Blagosklonny MV. Oncogenic resistance to growth-limiting conditions. Nat Rev Cancer 2002; 2(3):221–225.
10. Coussens LM, Werb Z. Inflammation and cancer. Nature 2002; 420(6917):860–867.
11. Kalluri R, Zeisberg M. Fibroblasts in cancer. Nat Rev Cancer 2006; 6(5):392–401.
12. Mueller MM, Fusenig NE. Friends or foes—bipolar effects of the tumour stroma in cancer. Nat Rev Cancer 2004; 4(11):839–849.
13. Boccaccio C, Medico E. Cancer and blood coagulation. Cell Mol Life Sci 2006; 63(9):1024–1027.
14. Trousseau A. Phlegmasia alba dolens. Clinique Médicale de l'Hotel-Dieu de Paris. Paris: JB Ballière et Fils, 1865:654–712.
15. Rickles FR, Levine MN. Epidemiology of thrombosis in cancer. Acta haematol 2001; 106:6–12.
16. Prandoni P, Falanga A, Piccioli A. Cancer and venous thromboembolism. Lancet Oncol 2005; 6(6):401–410.
17. Prandoni P, Piccioli A. Thrombosis as a harbinger of cancer. Curr Opin Hematol 2006; 13(5):362–365.
18. Sorensen HT, Mellemkjaer L, Olsen JH, Baron JA. Prognosis of cancers associated with venous thromboembolism. N Engl J Med 2000; 343(25):1846–1850.
19. Dvorak HF, Rickles FR. Malignancy and hemostasis. In: Colman RW, Hirsh J, Marder VJ, Clowes AW, George JN, eds. Hemostasis and Thrombosis. Philadelphia: Lippincott Williams & Wilkins, 2005:851–873.
20. Rickles FR. Mechanisms of cancer-induced thrombosis in cancer. Pathophysiol Haemost Thromb 2006; 35(1–2):103–110.
21. Wu KK, Thiagarajan P. Role of endothelium in thrombosis and hemostasis. Annu Rev Med 1996; 47:315–331.
22. Smith WL, De Witt DL, Garavito RM. Cyclooxygenases: structural, Cellular, and Molecular Biology. Annu Rev Biochem 2000; 69:145–182.
23 .Dahlback B. Blood coagulation. Lancet 2000; 355(9215):1627–1632.
24. Mann KG. Biochemistry and physiology of blood coagulation. Thromb Haemost 1999; 82(2):165–174.
25. Collen D. The plasminogen (fibrinolytic) system. Thromb Haemost 1999; 82:259–270.
26. Boccaccio C, Sabatino G, Medico E, et al. The MET oncogene drives a genetic programme linking cancer to haemostasis. Nature 2005; 434(7031):396–400.

27. Rong Y, Post DE, Pieper RO, Durden DL, Van Meir EG, Brat DJ. PTEN and hypoxia regulate tissue factor expression and plasma coagulation by glioblastoma. Cancer Res 2005; 65(4):1406–1413.
28. Yu JL, May L, Lhotak V, et al. Oncogenic events regulate tissue factor expression in colorectal cancer cells: implications for tumor progression and angiogenesis. Blood 2005; 105(4):1734–1741.
29. Trusolino L, Comoglio PM. Scatter-factor and semaphorin receptors: cell signalling for invasive growth. Nat Rev Cancer 2002; 2(4):289–300.
30. Boccaccio C, Comoglio PM. Invasive growth: a MET-driven genetic programme for cancer and stem cells. Nat Rev Cancer 2006; 6(8):637–645.
31. Trusolino L, Pugliese L, Comoglio PM. Interactions between scatter factors and their receptors: hints for therapeutic applications. FASEB J 1998; 12:1267–1280.
32. Birchmeier C, Birchmeier W, Gherardi E, Vande Woude GF. Met, metastasis, motility and more. Nat Rev Mol Cell Biol 2003; 4(12):915–925.
33. Pennacchietti S, Michieli P, Galluzzo M, Mazzone M, Giordano S, Comoglio PM. Hypoxia promotes invasive growth by transcriptional activation of the met protooncogene. Cancer Cell 2003; 3(4):347–361.
34. Denko NC, Giaccia AJ. Tumor hypoxia, the physiological link between Trousseau's syndrome (carcinoma-induced coagulopathy) and metastasis. Cancer Res 2001; 61(3):795–798.
35. Erickson LA, Fici GJ, Lund JE, Boyle TP, Polites HG, Marrott KR. Development of venous occlusions in mice transgenic for the plasminogen activator inhibitor-1 gene. Nature 1990; 346:74–76.
36. Kohler HP, Grant PJ. Plasminogen-activator inhibitor type 1 and coronary artery disease. NEJM 2000; 342:1792–1801.
37. Look MP, van Putten WL, Duffy MJ, et al. Pooled analysis of prognostic impact of urokinase-type plasminogen activator and its inhibitor PAI-1 in 8377 breast cancer patients. J Natl Cancer Inst 2002; 94:116–128.
38. Bajou K, Noel A, Gerard RD, et al. Absence of host plasminogen activator inhibitor 1 prevents cancer invasion and vascularization. Nat Med 1998; 4:923–928.
39. McMahon GA, Petitclerc E, Stefansson S, et al. Plasminogen activator inhibitor-1 regulates tumor growth and angiogenesis. J Biol Chem 2003; 276:33964–33968.
40. FitzGerald GA. COX-2 and beyond: approaches to prostaglandin inhibition in human disease. Nat Rev Drug Discov 2003; 2(11):879–890.
41. Oshima M, Murai N, Kargman S, et al. Chemoprevention of intestinal polyposis in the Apcdelta716 mouse by rofecoxib, a specific cyclooxygenase-2 inhibitor. Cancer Res 2001; 61(4):1733–1740.
42. Citri A, Yarden Y. EGF-ERBB signalling: towards the systems level. Nat Rev Mol Cell Biol 2006; 7(7):505–516.
43. Nicholson RI, Gee JM, Harper ME. EGFR and cancer prognosis. Eur J Cancer 2001; 37(suppl 4):S9–S15.
44. Downward J. Targeting RAS signalling pathways in cancer therapy. Nat Rev Cancer 2003; 3(1):11–22.
45. Lowe SW, Cepero E, Evan G. Intrinsic tumour suppression. Nature 2004; 432(7015):307–315.
46. Hollstein M, Rice K, Greenblatt MS, et al. Database of p53 gene somatic mutations in human tumors and cell lines. Nucleic Acids Res 1994; 22(17):3551–3555.
47. Cully M, You H, Levine AJ, Mak TW. Beyond PTEN mutations: the PI3K pathway as an integrator of multiple inputs during tumorigenesis. Nat Rev Cancer 2006; 6(3):184–192.
48. Cantley LC, Neel BG. New insights into tumor suppression: PTEN suppresses tumor formation by restraining the phosphoinositide 3-kinase/AKT pathway. Proc Natl Acad Sci USA 1999; 96(8):4240–4245.
49. Fernandez PM, Patierno SR, Rickles FR. Tissue factor and fibrin in tumor angiogenesis. Semin Thromb Hemost 2004; 30(1):31–44.
50. Winter PC. The pathogenesis of venous thromboembolism in cancer: emerging links with tumour biology. Hematol Oncol 2006; 24(3):126–133.

51. Rak J, Milsom C, May L, Klement P, Yu J. Tissue factor in cancer and angiogenesis: the molecular link between genetic tumor progression, tumor neovascularization, and cancer coagulopathy. Semin Thromb Hemost 2006; 32(1):54–70.
52. Koochekpour S, Jeffers M, Rulong S, et al. Met and hepatocyte growth factor/scatter factor expression in human gliomas. Cancer Res 1997; 57(23):5391–5398.
53. Dvorak HF. Tumors: wounds that do not heal. NEJM 1986; 315:1650–1659.
54. Browder T, Folkman J, Pirie-Shepherd S. The hemostatic system as a regulator of angiogenesis. J Biol Chem 2000; 275(3):1521–1524.
55. Mosesson MW. Fibrinogen and fibrin structure and functions. J Thromb Haemost 2005 3(8):1894–1904.
56. Costantini V, Zacharski LR. Fibrin and cancer. Thromb Haemost 1993; 69(5):406–414.
57. Palumbo JS, Potter JM, Kaplan LS, Talmage K, Jackson DG, Degen JL. Spontaneous hematogenous and lymphatic metastasis, but not primary tumor growth or angiogenesis, is diminished in fibrinogen-deficient mice. Cancer Res 2002; 62(23):6966–6972.
58. Palumbo JS, Talmage KE, Massari JV, et al. Platelets and fibrinogen increase metastatic potential by impeding natural killer cell-mediated elimination of tumor cells. Blood 2005; 105(1):178–185.
59. Bugge TH, Xiao Q, Kombrinck KW, et al. Fatal embryonic bleeding events in mice lacking tissue factor, the cell-associated initiator of blood coagulation. Proc Natl Acad Sci USA 1996; 93(13):6258–6263.
60. Carmeliet P, Mackman N, Moons L, et al. Role of tissue factor in embryonic blood vessel development. Nature 1996; 383(6595):73–75.
61. Ott I, Weigand B, Michl R, et al. Tissue factor cytoplasmic domain stimulates migration by activation of the GTPase Rac1 and the mitogen-activated protein kinase p38. Circulation 2005; 111(3):349–355.
62. Coughlin SR. Thrombin signalling and protease-activated receptors. Nature 2000; 407(6801):258–264.
63. Ruf W, Mueller BM. Thrombin generation and the pathogenesis of cancer. Semin Thromb Hemost 2006; 32(suppl 1):61–68.
64. Belting M, Dorrell MI, Sandgren S, et al. Regulation of angiogenesis by tissue factor cytoplasmic domain signaling. Nat Med 2004; 10(5):502–509.
65. Versteeg HH, Spek CA, Richel DJ, Peppelenbosch MP. Coagulation factors VIIa and Xa inhibit apoptosis and anoikis. Oncogene 2004; 23(2):410–417.
66. Hu L, Lee M, Campbell W, Perez-Soler R, Karpatkin S. Role of endogenous thrombin in tumor implantation, seeding, and spontaneous metastasis. Blood 2004; 104(9):2746–2751.
67. Sidenius N, Blasi F. The urokinase plasminogen activator system in cancer: recent advances and implication for prognosis and therapy. Cancer Metastasis Rev 2003; 22(2–3):205–222.
68. Durand MK, Bodker JS, Christensen A, et al. Plasminogen activator inhibitor-I and tumour growth, invasion, and metastasis. Thromb Haemost 2004; 91(3):438–449.
69. Stefansson S, Lawrence DA. The serpin PAI-1 inhibits cell migration by blocking integrin alpha V beta 3 binding to vitronectin. Nature 1996; 383(6599):441–443.
70. Czekay RP, Aertgeerts K, Curriden SA, Loskutoff DJ. Plasminogen activator inhibitor-1 detaches cells from extracellular matrices by inactivating integrins. J Cell Biol 2003; 160:781–791.
71. Stefansson S, Lawrence DA. Old dogs and new tricks: proteases, inhibitors, and cell migration. Sci STKE 2003; 2003(189):e24.
72. Fulton AM, Ma X, Kundu N. Targeting prostaglandin E EP receptors to inhibit metastasis. Cancer Res 2006; 66(20):9794–9797.
73. Mutoh M, Watanabe K, Kitamura T, et al. Involvement of prostaglandin E receptor subtype EP(4) in colon carcinogenesis. Cancer Res 2002; 62(1):28–32.
74. Ma X, Kundu N, Rifat S, Walser T, Fulton AM. Prostaglandin E receptor EP4 antagonism inhibits breast cancer metastasis. Cancer Res 2006; 66(6):2923–2927.

2
Hemostasis and Angiogenesis

Wolfram Ruf
Department of Immunology, The Scripps Research Institute, La Jolla, California, U.S.A.

- The hemostatic system, including coagulation proteases, fibrin, and platelets, influences multiple aspects of tumor angiogenesis.
- Expression of tissue factor by tumor or stromal cells renders the tumor microenvironment procoagulant due to local activation of extravascular plasma components following vascular endothelial growth factor (VEGF)-induced hyperpermeability.
- Matrix turnover, fibrin deposition, and degradation contribute to the immaturity of the tumor vasculature.
- Coagulation proteases through protease activated receptor (PAR) signaling upregulates key angiogenic regulators in the tumor microenvironment.
- Thrombin, plasmin, and matrix metalloproteinase 1 are potential activators of PAR1 on tumor or stromal cells.
- Tissue factor (TF)-VIIa activation of PAR2 may regulate tumor cell behavior as well as directly support host and stromal cell proangiogenic pathways.
- Platelets are a local source for angiogenic regulators and play a hemostatic role to seal the immature tumor vasculature.
- Hemostatic mechanisms contribute to endothelial cell barrier function and remodeling of the tumor vasculature to maintain functionality.
- Platelets and hemostatic mechanisms promote recruitment of proangiogenic progenitors to the tumor microenvironment.
- Coagulation inhibitors, proteases, and proteolytic fragments of hemostatic factors are key regulators of endothelial cell homeostasis.
- Pro- and antiangiogenic effects of the hemostatic system may be exploited for combination antiangiogenic therapy with other key angiogenic pathways.

INTRODUCTION

Cancer progression requires consecutive transformation events through which tumor cells escape proliferative checkpoint controls and regulatory cues from the extracellular milieu. In this process, tumor cells also acquire the ability to shape the tumor microenvironment for their survival advantage. Virtually, all clinically relevant carcinomas have undergone the "angiogenic switch" (1), i.e., developed mechanisms to sustain an appropriate blood supply for further tumor expansion. In principle, tumor cells utilize the same programs of angiogenesis that restore organ function after ischemic, mechanical, or microbial injury. Whereas regenerative angiogenesis typically progresses to restore a functional, organ-specific hierarchical vascular bed, tumor vessels retain various degrees of immaturity and tortuous architecture. Thus, tumor vessels have inconsistent directions of flow, imperfect vessel wall architecture including abnormal pericyte recruitment, and—most importantly for the current review—increased permeability and extravasation of blood plasma components.

Vascular endothelial growth factor (VEGF) is the major hypoxia-induced and tumor-derived cytokine that is responsible for angiogenic progenitor cell recruitment (2,3), endothelial cell proliferation and survival (4) as well as vascular hyperpermeability (5). Although VEGF-driven proliferation of tumor vessels is clearly beneficial for tumor expansion, the immature nature of the endothelial lining potentially exposes tumors to increased immune surveillance. However, tumor cells modulate immune responses by recruitment of immature dendritic cell and monocyte/macrophage populations that establish immunosuppressive cytokine networks. These antagonize antigen presentation and locally attenuate CD8-mediated, antigen-specific tumor killing (6). Moreover, immature myeloid populations and tumor-associated macrophages in the tumor microenvironment are increasingly appreciated as important facilitators of tumor metastatic niches and as local angiogenic regulators that support endothelial progenitors in neoangiogenesis (7). In addition to immune cells, the tumor environment is further shaped by reactive myofibroblasts that play important roles in the recruitment and retention of proangiogenic progenitors (8). As will be discussed in this review, both immune and mesenchymal cells are important participants in the interplay of the hemostatic system with angiogenesis.

Tumor and stromal cells express the initiator of the coagulation cascade, tissue factor (TF), which constitutes a strong procoagulant stimulus that activates coagulation factors extravasated from hyperpermeable tumor vessels (9). The deposition of fibrin is a well-characterized feature of the tumor stroma that enables functional cross talk of tumor and host cells. The hemostatic system not only shapes the tumor microenvironment but also organizes endothelial barriers by recruiting platelets at gaps in the hyperpermeable endothelium. This chapter will discuss pathways by which the hemostatic system regulates angiogenesis and contributes to endothelial homeostasis. These pathways show multiple synergies that may be relevant to sustain an immature angiogenic network with some degree of functionality. Conversely, regulatory mechanisms by which the hemostatic system controls angiogenesis are potential therapeutic modalities for antiangiogenic therapy.

COAGULATION ACTIVATION AND THE TUMOR MICROENVIRONMENT

Angiogenic regulators. The VEGF family of growth factors consists of several genes that undergo additional splicing to yield variants with distinct cell-surface and matrix-binding properties (10). VEGFA/vascular permeability factor is essential for developmental angiogenesis, signals through VEGF receptors 1 and 2, and thereby serves as the most important growth factor in the angiogenic switch induced by tumors. VEGF receptor 2 signaling achieves endothelial proliferation and survival. Targeting the VEGFA signaling pathways has proven to be of clinical antiangiogenic benefit, but other VEGF family members, such as placental growth factor (PlGF) (11), VEGFB, VEGFC, and VEGFD (12), may represent additional targets for tumor therapy. The VEGFC/VEGF receptor 3 axis regulates lymphangionesis (13) and expression of VEGFC in tumors establishes lymphatic routes of metastasis, for example, in breast cancer (14). VEGFA is frequently a component of regulatory networks by which other proangiogenic factors regulate tumor angiogenesis. Platelet-derived growth factor (PDGF) BB acts synergistically with VEGF to attract mural pericytes to stabilize neovessels (15,16). Pericyte recruitment is a highly dynamic process at endothelial sprouts and thus PDGF signaling is an accessory pathway that can be targeted to block angiogenesis (17). However, other growth factors or chemokines, such as basic fibroblast growth factor (bFGF) or interleukin (IL)-8, may compensate for loss of VEGF signaling (18) and thereby escape currently applied antiangiogenic therapy.

Angiogenic regulators are synthesized locally by tumor or stroma cells, including tumor-associated macrophages, or released from α-granules of activated platelets (19–21). However, these growth factors, chemokines, and cytokines have distinct molecular targets, a reflection of the complex cellular interactions that sustain tumor angiogenesis (Table 1). Several of the proangiogenic stimuli converge functionally in the recruitment of endothelial and hematopoietic progenitor population and tumor-associated macrophages. VEGFA gradients attract VEGF receptor 2 positive endothelial progenitors as well as VEGF receptor 1 positive hematopoietic, myeloid, and macrophage progenitors (7). The VEGF family member PlGF only activates VEGF receptor 1 and may thus play a more prominent role in the recruitment of certain progenitor populations (11). Motility and directed migration of progenitor populations is regulated by additional pathways. Stroma-derived factor-1 (SDF-1) is a CXC cytokine that is synthesized by stromal fibroblasts and endothelial cells. SDF-1 signaling through CXCR4 retains progenitor population in the tumor stroma (2,3). In addition, CXCR4 is upregulated in breast cancer cells and thereby reactive fibroblasts are involved in multiple cellular cross talks (8). The persistent activated state of myofibroblasts and the immaturity of myeloid populations determine by multiple pathways the overall character of pathological angiogenesis and of the tumor microenvironments as a "wound that does not heal."

Several cell types contribute to the procoagulant character of the tumor microenvironment. Local expression of TF activates a crucial axis in the cross talk of the hemostatic system and angiogenic mechanisms in the tumor microenvironment (Fig. 1). Hypoxia-induced VEGF secreted from tumor cells triggers TF expression in angiogenic endothelial

Table 1 Angiogenic Regulators

	Sources	Main functions
	Proangiogenic	
VEGFA	Tumor cells, platelets	Endothelial growth factor, hyperpermeability
VEGFC	Platelets	Growth factor, lymphangiogenesis
IL-8	Tumor cells, EC	CXC chemokine, TAM recruitment
bFGF (FGF-2)	Tumor cells, platelets	Growth factor, synergy with VEGF
PDGF	EC, platelets	Growth factor, pericyte recruitment
Cyr61, CTGF	Tumor cells, platelets	Cys knot angiogenic growth factor
	Antiangiogenic	
Thrombospondin	Platelets	Matrix protein, CD36 ligand
PF4	Platelets	CXC chemokine, heparin neutralizing
TGF-β	Fibroblasts, platelets	Antiproliferative growth factor
Angiostatin	TME, platelets	Plasminogen fragment
Endostatin	TME, platelets	Collagen XVII fragment

Abbreviations: VEGF, vascular endothelial growth factor; IL-8, interleukin-8; bFGF, basic fibroblast growth factor; PDGF, platelet-derived growth factor; CTGF, connective tissue growth factor; EC, endothelial cell; TME, tumor microenvironment; TAM, tumor-associated macrophages; TGF, transforming growth factor; PF4, platelet factor 4.

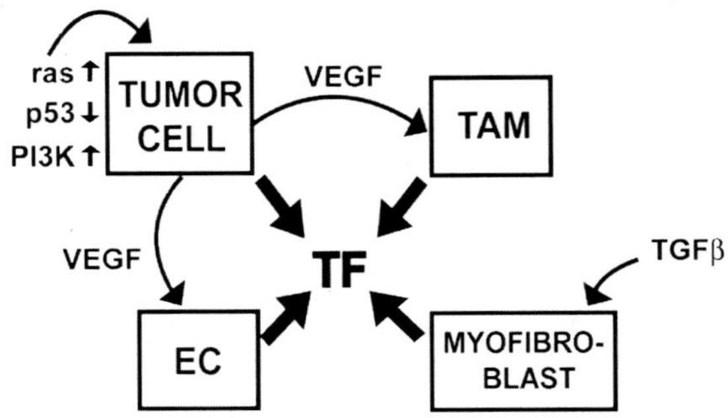

Figure 1 Multiple pathways converge to upregulate TF in the tumor microenvironment. VEGF produced by tumor cells not only triggers the angiogenic switch but also induces TF in ECs and monocytes that can mature into TAM. Transforming mutations in tumor cells and TGF-β activation of reactive myofibroblasts further contribute to local TF upregulation. *Abbreviations*: TF, tissue factor; VEGF, vascular endothelial growth factor; TAM, tumor-associated macrophages; TGF, transforming growth factor; ECs, endothelial cells.

cells and monocytes (22). Inflammatory cells further enhance endothelial cell TF expression by providing tumor necrosis factor that synergizes with VEGF to induce TF (23). However, tumor endothelium and tumor-associated macrophages are not the only TF-positive cell types in tumor tissues. Myofibroblasts and tumor cells stain positive to variable degrees (24,25). Tumor stroma myofibroblasts upregulate TF in response to transforming growth factor (TGF)-β stimulation (26). In tumor cells, transformation, including *ras* mutations and loss of *p53*, is associated with TF upregulation (27), and hypoxia induces TF in glioblastoma cells after loss of the tumor suppressor *PTEN*, a key regulator of the phosphatidylinositol-3 kinase pathway (28). Thus, nonoverlapping pathways on host and tumor cells produce sustained TF expression in the tumor microenvironment.

Role of fibrin in the tumor stroma. Coagulation activation in the tumor stroma leads to fibrin deposition, a key feature of the transitional extracellular matrix in tumors (24). Matrix interactions are important for localizing growth factors in order to establish concentration gradients that guide sprouting angiogenesis. Existing matrix may serve as "vascular memory," i.e., matrix guides the regeneration of vascular beads along existing basement structures after antiangiogenic therapy or vessel regression (29). Replacing an organ-specific, organized extracellular matrix by fibrin is a significant contributor to the immature and transitional character of the tumor microenvironment.

Fibrin stimulates angiogenesis by several mechanisms (30). Fibrin and fibronectin, which readily associates from the plasma with fibrin, serve as ligands for several integrins on tumor cells and angiogenic endothelial cells, thus orchestrating the dynamic interplay between tumor and host. Fibrin cooperates with activated platelets in the recruitment and differentiation of endothelial cell progenitors (31). The importance of coagulation activation in bone marrow–derived progenitor recruitment is further underscored by studies in which coagulation inhibitors were overexpressed at sites of vascular injury (32).

The β-chain sequence 15 to 42 binds heparin and vascular endothelial (VE)-cadherin and thereby regulates endothelial cell migration and tube formation. Fibrin particularly synergized with bFGF to promote angiogenesis (33). Fibrin recruits platelets through $\alpha IIb\beta 3$ that bind to RGD sites in the α-chain (Aα 572–575 and potentially 95–98) or

PAR2 signaling can induce similar cellular effects (71,87–89). PAR1 and PAR2 signaling also overlap in the ability to cross-activate the epidermal growth factor receptor to promote proliferation (90–92). Proangiogenic growth factors are upregulated by either PAR1 or 2 signaling in tumor or stromal cells, including IL-8 (54,55), VEGF (56), angiopoietin 2 (93), and the cysteine knot proteins Cyr61 and connective tissue growth factor (58,94,95).

Although PAR1 and 2 signaling show redundancy in the induction of proangiogenic mediators in tumor cells, it remains an important question which proteases are generated in sufficient concentrations to activate PARs in the tumor microenvironment. Protease coreceptors may further be expressed in a tumor-type specific manner and thus direct or amplify PAR signaling. Thrombin stimulates angiogenesis in certain angiogenesis models in vivo and PAR1 antagonists block these angiogenic responses (96–98). However, thrombin after binding to endothelial expressed thrombomodulin activates protein C. In turn, activated protein C (aPC) in complex with endothelial cell protein C receptor (EPCR) cleaves PAR1 of endothelial cells and PAR2 potentially on other cell types (99). The amount of local thrombin generation in combination with availability of the key receptors of the protein C pathway may determine whether thrombin activates PAR1 through direct cleavage or indirectly through the protein C pathway.

Importantly, PAR1 activation by thrombin and aPC/EPCR can produce opposing effects in endothelial cells exposed to inflammatory mediators (100). Direct thrombin signaling may produce apoptosis through upregulation of thrombospondin, whereas aPC/EPCR has profound endothelial protective, antiapoptotic effects (101). Indeed, aPC has proangiogenic properties in vivo (102,103). However, in certain tumor and angiogenesis models, coagulation inhibitors that target the upstream TF signaling complex have considerably higher potency compared to inhibitors to downstream coagulation proteases, which reduce thrombin and aPC generation (104). The complex contributions of PARs to tumor progression may result from nonredundant roles of PAR signaling on tumor versus host or stromal cells. It will be necessary to combine specific inhibitors, genetically engineered mice, and PAR-deficient tumor cell lines to clarify the proangiogenic effects of PARs and coagulation signaling complexes on host and tumor cells.

Role of direct TF signaling in angiogenesis. Evidence for a role of TF signaling in host cells came from the characterization of TF cytoplasmic domain–deleted mice that show deregulated angiogenesis (105). The complete knockout of TF had documented that the TF pathway maintains vasculature integrity in early embryonic development (106). Because PAR1 deficiency in endothelial cells showed a similar developmental phenotype (107), TF is likely upstream of vascular protective PAR1 signaling. In contrast, TF cytoplasmic domain–deleted mice have no developmental lethality. In postnatal mice, TF is expressed in the endothelium during inflammation and tumor progression (108,109). In mice that lack the TF cytoplasmic domain, we found significantly enhanced growth of TF-positive, syngeneic tumors. Because the tumor-expressed TF drives local thrombin generation, accelerated tumor development in mice that carried the TF cytoplasmatic domain deletion provided clear evidence for nonredundant and independent function of TF on host cells during tumor angiogenesis (105).

Angiogenesis in TF cytoplasmic domain–deleted mice was characterized by the in vitro aortic ring endothelial cell sprouting assay. These experiments showed that TF-VIIa drives PAR2-dependent angiogenesis specifically in the presence of PDGF BB. PAR2 deletion per se had little effect on angiogenesis. One possible explanation for normal angiogenesis of PAR2-deficient mice is a balanced signaling cross talk with the TF cytoplasmic domain. PAR2 signaling, but not PAR1 signaling, leads to TF cytoplasmic domain phosphorylation (110). Indeed, phosphorylation of the TF cytoplasmic domain was specifically observed in abnormal, proliferative neovasculature of the eye, whereas TF in normal vessels was not phosphorylated. Conceivably, dephosphorylation of the TF cytoplasmic domain may limit PAR2-dependent neovascularization, and hyperphosphorylation may lead to uncontrolled angiogenesis similar to that observed in TF cytoplasmic domain–deleted mice. Suppression of integrin α3β1-dependent migration is reversed by TF cytoplasmic domain phosphorylation (46) and integrin α3β1 has been shown to mediate antiangiogenic effects of tissue inhibitors of metalloproteinase 2 (111). In ongoing studies, we have validated in a relevant hypoxia-driven model that the proangiogenic phenotype of TF cytoplasmic domain–deleted mice is dependent on PAR2 and growth factor signaling pathways in vivo.

THE HEMOSTATIC SYSTEM AS REGULATOR OF ENDOTHELIAL HOMEOSTASIS (FIG. 2)

The hemostatic system participates in the dynamics of the tumor microenvironment by regulating angiogenic growth factor expression, cell proliferation, and matrix remodeling. These pathways may directly influence tumor cell proliferation, invasion, and metastasis. Examples for proliferative effects span from coagulation protease signaling through PARs to tumor cell stimulation by platelet-derived bioactive lipids, i.e., lysophosphatidic acid (112). Equally important for the mechanism of angiogenesis is the maintenance of endothelial functions by hemostatic mechanisms. The hemostatic system participates in the regulatory control of endothelial cell barrier integrity, apoptosis, and integration of signals that orchestrate the transit of cells and transmission of information across the endothelium.

Synergistic effects of hemostatic pathways on endothelial cell barrier function. Although VEGF results in upregulation of TF in endothelial cells, blockade of the VEGF pathway paradoxically increases thrombosis risk in combination with certain chemotherapies (113,114), emphasizing the persistent procoagulant character of the tumor microenvironment. The clinical use of inhibitors that target the VEGF receptor–signaling pathway in tumors further demonstrated the crucial role of elevated VEGF levels in maintaining the immature character of the tumor vasculature. Indeed, the remodeling and pruning of tortuous tumor vessels after VEGF blockade improves perfusion and delivery of cytostatic drugs in cancer therapy (115). There are several pathways by which the hemostatic system counteracts VEGF-dependent hyperpermeability and maintains tumor perfusion through enhanced endothelial barrier function and prevention of bleeding.

Although thrombin can acutely increase endothelial permeability through PAR1 signaling (116), the aPC/EPCR signaling pathway, by activating PAR1, can significantly increase endothelial cell barrier function through sphingosine-1 phosphate (S1P) production (117,118). S1P is a potent bioactive lipid that activates predominantly S1P receptor 1 on endothelial cells. Platelets also store and release S1P upon activation. Local synthesis of S1P is probably responsible for the tonic maintenance of barrier integrity, whereas acute release from platelets may acutely "seal off" endothelial cell barriers under increased stress.

Platelets stimulate angiogenesis by secretion of angiogenic growth factors VEGF, bFGF, and PDGF (20). The release of S1P may counteract VEGF-induced permeability increase and thereby contribute to the mechanisms by which platelets provide hemostatic protection during angiogenesis (119). Platelets also secrete platelet factor 4 (PF4), a CXC chemokine that interacts with IL-8 and thus regulates angiogenesis (120). PF4 plays roles in platelet thrombus formation and PF4 neutralizes heparin and thus attenuates antithrombin-dependent coagulation inhibition. PF4 also enhances thrombomodulin-dependent protein C activation and may thereby be integrated into pathways by which local platelet deposition initiates acute and sustained barrier protection of angiogenic endothelium.

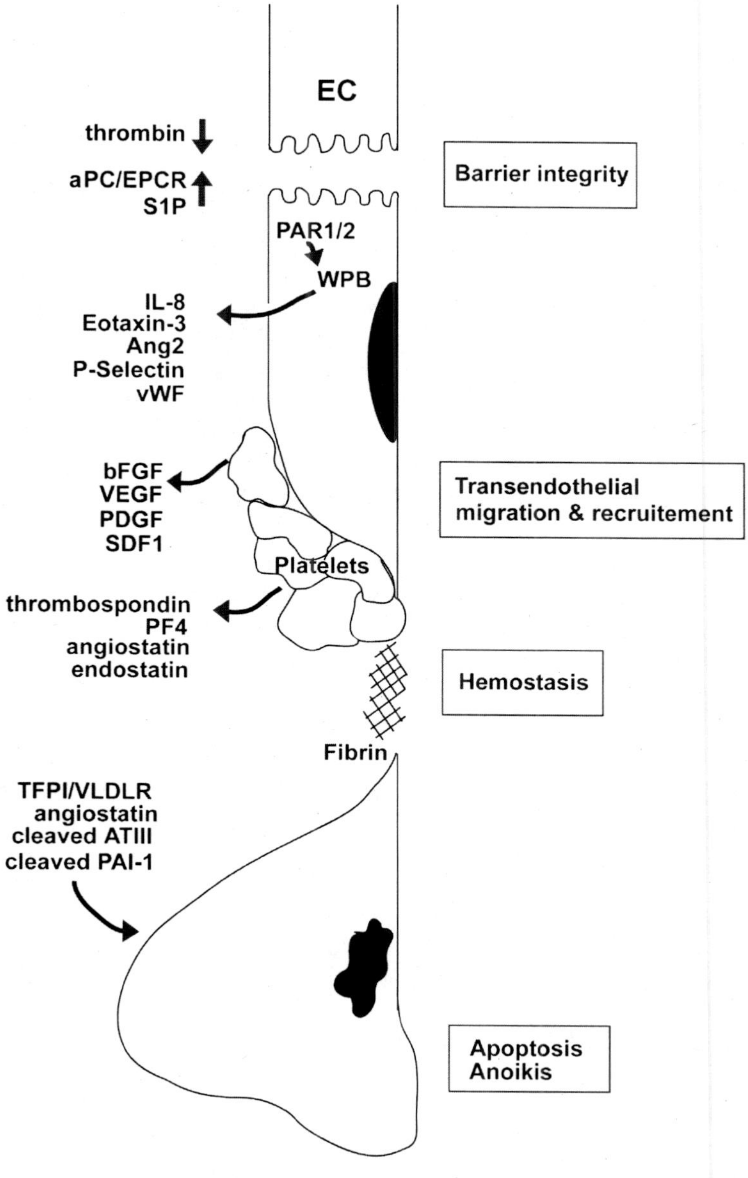

Figure 2 Regulation of endothelial homeostasis by hemostatic mechanisms. The key targets for proteases and S1P signaling are the regulation of endothelial cell barrier protection. Endothelial cells release angiogenic mediators from WPB and recruit inflammatory cells by P-selectin exposure and platelets through vWF release. Coagulation activation leads to turnover of inhibitors that act as proapoptotic signals for endothelial cells. *Abbreviations*: S1P, sphingosine-1 phosphate; WPB, Weibel–Palade bodies; PAR, protease-activated receptor; FGF, fibroblast growth factor; VEGF, vascular endothelial growth factor; PDGF, platelet-derived growth factor; SDF-1, stroma-derived factor-1; PF4, platelet factor 4; PAI, plasminogen activator inhibitor.

Hemostatic factors that induce endothelial cell apoptosis. Angiostatin has led the way in the identification of angiogenic regulators that are derived from the hemostatic system (121). This plasminogen-derived fragment is a ligand for integrins expressed by endothelial cells and induces endothelial apoptosis. Integrin αVβ3, which is expressed by angiogenic endothelia cells binds prothrombin in dependence of integrin activation, leading to prothrombin conversion (122). This may contribute to local accumulation of prothrombin kringle domains with antiangiogenic activities (123). Thrombin initiates fibrin deposition and subsequent proteolysis of fibrin exposes cryptic, proapoptotic epitopes that suppress angiogenesis (37,124). Kringle and fibrin fragments may exert antiangiogenic activities by concerted actions on integrin, VE-cadherin, and angiogenic growth factor pathways.

Cell surface proteoglycans are critical for angiogenic growth factor binding. Heparinase as well as heparin neutralization by, e.g., PF4, interfere with growth factor binding and attenuate VEGF- and bFGF-induced angiogenesis. Antiangiogenic antithrombin is a cleaved and latent form of this serine protease inhibitor (serpin) that blocks thrombin and factor Xa. The potent antiangiogenic activity of the latent serpin conformation (125) is due to preferential binding to proteoglycans involved in angiogenic growth factor binding, in comparison, to native antithrombin that interacts more tightly with anticoagulant heparins (126). A cleaved form of plasminogen activator inhibitor 1 also induces endothelia apoptosis (127), indicating a common theme of how protease action on serpins can produce feedback inhibition of angiogenesis.

TF pathway inhibitor (TFPI) is another coagulation inhibitor with antiangiogenic activity. TFPI has three Kunitz-type protease inhibitory domains and the third domain in conjunction with the basic carboxyl-terminus contributes to heparin binding (128). TFPI is the major inhibitor of the TF initiation complex and controls both TF-dependent initiation of coagulation and direct cell signaling (129). TFPI is tightly bound to endothelial cells by a glycosylphosphatidylinositol anchor attached either directly to an alternative spliced form of TFPI (130) or indirectly available through TPFI receptors (131). TFPI also interacts with versican (132) and the very-low-density lipoprotein receptor (VLDLR) (133). VLDLR is expressed on endothelial cells and the interaction was mapped to a sequence in the very carboxyl-terminus of TFPI (134). Interaction of this sequence with VLDLR triggers endothelial apoptosis and may thus regulate angiogenesis independent of the anticoagulant activity of TFPI.

The turnover of coagulation and fibrinolytic factors and their inhibitors thus either directly through endothelial receptor interaction or indirectly by angiogenic growth factor displacement induce endothelial cell apoptosis. This may contribute to pruning and partial maturation of the tumor vasculature. The resulting improved perfusion may benefit tumor growth and survival. Conversely, these mechanisms provide opportunities for improved antiangiogenic therapy in cancer.

The endothelium as a gatekeeper for inflammatory and stem cell recruitment. The endothelium is actively involved in recruiting and directing the transit of blood-derived inflammatory cells and precursors into the extravascular space. In addition to other agonists, coagulation protease–mediated PAR activation plays a key role in triggering the release of Weibel–Palade bodies, storage compartments specifically found in endothelial cells (135,136). PAR1 and PAR2 are involved in Weibel–Palade body release, but the intermediate signaling pathways appear to differ with PAR1 predominantly triggering calcium fluxes, whereas cAMP pathways play predominant roles in PAR2-mediated release. Weibel–Palade body release leads to P-selectin exposure that mediates leukocyte rolling and thus initiates the transendothelial migration and recruitment of tumor-associated macrophages. Weibel–Palade bodies also store angiogenic regulators IL-8 and angiopoietin 2, as well as eotaxin-3 (137). Furthermore, IL-8 synthesis and PAR2 expression in the endothelium are induced by inflammatory mediators. Resident macrophages in the tumor microenvironment may thereby maintain continuing influx of inflammatory cells in conjunction with protease-mediated activation of the endothelium.

Weibel–Palade body release triggers the local exposure of ultralarge von Willebrand Factor multimers that potently recruit platelets (138). The crucial role for platelets as hemostatic effectors in angiogenesis has been documented (119). However, platelets participate in multiple facets of the angiogenic process by locally releasing angiogenic mediators after activation (Table 1). Platelet activation also induces the release of microvesicles that are emerging as significant vehicles to transmit proangiogenic signals to the host.

Platelet-derived microparticles carry proangiogenic mediators VEGF, PDGF, and bFGF, and by dispersion into the circulation, microparticles serve as delivery vehicles for cargo to different areas of the tumor vasculature (139). Microparticles can alter the procoagulant properties of the endothelium, induce endothelial activation, and thus contribute to the recruitment of inflammatory cells (140). Release of microparticles from endothelial cells is conversely regulated by proteases and microparticles carry TF or EPCR as relevant protease receptors to modulate intravascular coagulation activation and control (141–143). In addition, microparticles derived from tumor cells can serve overlapping functions with platelet-derived microparticles (144) and by releasing tumor cell TF may contribute to the prothrombotic state of tumor patients.

A particularly important function of platelets in orchestrating proangiogenic progenitor recruitment is emerging. Fibrin and platelets provide a matrix for homing and differentiation of endothelial progenitor populations that are incorporated into newly formed vessels (31). Another relevant population of proangiogenic progenitors are integrin CD11b positive, immature myeloid cell populations that play important supportive roles in angiogenesis and revascularization. Platelets are intimately linked to the homing and retention of these progenitor populations in neoangiogenic vessels (3,7). In addition, evidence is emerging that hematopoietic and endothelial progenitors express coagulation receptors, such as EPCR (145) and PARs (85). The biology of proangiogenic progenitors cells may therefore be controlled and influenced directly by proteases of the coagulation cascade.

CONCLUSIONS

The hemostatic systems play crucial roles in maintaining the specific character of the tumor microenvironment and support angiogenesis by multiple mechanisms. Anticoagulant intervention has shown partial benefit to prolong survival in cancer patients (146–148) and it is reasonable to assume that part of the therapeutic effects relates to interference with angiogenic mechanisms. However, the complexity by which the hemostatic system participates in angiogenesis suggests a number of potential targets that have not been explored for therapeutic intervention. Targeting the TF-VIIa complex rather than thrombin in cancer will provide broader suppression of coagulation proteases and more importantly begin to intervene in the direct signaling pathways of TF. Antibody-based strategies to exosites, active site directed inhibitors of VIIa, or agents that suppress the expression of TF on tumor or host cells are strategies to be considered.

The hemostatic system makes contributions to and regulates angiogenesis distinct from and synergistic with the major proangiogenic growth factor pathways. Exploiting the prothrombotic character of the tumor microenvironment as a platform to induce thrombosis (149) remains a counterintuitive, but potentially feasible strategy to starve tumors of their blood supply. Additional studies are required to better define the overlap of proangiogenic pathways in order to identify true synergies that can be exploited for combination antiangiogenic therapy. Direct targeting of PARs and interference with platelet-induced angiogenic mechanism are potential avenues of interest. The unexpected association of thrombosis with antiangiogenic therapy has highlighted the close interdependence of angiogenesis and the hemostatic system. Continuing research in the cross talk of these pathways will be of critical importance for new advances as well as a safety consideration in antiangiogenic therapy.

REFERENCES

1. Hanahan D, Folkman J. Patterns and emerging mechanisms of the angiogenic switch during tumorigenesis. Cell 1996; 86:353–364.
2. Grunewald M, Avraham I, Dor Y, et al. VEGF-induced adult neovascularization: recruitment, retention, and role of accessory cells. Cell 2006; 124(1):175–189.
3. Jin DK, Shido K, Kopp HG, et al. Cytokine-mediated deployment of SDF-1 induces revascularization through recruitment of CXCR4+ hemangiocytes. Nat Med 2006; 12(5):557–567.
4. Gerber HP, Malik AK, Solar GP, et al. VEGF regulates haematopoietic stem cell survival by an internal autocrine loop mechanism. Nature 2002; 417(6892):954–958.
5. Dvorak HF, Brown LF, Detmar M, et al. Vascular permeability factor/vascular endothelial growth factor, microvascular hyperpermeability, and angiogenesis. Am J Pathol 1995; 146:1029–1038.
6. Zou W. Immunosuppressive networks in the tumour environment and their therapeutic relevance. Nat Rev Cancer 2005; 5(4):263–274.
7. Kopp HG, Ramos CA, Rafii S. Contribution of endothelial progenitors and proangiogenic hematopoietic cells to vascularization of tumor and ischemic tissue. Curr Opin Hematol 2006; 13(3):175–181.
8. Orimo A, Gupta PB, Sgroi DC, et al. Stromal fibroblasts present in invasive human breast carcinomas promote tumor growth and angiogenesis through elevated SDF-1/CXCL12 secretion. Cell 2005; 121(3):335–348.
9. Belting M, Ahamed J, Ruf W. Signaling of the Tissue Factor Coagulation Pathway in Angiogenesis and Cancer. Arterioscler Thromb Vasc Biol 2005; 25(8):1545–1550.
10. Ferrara N, Gerber HP, LeCouter J. The biology of VEGF and its receptors. Nat Med 2003; 9(6):669–676.
11. Autiero M, Luttun A, Tjwa M, et al. Placental growth factor and its receptor, vascular endothelial growth factor receptor-1: novel targets for stimulation of ischemic tissue revascularization and inhibition of angiogenic and inflammatory disorders. J Thromb Haemost 2003; 1(7):1356–1370.
12. Uutela M, Wirzenius M, Paavonen K, et al. PDGF-D induces macrophage recruitment, increased interstitial pressure, and blood vessel maturation during angiogenesis. Blood 2004; 104(10):3198–3204.
13. Mäkinen T, Jussila L, Veikkola T, et al. Inhibition of lymphangiogenesis with resulting lymphedema in transgenic mice expressing soluble VEGF receptor-3. Nature Med 2001; 7(2):199–205.
14. Skobe M, Hawighorst T, Jackson DG, et al. Induction of tumor lymphangiogenesis by VEGF-C promotes breast cancer metastasis. Nature Med 2001; 7(2):192–198.
15. Abramsson A, Lindblom P, Betsholtz C. Endothelial and nonendothelial sources of PDGF-B regulate pericyte recruitment and influence vascular pattern formation in tumors. J Clin Invest 2003; 112(8):1142–1151.
16. Jain RK. Molecular regulation of vessel maturation. Nat Med 2003; 9(6):685–693.
17. Bergers G, Song S, Meyer-Morse N, et al. Benefits of targeting both pericytes and endothelial cells in the tumor vasculature with kinase inhibitors. J Clin Invest 2003; 111(9):1287–1295.
18. Mizukami Y, Jo WS, Duerr EM, et al. Induction of interleukin-8 preserves the angiogenic response in HIF-1alpha-deficient colon cancer cells. Nat Med 2005; 11(9):992–997.

19. Sierko E, Wojtukiewicz MZ. Platelets and angiogenesis in malignancy. Semin Thromb Hemost 2004; 30(1):95–108.
20. Brill A, Elinav H, Varon D. Differential role of platelet granular mediators in angiogenesis. Cardiovasc Res 2004; 63(2):226–235.
21. Kubota S, Kawata K, Yanagita T, et al. Abundant retention and release of connective tissue growth factor (CTGF/CCN2) by platelets. J Biochem (Tokyo) 2004; 136(3):279–282.
22. Clauss M, Gerlach M, Gerlach H, et al. Vascular permeability factor: a tumor-derived polypeptide that induces endothelial cell and monocyte procoagulant activity, and promotes monocyte migration. J Exp Med 1990; 172:1535–1545.
23. Clauss M, Grell M, Fangmann C, et al. Synergistic induction of endothelial tissue factor by tumor necrosis factor and vascular endothelial growth factor: functional analysis of the tumor necrosis factor receptors. FEBS Lett 1996; 390:334–338.
24. Shoji M, Hancock WW, Abe K, et al. Activation of coagulation and angiogenesis in cancer. Immunohistochemical localization in situ of clotting proteins and vascular endothelial growth factor in human cancer. Am J Pathol 1998; 152:399–411.
25. Callander NS, Varki N, Rao LVM. Immunohistochemical identification of tissue factor in solid tumors. Cancer 1992; 70:1194–1201.
26. Vrana JA, Stang MT, Grande JP, et al. Expression of tissue factor in tumor stroma correlates with progression to invasive human breast cancer: paracrine regulation by carcinoma cell-derived members of the transforming growth factor β Family. Cancer Res 1996; 56:5063–5070.
27. Yu JL, May L, Lhotak V, et al. Oncogenic events regulate tissue factor expression in colorectal cancer cells: implications for tumor progression and angiogenesis. Blood 2005; 105(4):1734–1741.
28. Rong Y, Post DE, Pieper RO, et al. PTEN and hypoxia regulate tissue factor expression and plasma coagulation by glioblastoma. Cancer Res 2005; 65(4):1406–1413.
29. Red-Horse K, Ferrara N. Imaging tumor angiogenesis. J Clin Invest 2006; 116(10):2585–2587.
30. Mosesson MW. Fibrinogen and fibrin structure and functions. J Thromb Haemost 2005; 3(8):1894–1904.
31. de Boer HC, Verseyden C, Ulfman LH, et al. Fibrin and activated platelets cooperatively guide stem cells to a vascular injury and promote differentiation towards an endothelial cell phenotype. Arterioscler Thromb Vasc Biol 2006; 26(7):1653–1659.
32. Chen D, Weber M, Shiels PG, et al. Postinjury vascular intimal hyperplasia in mice is completely inhibited by CD34+ bone marrow-derived progenitor cells expressing membrane-tethered anticoagulant fusion proteins. J Thromb Haemost 2006; 4(10):2191–2198.
33. Sahni A, Khorana AA, Baggs RB, et al. FGF-2 binding to fibrin(ogen) is required for augmented angiogenesis. Blood 2006; 107(1):126–131.
34. Flick MJ, Du X, Witte DP, et al. Leukocyte engagement of fibrin(ogen) via the integrin receptor alphaMbeta2/Mac-1 is critical for host inflammatory response in vivo. J Clin Invest 2004; 113(11):1596–1606.
35. Palumbo JS, Potter JM, Kaplan LS, et al. Spontaneous hematogenous and lymphatic metastasis, but not primary tumor growth or angiogenesis, is diminished in fibrinogen-deficient mice. Cancer Res 2002; 62(23):6966–6972.
36. Palumbo JS, Talmage KE, Liu H, et al. Plasminogen supports tumor growth through a fibrinogen-dependent mechanism linked to vascular patency. Blood 2003; 102(8):2819–2827.
37. Akakura N, Hoogland C, Takada YK, et al. The COOH-Terminal Globular Domain of Fibrinogen {gamma} Chain Suppresses Angiogenesis and Tumor Growth. Cancer Res 2006; 66(19):9691–9697.
38. van Hinsbergh VW, Engelse MA, Quax PH. Pericellular proteases in angiogenesis and vasculogenesis. Arterioscler Thromb Vasc Biol 2006; 26(4):716–728.
39. Hynes RO. A reevaluation of integrins as regulators of angiogenesis. Nat Med 2002; 8(9):918–921.
40. Grant MA, Kalluri R. Structural basis for the functions of endogenous angiogenesis inhibitors. Cold Spring Harb Symp Quant Biol 2005; 70:399–410.

41. Dong ZY, Kumar R, Yang XL, et al. Macrophage-derived metalloelastase is responsible for the generation of angiostatin in Lewis lung carcinoma. Cell 1997; 88:801–810.
42. Pilch J, Brown DM, Komatsu M, et al. Peptides selected for binding to clotted plasma accumulate in tumor stroma and wounds. Proc Natl Acad Sci USA 2006; 103(8):2800–2804.
43. Dardik R, Loscalzo J, Inbal A. Factor XIII (FXIII) and angiogenesis. J Thromb Haemost 2006; 4(1):19–25.
44. Abe K, Shoji M, Chen J, et al. Regulation of vascular endothelial growth factor production and angiogenesis by the cytoplasmic tail of tissue factor. Proc Natl Acad Sci USA 1999; 96(15):8663–8668.
45. Zhang Y, Deng Y, Luther T, et al. Tissue factor controls the balance of angiogenic and antiangiogenic properties of tumor cells in mice. J Clin Invest 1994; 94:1320–1327.
46. Dorfleutner A, Hintermann E, Tarui T, et al. Crosstalk of integrin α3β1 and tissue factor in cell migration. Mol Biol Cell 2004; 15(10):4416–4425.
47. Ott I, Fischer EG, Miyagi Y, et al. A role for tissue factor in cell adhesion and migration mediated by interaction with actin binding protein 280. J Cell Biol 1998; 140:1241–1253.
48. Ott I, Weigand B, Michl R, et al. Tissue factor cytoplasmic domain stimulates migration by activation of the GTPase Rac1 and the mitogen-activated protein kinase p38. Circulation 2005; 111(3):349–355.
49. Randolph GJ, Luther T, Albrecht S, et al. Role of tissue factor in adhesion of mononuclear phagocytes to and trafficking through endothelium in vitro. Blood 1998; 92:4167–4177.
50. Siegbahn A, Johnell M, Sørensen BB, et al. Regulation of chemotaxis by the cytoplasmic domain of tissue factor. Thromb Haemost 2005; 93(1):27–34.
51. Wang H, Fu W, Im JH, et al. Tumor cell alpha3beta1 integrin and vascular laminin-5 mediate pulmonary arrest and metastasis. J Cell Biol 2004; 164(6):935–941.
52. Koizume S, Jin M-S, Miyagi E, et al. Activation of cancer cell migration and invasion by ectopic synthesis of coagulation factor VII. Cancer Res 2006; 66(19):9453–9460.
53. Riewald M, Ruf W. Mechanistic coupling of protease signaling and initiation of coagulation by tissue factor. Proc Natl Acad Sci USA 2001; 98:7742–7747.
54. Wang X, Gjernes E, Prydz H. Factor VIIa induces tissue factor-dependent up-regulation of Interleukin-8 in a human keratinocyte line. J Biol Chem 2002; 277:23620–23626.
55. Hjortoe GM, Petersen LC, Albrektsen T, et al. Tissue factor-factor VIIa specific up-regulation of IL-8 expression in MDA-MB-231 cells is mediated via PAR-2 and results in increased cell migration. Blood 2004; 103(8):3029–3037.
56. Liu Y, Mueller BM. Protease-activated receptor-2 regulates vascular endothelial growth factor expression in MDA-MB-231 cells via MAPK pathways. Biochem Biophys Res Commun 2006; 344(4):1263–1270.
57. Ahamed J, Versteeg HH, Kerver M, et al. Disulfide isomerization switches tissue factor from coagulation to cell signaling. Proc Natl Acad Sci USA 2006; 103(38):13932–13937.
58. Riewald M, Kravchenko VV, Petrovan RJ, et al. Gene induction by coagulation factor Xa is mediated by activation of PAR-1. Blood 2001; 97:3109–3116.
59. Camerer E, Kataoka H, Kahn M, et al. Genetic evidence that protease-activated receptors mediate factor Xa signaling in endothelial cells. J Biol Chem 2002; 277:16081–16087.
60. Coughlin SR. Protease-activated receptors in hemostasis, thrombosis and vascular biology. J Thromb Haemost 2005; 3(8):1800–1814.
61. O'Brien PJ, Prevost N, Molino M, et al. Thrombin responses in human endothelial cells. Contributions from receptors other than PAR1 include the transactivation of PAR2 by thrombin-cleaved PAR1. J Biol Chem 2000; 275:13502–13509.
62. Shi X, Gangadharan B, Brass LF, et al. Protease-activated receptor 1(PAR1) and PAR2 contribute to tumor cell motility and metastasis. Mol Cancer Res 2004; 2(7):395–402.
63. Lidington EA, Steinberg R, Kinderlerer AR, et al. A role for proteinase-activated receptor 2 and PKC-epsilon in thrombin-mediated induction of decay-accelerating factor on human endothelial cells. Am J Physiol Cell Physiol 2005; 289(6):C1437–C1447.
64. Majumdar M, Tarui T, Shi B, et al. Plasmin-induced migration requires signaling through protease-activated receptor 1 and integrin α9β1. J Biol Chem 2004; 279(36):37528–37534.

65. Jenkins RG, Su X, Su G, et al. Ligation of protease-activated receptor 1 enhances alpha(v)beta6 integrin-dependent TGF-beta activation and promotes acute lung injury. J Clin Invest 2006; 116(6):1606–1614.
66. Boire A, Covic L, Agarwal A, et al. PAR1 Is a matrix metalloprotease-1 receptor that promotes invasion and tumorigenesis of breast cancer cells. Cell 2005; 120(3):303–313.
67. Lourbakos A, Chinni C, Thompson P, et al. Cleavage and activation of proteinase-activated receptor-2 on human neutrophils by gingipain-R from Porphyromonas gingivalis. FEBS Lett 1998; 435(1):45–48.
68. Smith R, Jenkins A, Lourbakos A, et al. Evidence for the activation of PAR-2 by the sperm protease, acrosin: expression of the receptor on oocytes. FEBS Lett 2000; 484(3):285–290.
69. Molino M, Barnathan ES, Numerof R, et al. Interactions of mast cell tryptase with thrombin receptors and PAR-2. J Biol Chem 1997; 272:4043–4049.
70. Csernok E, Ai M, Gross WL, et al. Wegener autoantigen induces maturation of dendritic cells and licenses them for Th1 priming via the protease-activated receptor-2 pathway. Blood 2006; 107(11):4440–4448.
71. Miyata S, Koshikawa N, Yasumitsu H, et al. Trypsin stimulates integrin $\alpha_5\beta1$-dependent adhesion to fibronectin and proliferation of human gastric carcinoma cells through activation of proteinase-activated receptor-2. J Biol Chem 2000; 275:4592–4598.
72. Wilson S, Greer B, Hooper J, et al. The membrane-anchored serine protease, TMPRSS2, activates PAR-2 in prostate cancer cells. Biochem J 2005; 388(Pt 3):967–972.
73. Takeuchi T, Harris JL, Huang W, et al. Cellular localization of membrane-type serine protease 1 and identification of protease-activated receptor-2 and single-chain urokinase-type plasminogen activator as substrates. J Biol Chem 2000; 275:26333–26342.
74. Aimes RT, Zijlstra A, Hooper JD, et al. Endothelial cell serine proteases expressed during vascular morphogenesis and angiogenesis. Thromb Haemost 2003; 89(3):561–572.
75. Netzel-Arnett S, Hooper JD, Szabo R, et al. Membrane anchored serine proteases: a rapidly expanding group of cell surface proteolytic enzymes with potential roles in cancer. Cancer Metastasis Rev 2003; 22(2–3):237–258.
76. D'Andrea MR, Derian CK, Santulli RJ, et al. Differential expression of protease-activated receptors-1 and -2 in stromal fibroblasts of normal, benign, and malignant human tissues. Am J Pathol 2001; 158(6):2031–2041.
77. Colognato R, Slupsky JR, Jendrach M, et al. Differential expression and regulation of protease-activated receptors in human peripheral monocytes and monocyte-derived antigen-presenting cells. Blood 2003; 102(7):2645–2652.
78. Johansson U, Lawson C, Dabare M, et al. Human peripheral blood monocytes express protease receptor-2 and respond to receptor activation by production of IL-6, IL-8, and IL-1{beta}. J Leukoc Biol 2005; 78(4):967-975.
79. Fields RC, Schoenecker JG, Hart JP, et al. Protease-activated receptor-2 signaling triggers dendritic cell development. Am J Pathol 2003; 162(6):1817–1822.
80. Connolly AJ, Ishihara H, Kahn ML, et al. Role of the thrombin receptor in development and evidence for a second receptor. Nature 1996; 381:516–519.
81. Darrow AL, Fung-Leung W-P, Ye RD, et al. Biological consequences of thrombin receptor deficiency in mice. Thromb Haemost 1996; 76:860–866.
82. Tang H, Low B, Rutherford SA, et al. Thrombin induces endocytosis of endoglin and type-II TGF-beta receptor and down-regulation of TGF-beta signaling in endothelial cells. Blood 2005; 105(5):1977–1985.
83. Minami T, Horiuchi K, Miura M, et al. Vascular endothelial growth factor- and thrombin-induced termination factor, Down syndrome critical region-1, attenuates endothelial cell proliferation and angiogenesis. J Biol Chem 2004; 279(48):50537–50554.
84. Smadja DM, Bieche I, Uzan G, et al. PAR-1 activation on human late endothelial progenitor cells enhances angiogenesis in vitro with upregulation of the SDF-1/CXCR4 system. Arterioscler Thromb Vasc Biol 2005; 25(11):2321–2327.
85. Tarzami ST, Wang G, Li W, et al. Thrombin and PAR-1 stimulate differentiation of bone marrow-derived endothelial progenitor cells. J Thromb Haemost 2006; 4(3):656–663.

86. Flynn AN, Buret AG. Proteinase-activated receptor 1(PAR-1) and cell apoptosis. Apoptosis 2004; 9(6):729–737.
87. Versteeg HH, Arnold SC, Richel DJ, et al. Coagulation factors VIIa and Xa inhibit apoptosis and anoikis. Oncogene 2004; 23(2):410–417.
88. Sorensen BB, Rao LVM, Tornehave D, et al. Anti-apoptotic effect of coagulation factor VIIa. Blood 2003; 102(5):1708–1715.
89. Jiang X, Guo YL, Bromberg ME. Formation of tissue factor-factor VIIa-factor Xa complex prevents apoptosis in human breast cancer cells. Thromb Haemost 2006; 96(2):196–201.
90. Darmoul D, Gratio V, Devaud H, et al. Protease-activated receptor 2 in colon cancer: trypsin-induced MAPK phosphorylation and cell proliferation are mediated by epidermal growth factor receptor transactivation. J Biol Chem 2004; 279(20):20927–20934.
91. Prenzel N, Zwick E, Daub H, et al. EGF receptor transactivation by G-protein-coupled receptors requires metalloproteinase cleavage of proHB-EGF. Nature 2000; 402:884–888.
92. Wiiger MT, Prydz H. The epidermal growth factor receptor (EGFR) and proline rich tyrosine kinase 2(PYK2) are involved in tissue factor dependent factor VIIa signalling in HaCaT cells. Thromb Haemost 2004; 92(1):13–22.
93. Huang Y-Q, Li J-J, Hu L, et al. Thrombin induces increased expression and secretion of angiopoietin-2 from human umbilical vein endothelial cells. Blood 2002; 99:1646–1650.
94. Pendurthi UR, Allen KE, Ezban M, et al. Factor VIIa and thrombin induce the expression of cyr61 and connective tissue growth factor, extracellular matrix signaling proteins that could act as possible downstream mediators in factor VIIa tissue factor-induced signal transduction. J Biol Chem 2000; 275:14632–14641.
95. Pendurthi UR, Ngyuen M, Andrade-Gordon P, et al. Plasmin induces *Cyr61* gene expression in fibroblasts via protease-activated receptor-1 and p44/42 mitogen-activated protein kinase-dependent signaling pathway. Arterioscler Thromb Vasc Biol 2002; 22(9):1421–1426.
96. Caunt M, Huang YQ, Brooks PC, et al. Thrombin induces neoangiogenesis in the chick chorioallantoic membrane. J Thromb Haemost 2003; 1(10):2097–2102.
97. Haralabopoulos G, Grant D, Kleinman H, et al. Thrombin promotes endothelial cell alignment in Matrigel in vitro and angiogenesis in vivo. Am J Physiol 1997; 273:C239–C245.
98. Zania P, Kritikou S, Flordellis CS, et al. Blockade of angiogenesis by small molecule antagonists to protease-activated receptor-1 (PAR-1): association with endothelial cell growth suppression and induction of apoptosis. J Pharmacol Exp Ther 2006; 318:246–251.
99. Riewald M, Petrovan RJ, Donner A, et al. Activation of endothelial cell protease activated receptor 1 by the protein C pathway. Science 2002; 296:1880–1882.
100. Riewald M, Ruf W. Protease-activated receptor-1 signaling by activated protein C in cytokine-perturbed endothelial cells is distinct from thrombin signaling. J Biol Chem 2005; 280(20):19808–19814.
101. Mosnier LO, Griffin JH. Inhibition of staurosporine-induced apoptosis of endothelial cells by activated protein C requires protease-activated receptor-1 and endothelial cell protein C receptor. Biochem J 2003; 373(Pt 1):65–70.
102. Jackson CJ, Xue M, Thompson P, et al. Activated protein C prevents inflammation yet stimulates angiogenesis to promote cutaneous wound healing. Wound Repair Regen 2005; 13(3):284–294.
103. Uchiba M, Okajima K, Oike Y, et al. Activated protein C induces endothelial cell proliferation by mitogen-activated protein kinase activation in vitro and angiogenesis in vivo. Circ Res 2004; 95(1):34–41.
104. Hembrough TA, Swartz GM, Papathanassiu A, et al. Tissue factor/factor VIIa inhibitors block angiogenesis and tumor growth through a nonhemostatic mechanism. Cancer Res 2003; 63(11):2997–3000.
105. Belting M, Dorrell MI, Sandgren S, et al. Regulation of angiogenesis by tissue factor cytoplasmic domain signaling. Nature Med 2004; 10(5):502–509.
106. Carmeliet P, Mackman N, Moons L, et al. Role of tissue factor in embryonic blood vessel development. Nature 1996; 383:73–75.
107. Griffin CT, Srinavasan Y, Zheng Y-W, et al. A role for thrombin receptor signaling in endothelial cells during embryonic development. Science 2001; 293:1666–1670.

108. Drake TA, Cheng J, Chang A, et al. Expression of tissue factor, thrombomodulin, and E-selectin in baboons with lethal *E.coli* sepsis. Am J Pathol 1993; 142:1458–1470.
109. Contrino J, Hair G, Kreutzer DL, et al. *In situ* detection of tissue factor in vascular endothelial cells: correlation with the malignant phenotype of human breast disease. Nature Med 1996; 2:209–215.
110. Ahamed J, Ruf W. Protease-activated receptor 2-dependent phosphorylation of the tissue factor cytoplasmic domain. J Biol Chem 2004; 279:23038–23044.
111. Seo DW, Li H, Guedez L, et al. TIMP-2 mediated inhibition of angiogenesis: an MMP-independent mechanism. Cell 2003; 114(2):171–180.
112. Gupta GP, Massague J. Platelets and metastasis revisited: a novel fatty link. J Clin Invest 2004; 114(12):1691–1693.
113. Kuenen BC, Levi M, Meijers JCM, et al. Analysis of coagulation cascade and endothelial cell activation during inhibition of vascular endothelial growth factor/vascular endothelial growth factor receptor pathway in cancer patients. Arterioscler Thromb Vasc Biol 2002; 22(9):1500–1505.
114. Ma L, Francia G, Viloria-Petit A, et al. In vitro procoagulant activity induced in endothelial cells by chemotherapy and antiangiogenic drug combinations: modulation by lower-dose chemotherapy. Cancer Res 2005; 65(12):5365–5373.
115. Jain RK. Normalization of tumor vasculature: an emerging concept in antiangiogenic therapy. Science 2005; 307(5706):58–62.
116. Vogel SM, Gao X, Mehta D, et al. Abrogation of thrombin-induced increase in pulmonary microvascular permeability in PAR-1 knockout mice. Physiol Genomics 2000; 4(2):137–145.
117. Feistritzer C, Riewald M. Endothelial barrier protection by activated protein C through PAR1-dependent sphingosine 1-phosphate receptor-1 crossactivation. Blood 2005; 105(8):3178–3184.
118. Finigan JH, Dudek SM, Singleton PA, et al. Activated protein C mediates novel lung endothelial barrier enhancement: role of sphingosine 1-phosphate receptor transactivation. J Biol Chem 2005; 280(17):17286–17293.
119. Kisucka J, Butterfield CE, Duda DG, et al. Platelets and platelet adhesion support angiogenesis while preventing excessive hemorrhage. Proc Natl Acad Sci USA 2006; 103(4):855–860.
120. Slungaard A. Platelet factor 4: a chemokine enigma. Int J Biochem Cell Biol 2005; 37(6):1162–1167.
121. O'Reilly MS, Holmgren L, Shing Y, et al. Angiostatin: a novel angiogenesis inhibitor that mediates the suppression of metastases by a Lewis lung carcinoma. Cell 1994; 79:315–328.
122. Byzova TV, Plow EF. Activation of $\alpha_V\beta_3$ on vascular cells controls recognition of prothrombin. J Cell Biol 1998; 143(7):2081–2092.
123. Lee T-H, Rhim T, Kim SS. Prothrombin kringle-2 domain has a growth inhibitory activity against basic fibroblast growth factor-stimulated capillary endothelial cells. J Biol Chem 1998; 273:28805–28812.
124. Staton CA, Lewis CE. Angiogenesis inhibitors found within the haemostasis pathway. J Cell Mol Med 2005; 9(2):286–302.
125. O'Reilly MS, Pirie-Shepherd S, Lane WS, et al. Antiangiogenic activity of the cleaved conformation of the serpin antithrombin. Science 1999; 285(5435):1926–1928.
126. Zhang W, Swanson R, Xiong Y, et al. Antiangiogenic antithrombin blocks the heparan sulfate-dependent binding of proangiogenic growth factors to their endothelial cell receptors. Evidence for differential binding of antiangiogenic and anticoagulant forms of antithrombin to proangiogenic heparan sulfate domains. J Biol Chem 2006; 281:37302–37310.
127. Drinane M, Walsh J, Mollmark J, et al. The Anti-angiogenic Activity of rPAI-123 Inhibits Fibroblast Growth Factor-2 Functions. J Biol Chem 2006; 281(44):33336–33344.
128. Broze GJ. Tissue factor pathway inhibitor and the revised theory of coagulation. Annu Rev Med 1995; 46:103–112.
129. Ahamed J, Belting M, Ruf W. Regulation of tissue factor-induced signaling by endogenous and recombinant tissue factor pathway inhibitor 1. Blood 2005; 105(6):2384–2391.
130. Zhang J, Piro O, Lu L, et al. Glycosyl phosphatidylinositol anchorage of tissue factor pathway inhibitor. Circulation 2003; 108(5):623–627.

131. Sevinsky JR, Rao LVM, Ruf W. Ligand-induced protease receptor translocation into caveolae: a mechanism for regulating cell surface proteolysis of the tissue factor-dependent coagulation pathway. J Cell Biol 1996; 133:293–304.
132. Zheng PS, Reis M, Sparling C, et al. Versican G3 domain promotes blood coagulation through suppressing the activity of tissue factor pathway inhibitor-1. J Biol Chem 2006; 281(12):8175–8182.
133. Hembrough T, Ruiz J, Papathanassiu A, et al. Tissue factor pathway inhibitor inhibits endothelial cell proliferation via association with the very low density lipoprotein receptor. J Biol Chem 2001; 276(15):12241–12248.
134. Hembrough TA, Ruiz JF, Swerdlow BM, et al. Identification and characterization of a very low density lipoprotein receptor-binding peptide from tissue factor pathway inhibitor that has antitumor and antiangiogenic activity. Blood 2004; 103(9):3374–3380.
135. Cleator JH, Zhu WQ, Vaughan DE, et al. Differential regulation of endothelial exocytosis of P-selectin and von Willebrand factor by protease-activated receptors and cAMP. Blood 2006; 107(7):2736–2744.
136. Klarenbach SW, Chipiuk A, Nelson RC, et al. Differential actions of PAR2 and PAR1 in stimulating human endothelial cell exocytosis and permeability: the role of Rho-GTPases. Circ Res 2003; 92(3):272–278.
137. Rondaij MG, Bierings R, Kragt A, et al. Dynamics and plasticity of Weibel-Palade bodies in endothelial cells. Arterioscler Thromb Vasc Biol 2006; 26(5):1002–1007.
138. Lopez JA, Dong JF. Shear stress and the role of high molecular weight von Willebrand factor multimers in thrombus formation. Blood Coagul Fibrinolysis 2005; 16(suppl 1):S11–S16.
139. Brill A, Dashevsky O, Rivo J, et al. Platelet-derived microparticles induce angiogenesis and stimulate post-ischemic revascularization. Cardiovasc Res 2005; 67(1):30–38.
140. Mesri M, Altieri DC. Leukocyte microparticles stimulate endothelial cell cytokine release and tissue factor induction in a JNK1 signaling pathway. J Biol Chem 1999; 274:23111–23118.
141. Sapet C, Simoncini S, Loriod B, et al. Thrombin-induced endothelial microparticle generation: identification of a novel pathway involving ROCK-II activation by caspase-2. Blood 2006; 108(6):1868–1876.
142. Perez-Casal M, Downey C, Fukudome K, et al. Activated protein C induces the release of microparticle-associated endothelial protein C receptor. Blood 2005; 105(4):1515–1522.
143. Morel O, Toti F, Hugel B, et al. Cellular microparticles: a disseminated storage pool of bioactive vascular effectors. Curr Opin Hematol 2004; 11(3):156–164.
144. Baj-Krzyworzeka M, Szatanek R, Weglarczyk K, et al. Tumour-derived microvesicles carry several surface determinants and mRNA of tumour cells and transfer some of these determinants to monocytes. Cancer Immunol Immunother 2006; 55(7):808–818.
145. Balazs AB, Fabian AJ, Esmon CT, et al. Endothelial protein C receptor (CD201) explicitly identifies hematopoietic stem cells in murine bone marrow. Blood 2005; 107(6):2317–2321.
146. Schulman S, Lindmarker P. Incidence of cancer after prophylaxis with warfarin against recurrent venous thromboembolism. Duration of Anticoagulation Trial. N Engl J Med 2000; 342(26):1953–1958.
147. Klerk CP, Smorenburg SM, Otten HM, et al. The effect of low molecular weight heparin on survival in patients with advanced malignancy. J Clin Oncol 2005; 23(10):2130–2135.
148. Zacharski LR, Henderson WG, Rickles FR, et al. Effect of warfarin anticoagulation on survival in carcinoma of the lung, colon, head and neck, and prostate. Cancer 1984; 53:2046–2052.
149. Huang XM, Molema G, King S, et al. Tumor infarction in mice by antibody-directed targeting of tissue factor to tumor vasculature. Science 1997; 275:547–550.

3

Tissue Factor in Cancer Angiogenesis and Coagulopathy

Mark B. Taubman

Department of Medicine and Cardiovascular Research Institute, University of Rochester, Rochester, New York, U.S.A.

- Tissue factor (TF) is a transmembrane glycoprotein that initiates the coagulation cascade.
- TF is highly expressed in many tumors and in most angiogenic endothelium. This may be in part responsible for the prothrombotic state associated with cancer and cancer chemotherapy.
- In addition to its role in thrombosis, TF has also been implicated in angiogenesis and tumor metastasis.
- The nonthrombotic roles of TF may in part be mediated by the generation of thrombin and the resulting activation of protease-activated receptors (PARs).
- TF also appears to have a "direct" signaling function, mediated in part by the phosphorylation of its cytoplasmic domain.
- Factor (F) VIIa and FXa also appear to signal through the PARs, alone or as part of TF:FVIIa and TF:FVIIa:FXa complexes.
- TF-containing microparticles are released from cells and are present in the circulation. These may contribute to thrombosis.

INTRODUCTION

Tissue factor (TF) is a transmembrane glycoprotein that initiates coagulation (1,2) and plays a critical role in regulating hemostasis and thrombosis (3,4). Human TF consists of three domains: a short cytoplasmic domain of 21 residues, a single transmembrane domain of 23 residues, and an extracellular domain of 219 residues. TF binds to factor (F) VIIa, and the resulting complex acts as a catalyst for the conversion of FIX and FX to FIXa and FXa, respectively, triggering the clotting cascade and leading to the generation of thrombin. Thrombin cleaves fibrinogen to fibrin, a major ingredient of thrombus. Thrombin is also a potent cell activator that has been implicated in inflammation, growth, migration, and angiogenesis. TF is highly expressed in many tumors and in angiogenic endothelium, and it is inducible in vascular cells by many tumor-related agonists. TF expression is also coupled to vascular endothelial growth factor (VEGF), a potent angiogenic factor. TF has been implicated in the thrombotic complications of cancer and in enhancing tumor growth, migration, metastasis, and angiogenesis. This chapter will summarize the multiple roles of TF in malignancy.

The TF gene is a member of the class of "primary response" genes that are expressed at low levels in quiescent cells, are rapidly induced by serum, and are "superinduced" in the presence of protein synthesis inhibitors, such as cycloheximide. TF transcription is regulated by common transcription factors (5), including nuclear factor (NF)κB, *egr-1*, AP-1, and SP-1. As a result, TF is induced by numerous cytokines, chemokines, and growth factors (1,6), some of which, such as tumor necrosis factor-α, transforming growth factor-β, and VEGF, are elevated in many tumors and can act additively and in some cases synergistically to increase TF expression (7). Chemotherapeutic agents, such as cisplatin and doxorubicin, have been shown to induce TF expression (8). The VEGF inhibitor, SU5416, one of a group of antiangiogenic factors being examined for cancer chemotherapy, also induces TF expression in endothelial cells (EC) (9).

TF EXPRESSION AND HUMAN CANCER: IMMUNOHISTOCHEMICAL STUDIES

Increased TF expression has been detected in a variety of human tumors (10), including glioma (11), breast cancer (12,13), non–small cell lung cancer (14,15), leukemia (16,17), colorectal cancer (18–21), hepatocellular cancer (22), prostate cancer (23,24), and pancreatic cancer (25–28). Even more widespread than in tumor cells, enhanced TF expression has been seen consistently in angiogenic endothelium, presumably due to its induction by local factors released from malignant cells. High TF levels correlate with VEGF expression, increased angiogenesis, vascular density, more advanced stage, and in some cases, unfavorable prognosis (12–14,17,19,22,23,25,27,28). In addition, increased tumor TF expression has been correlated with the incidence of metastasis (13,15,19–21,27). Although less well studied, a few reports have suggested that high levels of tumor TF are associated with an enhanced prothrombotic state and increased incidence of thromboembolic events (28,29).

TF AND METASTASIS

In addition to the immunohistochemical studies described above, experiments involving cell culture and animal models of cancer have provided evidence that TF expression is linked to metastasis. TF was found to be highly expressed in metastatic breast carcinoma cells in contrast to nonmetastatic breast carcinoma cells (30). Similarly TF expression was 1000-fold higher in metastatic than nonmetastatic human melanoma cells (31). Injection of these melanoma cells into severe combined immunodeficient (SCID) mice resulted in extensive pulmonary metastases. However, the growth of these metastases was significantly inhibited by a blocking antibody to TF, but not by a noninhibitory TF antibody, suggesting that tumor TF enzymatic activity was essential. The same laboratory also showed that in SCID mice, the metastatic potential of Chinese hamster ovary cells, transfected with various forms of TF, was dependent upon both TF enzymatic activity and the cytoplasmic domain (32). Bromberg et al. also examined the development of pulmonary metastases in SCID mice injected with human melanoma cells expressing different forms of TF (33). They found that the number and size of metastases was dependent upon the extent of TF expression and the presence of the cytoplasmic domain, but not dependent upon TF enzymatic activity. In subsequent studies, the metastatic potential of human melanoma cells was found to be dependent upon the presence of active phosphorylation sites on the cytoplasmic domain and upon FVIIa binding (34), but not on the expression of the thrombin receptor [protease-activated receptor (PAR)-1; see below] (35). In a mouse melanoma model, metastases and tumor growth were reduced by inhibitors of the TF:FVIIa or TF:FVIIa:FXa complex but not by inhibitors of FXa (36).

TF, VEGF, AND ANGIOGENESIS

There has been considerable interest in the role of TF in promoting tumor angiogenesis (37–40). $TF^{-/-}$ mice display embryonic lethality at days 7.5 to 10.5 in association with severe bleeding and abnormal development of the yolk sac vasculature (41,42). Interestingly, VEGF-deficient embryos have a similar yolk sac defect (43,44). As noted above, TF and VEGF antigens colocalize by immunostaining in human tumors (14,19,45,46), and there is a correlation between TF expression and microvessel density (14,23,28). VEGF is a potent inducer of TF in a variety of cells, including EC. Several studies have demonstrated a correlation between TF and VEGF expression in tumor cells (45,47). In human fibroblasts, FVIIa-induced VEGF expression was dependent upon TF binding and subsequent generation of FXa and thrombin (48,49).

VEGF expression was enhanced in Meth-A sarcoma cells overexpressing TF and decreased in cells with antisense-mediated deficiency of TF (50). In addition, cells overexpressing TF grew more rapidly and established larger and more vascularized tumors in mice, whereas cells expressing antisense TF grew the slowest and produced the least vascularized tumors. Human melanoma cells overexpressing TF cDNA had high levels of VEGF expression, whereas those expressing a mutant TF cDNA lacking the cytoplasmic domain had minimal levels of TF expression (47), suggesting the involvement of direct TF signaling (see below). Transfection of low-VEGF lines with TF cDNA resulted in enhanced VEGF expression. Interestingly, inoculation of a high TF and VEGF–producing melanoma line in SCID mice yielded highly vascular tumors, whereas tumors produced by a low TF and VEGF cell were avascular.

MECHANISMS OF TF-MEDIATED TUMORIGENESIS

There are a number of mechanisms by which TF may mediate tumor growth, migration, and angiogenesis. These are both dependent on and independent of TF procoagulant activity and in addition may involve direct and indirect effects of TF binding. These pathways are summarized in Figure 1.

"DIRECT" SIGNALING MEDIATED BY THE TF CYTOPLASMIC TAIL

Because TF has a transmembrane-spanning domain and a cytoplasmic tail, it has the potential to be involved in cell signaling. Although the presence and importance of "direct" TF signaling remains controversial, a number of observations support the role of the TF cytoplasmic domain in mediating signal transduction. The TF cytoplasmic tail has two serine phosphorylation sites. Upon ligand binding (e.g., FVIIa), these serine residues are phosphorylated by a protein kinase C (PKC)–dependent mechanism (51,52). Ruf et al. demonstrated, by yeast two-hybrid analysis, that the carboxyl terminus of the actin-binding

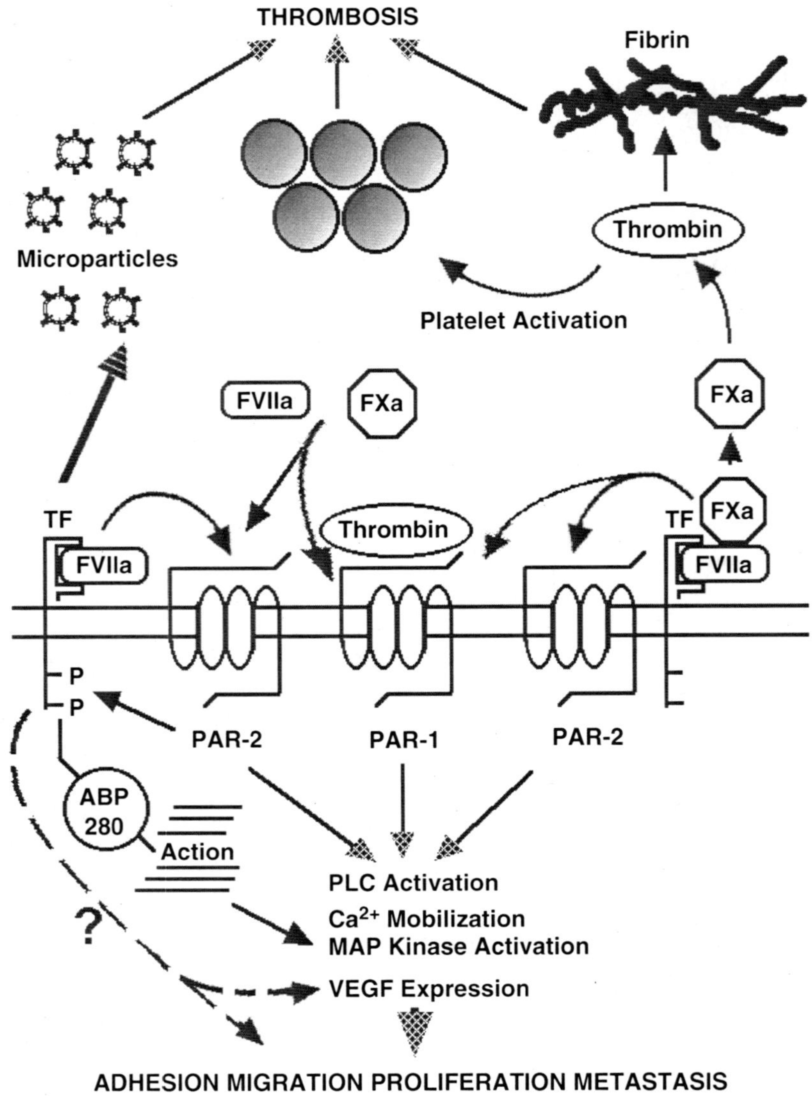

Figure 1 TF-mediated pathways in cancer and thrombosis. TF anchored in the cell membrane forms a tripartite complex with FVIIa and FX to generate FXa, leading to the generation of thrombin. Thrombin catalyzes the formation of fibrin and activates platelets, thereby promoting thrombosis. TF is also released from cell surfaces as microparticles, which may also contribute to thrombosis. In addition to its role in thrombosis, thrombin binds to PAR-1, initiating several important signals (PLC activation, MAP kinase activation, Ca^{2+} mobilization, and VEGF expression) that promote cell adhesion, migration, proliferation, and metastasis. TF appears to have a "direct" signaling function that involves the phosphorylation (P) of two serine residues on the cytoplasmic domain and may active several signaling pathways, one of which is mediated by interaction with the ABP 280 and stimulates cell migration. The activation of PAR-2 may facilitate phosphorylation of the cytoplasmic domain. FVIIa and FXa, alone or as part of TF:FVIIa and TF:FVIIa:FXa complexes, also signal via PAR-1 and PAR-2, inducing pathways linked to adhesion, migration, proliferation, and metastasis. In addition to its role in thrombosis, fibrin acts as a surface that facilitates cell migration, adhesion, and metastasis. *Abbreviations*: TF, tissue factor; PAR, protease-activated receptor; PLC, phospholipase C; MAP, mitogen-activated protein; VEGF, vascular endothelial growth factor; ABP, actin-binding protein.

protein-280 binds the TF cytoplasmic tail (53). Concomitant with TF binding, the amino terminus of the actin-binding protein-280 interacts with actin filaments (53,54). This leads to mitogen-activated protein kinase (MAPK) signaling and phosphorylation of focal adhesion kinases, which are known to promote cell adhesion and migration. Additional studies using human melanoma cell lines have suggested that the cytoplasmic tail is required for the generation of intracellular Ca^{2+} transients and the generation of VEGF (47) and for promoting metastases in mice (34). Most recently, an inactivated FVIIa was shown to mediate TF cytoplasmic tail–dependent induction of the GTPase Rac1 and p38 MAPK in J82 bladder carcinoma cells (55). Importantly, this pathway was linked to cell migration.

THROMBIN-DEPENDENT MECHANISMS

Thrombin regulates the growth, migration, and synthesis of inflammatory mediators and receptors in a variety of cells, including EC and tumor cells. The direct effects of thrombin occur via interactions with members of the PAR family, and in particular PAR-1. The vascular effects of thrombin and the biology of the PARs have been recently reviewed in Refs. 56 and 57, respectively. Interestingly, the PAR-$1^{-/-}$ mice have a deficiency in yolk sac blood vessel formation similar to that of the $TF^{-/-}$ mice. Unlike the $TF^{-/-}$ mice, it is only partially lethal and can be rescued by EC expression of PAR-1 (58).

Thrombin may promote angiogenesis through a variety of mechanisms. Thrombin interacts directly with EC. Attachment of EC to thrombin is mediated in part by the $\alpha^{v}\beta^{3}$ integrin, which itself is induced by thrombin. Thrombin functions as a potent EC chemoattractant and also provides EC with survival signals during anchorage-independent migration (59). In addition to its effects on EC, thrombin facilitates cell invasion through the basement membrane by activating matrix metalloproteinase-2 (60). By inducing cell surface adhesion molecules, such as the $\alpha II^{b}\beta^{3}$ integrin (61,62), P-selectin (63,64), and CD40 ligand (65), thrombin enhances adhesion of tumor cells to platelets, EC, and the extracellular matrix. Thrombin stimulates the synthesis of VEGF and other growth factors (66), cytokines, chemokines, and extracellular proteins (67) that promote the proliferation and migration of tumor cells (68,69). Thrombin also promotes the release of VEGF and other growth- and migration-promoting factors from platelet granules (70,71).

Thrombin also appears to have direct effects on the proliferation of metastatic tumor cells (72) and on tumor cell survival (73). Thrombin also enhances tumor cell motility, perhaps involving cross-talk of the PAR-1 cytoplasmic tail with the $\alpha^{v}\beta^{5}$ integrin (74). A direct correlation has been reported between PAR-1 expression and tumor cell invasiveness (69). Importantly, reduction of PAR-1 levels with antisense cDNA significantly reduces the invasive potential of MDA-435 breast cancer cells. In experimental pulmonary metastasis models, thrombin-treated tumor cells produce a marked increase in lung metastases, as compared to untreated tumor cells (61,75). These effects are mediated by PAR-1 signaling and not procoagulant activity (76), in that metastasis is enhanced by non–enzymatically active thrombin peptides. Because tumor cells metastasize with high efficiency in PAR-1–deficient mice (77), tumor cell–derived, rather than host cell, PAR-1 appears to be of paramount importance.

In addition to effects mediated by the activation of the PARs, thrombin also exerts its effects through its procoagulant activity. Thrombin enzymatic activity leads to the deposition of cross-linked fibrin. Fibrinogen serves as a scaffolding molecule for binding promigratory and angiogenic growth factors, particularly VEGF (78). Cleavage and degradation of fibrinogen and fibrin expose cryptic sites that facilitate adhesion to cell-surface receptors (79). Fibrinogen has been shown to play a role in tumor metastasis to lymph nodes and the lung (80). In addition, cross-linked fibrin facilitates critical cell–matrix interactions that mediate inflammation, EC proliferation and migration, and new vessel formation (81,82). In at least one study, fibrin generation in metastasis was shown to result from tumor cell–expressed TF (31). In addition to the role of fibrin/fibrinogen as a scaffolding, several biologically active plasmin and/or thrombin cleavage fragments of fibrinogen have been shown to induce proangiogenic or antiangiogenic effects (83,84). Plasma levels of fibrinopeptide A, a cleavage product of fibrinogen, correlate with tumor growth and regression in patients with cancer (85). Many cancers are associated with the deposition of cross-linked fibrin (86), including breast (12), lung (45), brain (87), and prostate (88). Fibrin also stimulates the synthesis and secretion of proangiogenic factors, such as interleukin-8, from tumor cells (89). In spite of these properties, it is worth noting that fibrinogen-deficient mice do not show differences in tumor growth (90) or in angiogenesis.

SIGNALING MEDIATED BY FVIIa AND FXa

FVIIa and FXa induce cell signaling, either independently or as part of a complex with TF. FVIIa mobilizes intracellular Ca^{2+} in various cell types (91), induces the production of inositol-1,4,5-trisphosphate (92), activates phospholipase C (93), and activates MAPKs (94–97), c-Jun N-terminal kinase (96), and members of the Src family of kinases (98). Although most of these effects are dependent upon the expression of TF, they appear to be independent of the presence of the TF cytoplasmic domain (91,95,96). Several studies have implicated PAR-2 in VIIa-mediated cell activation (99,100) and have suggested that PAR2 is activated directly by TF:FVIIa complexes (101).

In addition to TF:VIIa, the TF:FVIIa:FXa ternary complex has been shown to induce cell signaling (102). In this study, the TF:FVIIa complex was immobilized using a nematode anticoagulant protein C2 backbone, resulting in the inhibition of FVIIa enzymatic activity. Nevertheless, the addition of FXa activated both PAR-1 and PAR-2, suggesting that in addition to direct activation of PAR-2, the TF:FVIIa complex may act as a docking site for FXa, allowing for activation of PAR-1 and PAR-2. Additional evidence for TF:FVIIa:Xa signaling has come from studies on the human breast cancer adriamycin-resistant-MCF-7 cell line (103). Induction of MAPK phosphorylation involved the formation of a TF–FVIIa–FXa complex, did not require thrombin generation, and was independent of PAR-1 activation. The induction of MAPK phosphorylation by the TF:FVIIa:FXa complex was necessary for cell migration. Other studies have suggested that TF:FVIIa-mediated signaling may also involve receptors distinct from the PARs (91,97).

FXa also has direct effects on cell signaling, particularly in vascular smooth muscle cells. These effects include stimulation of proliferation, activation of MAPK, phosphoinositol turnover, and Ca^{2+} mobilization (101,104–108). FXa also induces $NF_{K}B$ and the angiogenesis-related gene Cyr61 (109). Several receptors have been implicated in the direct effects of FXa, including effector protease receptor 1 (106,110), and PAR-1 (108,109) and PAR-2 (96,99,101,108).

Recent data suggest that PAR-2 may play a dual role by mediating cell signaling induced by TF:FVIIa and TF:FVIIa:FXa complexes and by facilitating signaling through the TF cytoplasmic tail. The TF–FVIIa–FXa complex induced TF cytoplasmic tail phosphorylation specifically by activating PAR-2, but not PAR-1, and was dependent upon the activation of PKCα (111). In addition, expression of TF suppressed a3b1-dependent migration on laminin 5, but only when the TF cytoplasmic domain was not phosphorylated (52). Suppression of migration was reversed by a specific antibody to the extracellular domain of TF, likely due to blocking the $\alpha^3\beta^1$ interaction, and by addition of VIIa. In both cases, suppression of a3b1-dependent migration was blocked by mutation of the phosphorylation sites in the TF cytoplasmic domain.

TF, CIRCULATING MICROPARTICLES, AND CANCER-RELATED THROMBOSIS

As discussed in other chapters, cancer is associated with high rates of venous and arterial thromboembolic events. TF is thought to be a key mediator of cancer-related thrombosis. TF has been found in whole blood and plasma (112–119), and elevated levels have been reported in patients with sickle cell disease (114), diffuse intravascular coagulopathy (112), sepsis (119), and acute myocardial infarction (118). Most recently, blood TF levels have been shown to be elevated in patients with ovarian cancer, and the highest levels (>190 pg/mL) correlated with poorer prognosis (120). Although the study was too small to reach statistical significance, levels of blood TF were higher in patients whose tumors stained most heavily for TF.

The source and structure of circulating TF remains to be determined. Studies have demonstrated that cultured cells release TF into the culture medium in microparticles (121–127). Immunohistochemical studies on circulating TF from human blood have identified TF-containing microparticles that also possess EC-, platelet-, and macrophage-derived surface antigens (115,122,128). Platelet-derived microparticles have received considerable interest as mediators of thrombosis (129,130), particularly in the light of recent studies by Furie et al. demonstrating the role of P-selectin–containing microparticles (MPs)in propagating thrombosis (see below). Beginning with the work of Dvorak et al., many studies have demonstrated that cancer cells also shed procoagulant MPs into the circulation (131–135). In addition to being procoagulant, microparticles may themselves act as agonists for EC, promoting angiogenesis and endothelial inflammation (136,137).

The role of circulating TF in cancer-mediated thrombosis remains to be determined. It has been argued that under normal conditions, the concentration of blood TF is too low to play much of a role in thrombosis (138). In addition, were there "significant" levels of circulating TF activity, it would likely create an unacceptable procoagulant state. More likely, the circulating TF is "encrypted" or complexed with inhibitors and becomes activated only at local sites of thrombus formation. Because TF appears to be associated chiefly with platelets at sites of thrombus formation (113), activation may be platelet dependent.

Recent data have suggested that circulating TF is thrombogenic. Using an ex vivo system, Giesen et al. demonstrated that TF-containing microthrombi formed on TF-naïve surfaces when perfused with human blood (113). Most importantly, microthrombus formation was inhibited by blocking TF. In a series of elegant studies employing intravital microscopy in a model of microvascular thrombosis, Furie et al. demonstrated that TF-containing MPs accumulate at the site of injury in a P-selectin–dependent manner and are critical to thrombus size (139–144). This supports the hypothesis that low concentrations of TF may accumulate at sites of injury and thereby mediate thrombus progression. The model used for these studies was laser injury to the microvasculature and may not reflect the same process that occurs in large vessels. Indeed, a recent study using mouse carotid arterial injury and inferior vena cava ligation models, in concert with bone marrow transplantation from normal and TF-deficient mice, demonstrated that bone marrow–derived TF did not contribute significantly to thrombosis, suggesting that arterial wall TF may be more important (145). However, because bone marrow–derived cells may not be the major source of circulating TF–containing MPs and levels of circulating TF activity were not determined in all of the experimental states, one cannot reach a conclusion about the role of circulating TF in mediating macrovascular thrombosis.

Very high levels of circulating TF have been found in some patients with cancer (120), and we have recently identified several patients with metastatic pancreatic cancer whose levels of circulating TF were >10-fold those of normals (unpublished observations). Chemotherapy might further enhance circulating TF levels by releasing TF into the blood from necrotic tumor cells and angiogenic endothelium. In contrast to the normal state, such high levels may play a direct role in mediating a prothrombotic state. Given the current interest in the biologic role of circulating TF, it is likely that considerable new information will be available concerning the role of circulating TF in mediating cancer-related thromboembolic events.

CONCLUSIONS AND PERSPECTIVES

TF expression is upregulated in many cancers and in most angiogenic endothelium. TF-containing MPs may also be increased in the blood of patients with cancer and may be increased in the early stages of chemotherapy. The increased expression of TF may play an important role in the enhanced thromboembolic complications seen in cancer. In addition, TF may play a role in mediating tumor growth, metastasis, and angiogenesis. These effects appear to be related to multiple mechanisms of action, including "direct" signaling mediated by the cytoplasmic tail of TF, the activation of cell surface receptors by TF complexed to FVIIa and FXa, and by activation of PARs by downstream products of TF enzymatic activity, such as thrombin and FXa. TF or TF-related signaling may therefore be a target not only for attenuating cancer-related thrombosis, but also for inhibiting tumor growth and metastasis. Although the animal studies described above have linked TF with these processes, considerably more information is required to firmly establish the relationship between TF and cancer and to determine the utility of targeting TF. The role of circulating TF in mediating thrombosis remains unclear and needs to be further explored in more animal models. Independent of its role in mediating thrombosis, circulating TF may serve as a marker for thrombosis in high-risk populations and may be useful in determining which patients should receive aggressive antithrombotic therapies, perhaps involving TF inhibition. Given the availability of animal models with altered TF expression and reagents that act on TF, it is likely that this information will be forthcoming and may lead to clinical trials in patients with cancer.

REFERENCES

1. Edgington TS, Mackman N, Brand K, Ruf W. The structural biology of expression and function of tissue factor. Thromb Haemost 1991; 66(1):67–79.
2. Nemerson Y. Tissue factor and hemostasis. Blood 1988; 71(1):1–8.
3. Nemerson Y. Tissue factor: then and now. Thromb Haemost 1995; 74(1):180–184.
4. Rapaport SI, Rao LV. The tissue factor pathway: how it has become a "prima ballerina". Thromb Haemost 1995; 74(1):7–17.
5. Mackman N. Regulation of the tissue factor gene. FASEB J 1995; 9(10):883–889.
6. Taubman MB. Thrombosis, arteriosclerosis, and coronary artery disease. In: Beutler E, Lichtman MA, Coller BS, Kipps TJ, Seligsohn U, eds. Williams' Hematology. New York: McGraw Hill, 2001:1743–1762.
7. Camera M, Giesen PL, Fallon J, et al. Cooperation between VEGF and TNF-alpha is necessary for exposure of active tissue factor on the surface of human endothelial cells. Arterioscler Thromb Vasc Biol 1999; 19(3):531–537.

8. Walsh J, Wheeler HR, Geczy CL. Modulation of tissue factor on human monocytes by cisplatin and adriamycin. Br J Haematol 1992; 81(4):480–488.
9. Ma L, Francia G, Viloria-Petit A, et al. In vitro procoagulant activity induced in endothelial cells by chemotherapy and antiangiogenic drug combinations: modulation by lower-dose chemotherapy. Cancer Res 2005; 65(12):5365–5373.
10. Khorana AA, Fine RL. Pancreatic cancer and thromboembolic disease. Lancet Oncol 2004; 5(11):655–663.
11. Guan M, Jin J, Su B, Liu WW, Lu Y. Tissue factor expression and angiogenesis in human glioma. Clin Biochem 2002; 35(4):321–325.
12. Contrino J, Hair G, Kreutzer DL, Rickles FR. In situ detection of tissue factor in vascular endothelial cells: correlation with the malignant phenotype of human breast disease. Nat Med 1996; 2(2):209–215.
13. Ueno T, Toi M, Koike M, Nakamura S, Tominaga T. Tissue factor expression in breast cancer tissues: its correlation with prognosis and plasma concentration. Br J Cancer 2000; 83(2):164–170.
14. Koomagi R, Volm M. Tissue-factor expression in human non-small-cell lung carcinoma measured by immunohistochemistry: correlation between tissue factor and angiogenesis. Int J Cancer 1998; 79(1):19–22.
15. Sawada M, Miyake S, Ohdama S, et al. Expression of tissue factor in non-small-cell lung cancers and its relationship to metastasis. Br J Cancer 1999; 79(3–4):472–477.
16. Hair GA, Padula S, Zeff R, et al. Tissue factor expression in human leukemic cells. Leuk Res 1996; 20(1):1–11.
17. Lopez-Pedrera C, Barbarroja N, Dorado G, Siendones E, Velasco F. Tissue factor as an effector of angiogenesis and tumor progression in hematological malignancies. Leukemia 2006; 20(8):1331–1340.
18. Kataoka H, Uchino H, Asada Y, et al. Analysis of tissue factor and tissue factor pathway inhibitor expression in human colorectal carcinoma cell lines and metastatic sublines to the liver. Int J Cancer 1997; 72(5):878–884.
19. Nakasaki T, Wada H, Shigemori C, et al. Expression of tissue factor and vascular endothelial growth factor is associated with angiogenesis in colorectal cancer. Am J Hematol 2002; 69(4):247–254.
20. Seto S, Onodera H, Kaido T, et al. Tissue factor expression in human colorectal carcinoma: correlation with hepatic metastasis and impact on prognosis. Cancer 2000; 88(2):295–301.
21. Shigemori C, Wada H, Matsumoto K, Shiku H, Nakamura S, Suzuki H. Tissue factor expression and metastatic potential of colorectal cancer. Thromb Haemost 1998; 80(6):894–898.
22. Poon RT, Lau CP, Ho JW, Yu WC, Fan ST, Wong J. Tissue factor expression correlates with tumor angiogenesis and invasiveness in human hepatocellular carcinoma. Clin Cancer Res 2003; 9(14):5339–5345.
23. Abdulkadir SA, Carvalhal GF, Kaleem Z, et al. Tissue factor expression and angiogenesis in human prostate carcinoma. Hum Pathol 2000; 31(4):443–447.
24. Ohta S, Wada H, Nakazaki T, et al. Expression of tissue factor is associated with clinical features and angiogenesis in prostate cancer. Anticancer Res 2002; 22(5):2991–2996.
25. Kakkar AK, Lemoine NR, Scully MF, Tebbutt S, Williamson RC. Tissue factor expression correlates with histological grade in human pancreatic cancer. Br J Surg 1995; 82(8):1101–1104.
26. Ueda C, Hirohata Y, Kihara Y, et al. Pancreatic cancer complicated by disseminated intravascular coagulation associated with production of tissue factor. J Gastroenterol 2001; 36(12):848–850.
27. Nitori N, Ino Y, Nakanishi Y, et al. Prognostic significance of tissue factor in pancreatic ductal adenocarcinoma. Clin Cancer Res 2005; 11(7):2531–2539.
28. Khorana AA, Ahrendt SA, Ryan CK, et al. Tissue factor expression, angiogenesis, and thrombosis in pancreatic cancer. Clin Cancer Res 2007; 13(10):2870–2875.
29. Tallman MS, Lefebvre P, Baine RM, et al. Effects of all-trans retinoic acid or chemotherapy on the molecular regulation of systemic blood coagulation and fibrinolysis in patients with acute promyelocytic leukemia. J Thromb Haemost 2004; 2(8):1341–1350.

30. Zhou JN, Ljungdahl S, Shoshan MC, Swedenborg J, Linder S. Activation of tissue-factor gene expression in breast carcinoma cells by stimulation of the RAF-ERK signaling pathway. Mol Carcinog 1998; 21(4):234–243.
31. Mueller BM, Reisfeld RA, Edgington TS, Ruf W. Expression of tissue factor by melanoma cells promotes efficient hematogenous metastasis. Proc Natl Acad Sci USA 1992; 89(24):11832–11836.
32. Mueller BM, Ruf W. Requirement for binding of catalytically active factor VIIa in tissue factor-dependent experimental metastasis. J Clin Invest 1998; 101(7):1372–1378.
33. Bromberg ME, Konigsberg WH, Madison JF, Pawashe A, Garen A. Tissue factor promotes melanoma metastasis by a pathway independent of blood coagulation. Proc Natl Acad Sci USA 1995; 92(18):8205–8209.
34. Bromberg ME, Sundaram R, Homer RJ, Garen A, Konigsberg WH. Role of tissue factor in metastasis: functions of the cytoplasmic and extracellular domains of the molecule. Thromb Haemost 1999; 82(1):88–92.
35. Bromberg ME, Bailly MA, Konigsberg WH. Role of protease-activated receptor 1 in tumor metastasis promoted by tissue factor. Thromb Haemost 2001; 86(5):1210–1214.
36. Hembrough TA, Swartz GM, Papathanassiu A, et al. Tissue factor/factor VIIa inhibitors block angiogenesis and tumor growth through a nonhemostatic mechanism. Cancer Res 2003; 63(11):2997–3000.
37. Fernandez PM, Rickles FR. Tissue factor and angiogenesis in cancer. Curr Opin Hematol 2002; 9(5):401–406.
38. Belting M, Ahamed J, Ruf W. Signaling of the tissue factor coagulation pathway in angiogenesis and cancer. Arterioscler Thromb Vasc Biol 2005; 25(8):1545–1550.
39. Versteeg HH, Spek CA, Peppelenbosch MP, Richel DJ. Tissue factor and cancer metastasis: the role of intracellular and extracellular signaling pathways. Mol Med 2004; 10(1–6):6–11.
40. Ruf W, Mueller BMf. Tissue factor in cancer angiogenesis and metastasis. Curr Opin Hematol 1996; 3(5):379–384.
41. Carmeliet P, Mackman N, Moons L, et al. Role of tissue factor in embryonic blood vessel development. Nature 1996; 383(6595):73–75.
42. Toomey JR, Kratzer KE, Lasky NM, Stanton JJ, Broze GJ Jr. Targeted disruption of the murine tissue factor gene results in embryonic lethality. Blood 1996; 88(5):1583–1587.
43. Carmeliet P, Ferreira V, Breier G, et al. Abnormal blood vessel development and lethality in embryos lacking a single VEGF allele. Nature 1996; 380(6573):435–439.
44. Ferrara N, Carver-Moore K, Chen H, et al. Heterozygous embryonic lethality induced by targeted inactivation of the VEGF gene. Nature 1996; 380(6573):439–442.
45. Shoji M, Hancock WW, Abe K, et al. Activation of coagulation and angiogenesis in cancer: immunohistochemical localization in situ of clotting proteins and vascular endothelial growth factor in human cancer. Am J Pathol 1998; 152(2):399–411.
46. Takano S, Tsuboi K, Tomono Y, Mitsui Y, Nose T. Tissue factor, osteopontin, alphavbeta3 integrin expression in microvasculature of gliomas associated with vascular endothelial growth factor expression. Br J Cancer 2000; 82(12):1967–1973.
47. Abe K, Shoji M, Chen J, et al. Regulation of vascular endothelial growth factor production and angiogenesis by the cytoplasmic tail of tissue factor. Proc Natl Acad Sci USA 1999; 96(15):8663–8668.
48. Ollivier V, Bentolila S, Chabbat J, Hakim J, de Prost D. Tissue factor-dependent vascular endothelial growth factor production by human fibroblasts in response to activated factor VII. Blood 1998; 91(8):2698–2703.
49. Ollivier V, Chabbat J, Herbert JM, Hakim J, de Prost D. Vascular endothelial growth factor production by fibroblasts in response to factor VIIa binding to tissue factor involves thrombin and factor Xa. Arterioscler Thromb Vasc Biol 2000; 20(5):1374–1381.
50. Zhang Y, Deng Y, Luther T, et al. Tissue factor controls the balance of angiogenic and antiangiogenic properties of tumor cells in mice. J Clin Invest 1994; 94(3):1320–1327.
51. Zioncheck TF, Roy S, Vehar GA. The cytoplasmic domain of tissue factor is phosphorylated by a protein kinase C-dependent mechanism. J Biol Chem 1992; 267(6):3561–3564.

52. Dorfleutner A, Hintermann E, Tarui T, Takada Y, Ruf W. Cross-talk of integrin alpha3beta1 and tissue factor in cell migration. Mol Biol Cell 2004; 15(10):4416–4425.
53. Ott I, Fischer EG, Miyagi Y, Mueller BM, Ruf W. A role for tissue factor in cell adhesion and migration mediated by interaction with actin-binding protein 280. J Cell Biol 1998; 140(5):1241–1253.
54. Muller M, Albrecht S, Golfert F, et al. Localization of tissue factor in actin-filament-rich membrane areas of epithelial cells. Exp Cell Res 1999; 248(1):136–147.
55. Ott I, Weigand B, Michl R, et al. Tissue factor cytoplasmic domain stimulates migration by activation of the GTPase Rac1 and the mitogen-activated protein kinase p38. Circulation 2005; 111(3):349–355.
56. Patterson C, Stouffer GA, Madamanchi N, Runge MS. New tricks for old dogs: nonthrombotic effects of thrombin in vessel wall biology. Circ Res 2001; 88(10):987–997.
57. Macfarlane SR, Seatter MJ, Kanke T, Hunter GD, Plevin R. Proteinase-activated receptors. Pharmacol Rev 2001; 53(2):245–282.
58. Griffin CT, Srinivasan Y, Zheng YW, Huang W, Coughlin SR. A role for thrombin receptor signaling in endothelial cells during embryonic development. Science 2001; 293(5535):1666–1670.
59. Haralabopoulos GC, Grant DS, Kleinman HK, Maragoudakis ME. Thrombin promotes endothelial cell alignment in Matrigel in vitro and angiogenesis in vivo. Am J Physiol 1997; 273(1 Pt 1):C239–C245.
60. Maragoudakis ME, Kraniti N, Giannopoulou E, Alexopoulos K, Matsoukas J. Modulation of angiogenesis and progelatinase a by thrombin receptor mimetics and antagonists. Endothelium 2001; 8(3):195–205.
61. Wojtukiewicz MZ, Tang DG, Ciarelli JJ, et al. Thrombin increases the metastatic potential of tumor cells. Int J Cancer 1993; 54(5):793–806.
62. Wojtukiewicz MZ, Tang DG, Nelson KK, Walz DA, Diglio CA, Honn KV. Thrombin enhances tumor cell adhesive and metastatic properties via increased alpha IIb beta 3 expression on the cell surface. Thromb Res 1992; 68(3):233–245.
63. Hattori R, Hamilton KK, Fugate RD, McEver RP, Sims PJ. Stimulated secretion of endothelial von Willebrand factor is accompanied by rapid redistribution to the cell surface of the intracellular granule membrane protein GMP-140. J Biol Chem 1989; 264(14):7768–7771.
64. Stenberg PE, McEver RP, Shuman MA, Jacques YV, Bainton DF. A platelet alpha-granule membrane protein (GMP-140) is expressed on the plasma membrane after activation. J Cell Biol 1985; 101(3):880–886.
65. Henn V, Slupsky JR, Grafe M, et al. CD40 ligand on activated platelets triggers an inflammatory reaction of endothelial cells. Nature 1998; 391(6667):591–594.
66. Daniel TO, Gibbs VC, Milfay DF, Garovoy MR, Williams LT. Thrombin stimulates c-sis gene expression in microvascular endothelial cells. J Biol Chem 1986; 261(21):9579–9582.
67. Papadimitriou E, Manolopoulos VG, Hayman GT, et al. Thrombin modulates vectorial secretion of extracellular matrix proteins in cultured endothelial cells. Am J Physiol 1997; 272(4 Pt 1):C1112–C1122.
68. Tsopanoglou NE, Maragoudakis ME. On the mechanism of thrombin-induced angiogenesis. Potentiation of vascular endothelial growth factor activity on endothelial cells by up-regulation of its receptors. J Biol Chem 1999; 274(34):23969–23976.
69. Even-Ram S, Uziely B, Cohen P, et al. Thrombin receptor overexpression in malignant and physiological invasion processes. Nat Med 1998; 4(8):909–914.
70. Maloney JP, Silliman CC, Ambruso DR, Wang J, Tuder RM, Voelkel NF. In vitro release of vascular endothelial growth factor during platelet aggregation. Am J Physiol 1998; 275(3 Pt 2):H1054–H1061.
71. Mohle R, Green D, Moore MA, Nachman RL, Rafii S. Constitutive production and thrombin-induced release of vascular endothelial growth factor by human megakaryocytes and platelets. Proc Natl Acad Sci USA 1997; 94(2):663–668.
72. Fischer EG, Riewald M, Huang HY, et al. Tumor cell adhesion and migration supported by interaction of a receptor-protease complex with its inhibitor. J Clin Invest 1999; 104(9):1213–1221.

73. Karpatkin S. Does hypercoagulability awaken dormant tumor cells in the host? J Thromb Haemost 2004; 2(12):2103–2106.
74. Yin YJ, Salah Z, Grisaru-Granovsky S, et al. Human protease-activated receptor 1 expression in malignant epithelia: a role in invasiveness. Arterioscler Thromb Vasc Biol 2003; 23(6):940–944.
75. Nierodzik ML, Plotkin A, Kajumo F, Karpatkin S. Thrombin stimulates tumor-platelet adhesion in vitro and metastasis in vivo. J Clin Invest 1991; 87(1):229–236.
76. Nierodzik ML, Chen K, Takeshita K, et al. Protease-activated receptor 1 (PAR-1) is required and rate-limiting for thrombin-enhanced experimental pulmonary metastasis. Blood 1998; 92(10):3694–3700.
77. Camerer E, Qazi AA, Duong DN, Cornelissen I, Advincula R, Coughlin SR. Platelets, protease-activated receptors, and fibrinogen in hematogenous metastasis. Blood 2004; 104(2):397–401.
78. Rickles FR, Patierno S, Fernandez PM. Tissue factor, thrombin, and cancer. Chest 2003; 124(3 suppl):58S–68S.
79. Medved L, Tsurupa G, Yakovlev S. Conformational changes upon conversion of fibrinogen into fibrin. The mechanisms of exposure of cryptic sites. Ann N Y Acad Sci 2001; 936:185–204.
80. Palumbo JS, Kombrinck KW, Drew AF, et al. Fibrinogen is an important determinant of the metastatic potential of circulating tumor cells. Blood 2000; 96(10):3302–3309.
81. van Hinsbergh VW, Collen A, Koolwijk P. Role of fibrin matrix in angiogenesis. Ann N Y Acad Sci 2001; 936:426–437.
82. Degen JL, Drew AF, Palumbo JS, et al. Genetic manipulation of fibrinogen and fibrinolysis in mice. Ann N Y Acad Sci 2001; 936:276–290.
83. Bootle-Wilbraham CA, Tazzyman S, Marshall JM, Lewis CE. Fibrinogen E-fragment inhibits the migration and tubule formation of human dermal microvascular endothelial cells in vitro. Cancer Res 2000; 60(17):4719–4724.
84. Thompson WD, Smith EB, Stirk CM, Marshall FI, Stout AJ, Kocchar A. Angiogenic activity of fibrin degradation products is located in fibrin fragment E. J Pathol 1992; 168(1):47–53.
85. Rickles FR, Falanga A. Molecular basis for the relationship between thrombosis and cancer. Thromb Res 2001; 102(6):V215–V224.
86. Dvorak HF, Senger DR, Dvorak AM. Fibrin as a component of the tumor stroma: origins and biological significance. Cancer Metastasis Rev 1983; 2(1):41–73.
87. Bardos H, Molnar P, Csecsei G, Adany R. Fibrin deposition in primary and metastatic human brain tumours. Blood Coagul Fibrinolysis 1996; 7(5):536–548.
88. Wojtukiewicz MZ, Zacharski LR, Memoli VA, et al. Fibrin formation on vessel walls in hyperplastic and malignant prostate tissue. Cancer 1991; 67(5):1377–1383.
89. Lalla RV, Goralnick SJ, Tanzer ML, Kreutzer DL. Fibrin induces IL-8 expression from human oral squamous cell carcinoma cells. Oral Oncol 2001; 37(3):234–242.
90. Palumbo JS, Potter JM, Kaplan LS, Talmage K, Jackson DG, Degen JL. Spontaneous hematogenous and lymphatic metastasis, but not primary tumor growth or angiogenesis, is diminished in fibrinogen-deficient mice. Cancer Res 2002; 62(23):6966–6972.
91. Petersen LC, Freskgard P, Ezban M. Tissue factor-dependent factor VIIa signaling. Trends Cardiovasc Med 2000; 10(2):47–52.
92. Siegbahn A, Johnell M, Rorsman C, Ezban M, Heldin CH, Ronnstrand L. Binding of factor VIIa to tissue factor on human fibroblasts leads to activation of phospholipase C and enhanced PDGF-BB-stimulated chemotaxis. Blood 2000; 96(10):3452–3458.
93. Cunningham MA, Romas P, Hutchinson P, Holdsworth SR, Tipping PG. Tissue factor and factor VIIa receptor/ligand interactions induce proinflammatory effects in macrophages. Blood 1999; 94(10):3413–3420.
94. Poulsen LK, Jacobsen N, Sorensen BB, et al. Signal transduction via the mitogen-activated protein kinase pathway induced by binding of coagulation factor VIIa to tissue factor. J Biol Chem 1998; 273(11):6228–6232.
95. Sorensen BB, Freskgard PO, Nielsen LS, Rao LV, Ezban M, Petersen LC. Factor VIIa-induced p44/42 mitogen-activated protein kinase activation requires the proteolytic activity of fac-

tor VIIa and is independent of the tissue factor cytoplasmic domain. J Biol Chem 1999; 274(30):21349–21354.
96. Camerer E, Rottingen JA, Gjernes E, et al. Coagulation factors VIIa and Xa induce cell signaling leading to up- regulation of the egr-1 gene. J Biol Chem 1999; 274(45):32225–32233.
97. Petersen LC, Thastrup O, Hagel G, et al. Exclusion of known protease-activated receptors in factor VIIa-induced signal transduction. Thromb Haemost 2000; 83(4):571–576.
98. Versteeg HH, Hoedemaeker I, Diks SH, et al. Factor VIIa/tissue factor-induced signaling via activation of Src-like kinases, phosphatidylinositol 3-kinase, and Rac. J Biol Chem 2000; 275(37):28750–28756.
99. Camerer E, Huang W, Coughlin SR. Tissue factor- and factor X-dependent activation of protease-activated receptor 2 by factor VIIa. Proc Natl Acad Sci USA 2000; 97(10):5255–5260.
100. Hjortoe GM, Petersen LC, Albrektsen T, et al. Tissue factor-factor VIIa-specific up-regulation of IL-8 expression in MDA-MB-231 cells is mediated by PAR-2 and results in increased cell migration. Blood 2004; 103(8):3029–3037.
101. Bono F, Schaeffer P, Herault JP, et al. Factor Xa activates endothelial cells by a receptor cascade between EPR-1 and PAR-2. Arterioscler Thromb Vasc Biol 2000; 20(11):E107–E112.
102. Riewald M, Ruf W. Mechanistic coupling of protease signaling and initiation of coagulation by tissue factor. Proc Natl Acad Sci USA 2001; 98(14):7742–7747.
103. Jiang X, Bailly MA, Panetti TS, Cappello M, Konigsberg WH, Bromberg ME. Formation of tissue factor-factor VIIa-factor Xa complex promotes cellular signaling and migration of human breast cancer cells. J Thromb Haemost 2004; 2(1):93–101.
104. Bretschneider E, Braun M, Fischer A, Wittpoth M, Glusa E, Schror K. Factor Xa acts as a PDGF-independent mitogen in human vascular smooth muscle cells. Thromb Haemost 2000; 84(3):499–505.
105. Gasic GP, Arenas CP, Gasic TB, Gasic GJ. Coagulation factors X, Xa, and protein S as potent mitogens of cultured aortic smooth muscle cells. Proc Natl Acad Sci USA 1992; 89(6):2317–2320.
106. Herbert J, Bono F, Herault J, Avril C, Dol F, Mares A, Schaeffer P. Effector protease receptor 1 mediates the mitogenic activity of factor Xa for vascular smooth muscle cells in vitro and in vivo. J Clin Invest 1998; 101(5):993–1000.
107. Ko FN, Yang YC, Huang SC, Ou JT. Coagulation factor Xa stimulates platelet-derived growth factor release and mitogenesis in cultured vascular smooth muscle cells of rat. J Clin Invest 1996; 98(6):1493–1501.
108. McLean K, Schirm S, Johns A, Morser J, Light DR. FXa-induced responses in vascular wall cells are PAR-mediated and inhibited by ZK-807834. Thromb Res 2001; 103(4):281–297.
109. Riewald M, Kravchenko VV, Petrovan RJ, et al. Gene induction by coagulation factor Xa is mediated by activation of protease-activated receptor 1. Blood 2001; 97(10):3109–3116.
110. Altieri DC. Xa receptor EPR-1. Faseb J 1995; 9(10):860–865.
111. Ahamed J, Ruf W. Protease-activated receptor 2-dependent phosphorylation of the tissue factor cytoplasmic domain. J Biol Chem 2004; 279(22):23038–23044.
112. Fukuda C, Iijima K, Nakamura K. Measuring tissue factor (factor III) activity in plasma. Clin Chem 1989; 35(9):1897–1900.
113. Giesen PLA, Rauch U, Bohrmann B, et al. Blood-borne tissue factor: a new view of thrombosis. Proc Natl Acad Sci USA 1999; 96(5):2311–2315.
114. Key NS, Slungaard A, Dandelet L, et al. Whole blood tissue factor procoagulant activity is elevated in patients with sickle cell disease. Blood 1998; 91(11):4216–4223.
115. Mallat Z, Benamer H, Hugel B, et al. Elevated levels of shed membrane microparticles with procoagulant potential in the peripheral circulating blood of patients with acute coronary syndromes. Circulation 2000; 101(8):841–843.
116. Santucci RA, Erlich J, Labriola J, et al. Measurement of tissue factor activity in whole blood. Thromb Haemost 2000; 83(3):445–454.
117. Soejima H, Ogawa H, Yasue H, et al. Heightened tissue factor associated with tissue factor pathway inhibitor and prognosis in patients with unstable angina. Circulation 1999; 99(22):2908–2913.

118. Suefuji H, Ogawa H, Yasue H, et al. Increased plasma tissue factor levels in acute myocardial infarction. Am Heart J 1997; 134(2 Pt 1):253–259.
119. te Velthuis H, van den Brink HG, de Groot ER, Creasey AA, Aarden LA. Soluble tissue factor in plasma [abstr]. Thromb Haemost 1999;
120. Han LY, Landen CN Jr, Kamat AA, et al. Preoperative serum tissue factor levels are an independent prognostic factor in patients with ovarian carcinoma. J Clin Oncol 2006; 24(5):755–761.
121. Carson SD, Perry GA, Pirruccello SJ. Fibroblast tissue factor: calcium and ionophore induce shape changes, release of membrane vesicles, and redistribution of tissue factor antigen in addition to increased procoagulant activity. Blood 1994; 84(2):526–534.
122. Combes V, Simon AC, Grau GE, et al. In vitro generation of endothelial microparticles and possible prothrombotic activity in patients with lupus anticoagulant. J Clin Invest 1999; 104(1):93–102.
123. Kagawa H, Komiyama Y, Nakamura S, et al. Expression of functional tissue factor on small vesicles of lipopolysaccharide-stimulated human vascular endothelial cells [in process citation]. Thromb Res 1998; 91(6):297–304.
124. Mallat Z, Hugel B, Ohan J, Leseche G, Freyssinet JM, Tedgui A. Shed membrane microparticles with procoagulant potential in human atherosclerotic plaques: a role for apoptosis in plaque thrombogenicity. Circulation 1999; 99(3):348–353.
125. Maynard JR, Heckman CA, Pitlick FA, Nemerson Y. Association of tissue factor activity with the surface of cultured cells. J Clin Invest 1975; 55(4):814–824.
126. Satta N, Toti F, Feugeas O, et al. Monocyte vesiculation is a possible mechanism for dissemination of membrane-associated procoagulant activities and adhesion molecules after stimulation by lipopolysaccharide. J Immunol 1994; 153(7):3245–3255.
127. Schecter AD, Spirn B, Rossikhina M, et al. Release of active tissue factor by human arterial smooth muscle cells [see comments]. Circ Res 2000; 87(2):126–132.
128. Siddiqui FA, Desai H, Amirkhosravi A, Amaya M, Francis JL. The presence and release of tissue factor from human platelets. Platelets 2002; 13(4):247–253.
129. Morel O, Toti F, Hugel B, Freyssinet JM. Cellular microparticles: a disseminated storage pool of bioactive vascular effectors. Curr Opin Hematol 2004; 11(3):156–164.
130. Polgar J, Matuskova J, Wagner DD. The P-selectin, tissue factor, coagulation triad. J Thromb Haemost 2005; 3(8):1590–1596.
131. Dvorak HF, Quay SC, Orenstein NS, et al. Tumor shedding and coagulation. Science 1981; 212(4497):923–924.
132. Carr JM, Dvorak AM, Dvorak HF. Circulating membrane vesicles in leukemic blood. Cancer Res 1985; 45(11 Pt 2):5944–5951.
133. Bastida E, Ordinas A, Escolar G, Jamieson GA. Tissue factor in microvesicles shed from U87MG human glioblastoma cells induces coagulation, platelet aggregation, and thrombogenesis. Blood 1984; 64(1):177–184.
134. VanDeWater L, Tracy PB, Aronson D, Mann KG, Dvorak HF. Tumor cell generation of thrombin via functional prothrombinase assembly. Cancer Res 1985; 45(11 Pt 1):5521–5525.
135. Yu JL, Rak JW. Shedding of tissue factor (TF)-containing microparticles rather than alternatively spliced TF is the main source of TF activity released from human cancer cells. J Thromb Haemost 2004; 2(11):2065–2067.
136. Kim HK, Song KS, Chung JH, Lee KR, Lee SN. Platelet microparticles induce angiogenesis in vitro. Br J Haematol 2004; 124(3):376–384.
137. Martinez MC, Tesse A, Zobairi F, Andriantsitohaina R. Shed membrane microparticles from circulating and vascular cells in regulating vascular function. Am J Physiol Heart Circ Physiol 2005; 288(3):H1004–H1009.
138. Butenas S, Bouchard BA, Brummel-Ziedins KE, Parhami-Seren B, Mann KG. Tissue factor activity in whole blood. Blood 2005; 105(7):2764–2770.
139. Falati S, Patil S, Gross PL, et al. Platelet PECAM-1 inhibits thrombus formation in vivo. Blood 2006; 107: 535–541.
140. Falati S, Gross PL, Merrill-Skoloff G, et al. In vivo models of platelet function and thrombosis: study of real-time thrombus formation. Methods Mol Biol 2004; 272:187–197.

141. Celi A, Merrill-Skoloff G, Gross P, et al. Thrombus formation: direct real-time observation and digital analysis of thrombus assembly in a living mouse by confocal and widefield intravital microscopy. J Thromb Haemost 2003; 1(1):60–68.
142. Falati S, Liu Q, Gross P, Merrill-Skoloff G, et al. Accumulation of tissue factor into developing thrombi in vivo is dependent upon microparticle P-selectin glycoprotein ligand 1 and platelet P-selectin. J Exp Med 2003; 197(11):1585–1598.
143. Falati S, Gross P, Merrill-Skoloff G, Furie BC, Furie B. Real-time in vivo imaging of platelets, tissue factor and fibrin during arterial thrombus formation in the mouse. Nat Med 2002; 8(10):1175–1181.
144. Chou J, Mackman N, Merrill-Skoloff G, Pedersen B, Furie BC, Furie B. Hematopoietic cell-derived microparticle tissue factor contributes to fibrin formation during thrombus propagation. Blood 2004; 104(10):3190–3197.
145. Day SM, Reeve JL, Pedersen B, et al. Macrovascular thrombosis is driven by tissue factor derived primarily from the blood vessel wall. Blood 2005; 105(1):192–198.

4

Genetic Analysis of Hemostatic Factors and Cancer

Joseph S. Palumbo and Eric S. Mullins
Divisions of Hematology/Oncology, Cincinnati Children's Hospital Research Foundation, and University of Cincinnati College of Medicine, Cincinnati, Ohio, U.S.A.

Jay L. Degen
Division of Developmental Biology, Cincinnati Children's Hospital Research Foundation, and University of Cincinnati College of Medicine, Cincinnati, Ohio, U.S.A.

- Hemostatic system components actively contribute to the process of tumor dissemination.
- Multiple procoagulant factors are determinants of metastatic potential.
- Tumor cell–associated tissue factor (TF) promotes metastatic potential primarily, although not exclusively, through thrombin generation and ultimately thrombin-mediated proteolysis.
- Platelets and fibrinogen support metastasis by impeding the clearance of newly formed micrometastases by natural killer (NK) cells.
- Tumor cell–associated TF and prothrombin influence metastasis by an additional mechanism independent of NK cell function.

INTRODUCTION

A link between cancer and the hemostatic system was first recognized more than a century ago with the observation that cancer patients are prone to hemostatic derangements, such as thrombophlebitis and disseminated intravascular coagulation. Malignant human and experimental animal tumor cells frequently express procoagulant and fibrinolytic factors [e.g., tissue factor (TF), plasminogen activator (PA), plasminogen activator receptor] that are either absent or minimally expressed in the normal cells from which the transformed cell is derived (1–3). Additionally, tumor stromal cells often express either cell-associated or secreted hemostatic factors (e.g., PA) that may contribute to tumor growth and/or dissemination (4,5). Multiple clinical studies have shown that the expression of hemostatic factors by malignant and/or stromal cells is associated with more advanced disease and a worse prognosis for a variety of human cancers (1,2,4). These correlative findings have suggested that the pattern of hemostatic factor expression might be useful for establishing both clinical prognosis and optimal therapy. However, expression data alone provided no insight into whether there was a causal relationship between specific hemostatic factors and the malignant phenotype. This gap in our understanding of tumor biology has begun to be filled through detailed studies of animal models of cancer. It is increasingly clear that the relationship between hemostatic system components and cancer is not merely an epiphenomenon. Rather, hemostatic factors actively contribute to tumor progression. Much of the data supporting this view has come from analyses of gene-targeted mice with defects in specific hemostatic factors. Nearly all of the known coagulation and fibrinolytic factors as well as their receptors and inhibitors have been genetically disrupted or modified in mice. Similarly, many genes essential for either platelet development or function have been selectively disrupted. Since many of these mutant animals are viable and can be studied well into adulthood, they have been an extraordinary resource in establishing the precise contribution of the hemostatic system to tumor growth and dissemination.

THE HEMOSTATIC SYSTEM AND TUMOR GROWTH

The Role of Thrombin Generation in Tumor Growth

Tumor growth is critically dependent on the development of a complex supportive stroma. More than two decades ago, Dvorak and colleagues made the provocative observation that tumor stroma and the stroma of healing wounds bear many striking similarities (6). Tumors and healing wounds require similar types of support cells, including fibroblasts, endothelial cells, and inflammatory cells. It was also recognized that wound fields and tumor stroma are rich in provisional fibrin matrices and are active in fibrin deposition and dissolution (7,8). Based on the importance of hemostatic factors in tissue remodeling/repair (9–11), angiogenesis, and the regulation of inflammatory processes (12–14), a reasonable hypothesis that emerged was that hemostatic system components are likely to be important determinants of tumor stroma formation, tumor growth, and/or tumor cell dissemination.

A potential role for hemostatic system components in tumor angiogenesis has been supported by many observations, including the well-known proangiogenic properties of fibrin. However, procoagulant expression in the tumor microenvironment could influence angiogenesis through mechanisms that are independent of fibrin formation. Consistent with this notion, TF and prothrombin are important in embryonic vascular development through mechanisms that are independent of the capacity to form thrombi (13,15–21). The binding of fVII to TF has been proposed to initiate cell-autologous signaling events through the TF cytoplasmic domain that are capable of affecting angiogenesis (22). However, other studies have suggested that TF expression by malignant cells is not a determinant of tumor angiogenesis (23). It is also notable that tumors established with teratocarcinomas derived from either TF-deficient or wild-type embryonic stem cells were shown to grow similarly in mice (15). Corroborating these findings, more recent analyses of Ras-transformed tumor cells engineered to express no TF, wild-type TF, or a truncated form of TF lacking the cytoplasmic domain showed that neither TF expression nor signaling events coupled to the TF cytoplasmic domain were required for rapid tumor growth and tumor angiogenesis in immunocompetent mice (24). While these studies unambiguously show that tumor cell–derived TF is not strictly required for tumor growth or stroma formation, the available data do not exclude an important role of TF in tumor growth in certain contexts, such as specific tumor types.

The importance of TF in tumor growth may depend on which cells within the tumor microenvironment produce this fVII/fX receptor. Recent studies have suggested that TF expression by stromal cells, rather than malignant cells, may be a key determinant of tumor angiogenesis. In these studies, the growth of subcutaneously transplanted tumors was compared in wild-type mice and "knock in" mice constitutively expressing a truncated form of TF lacking the cytoplasmic domain ($TF^{\Delta CT}$ mice) (25). Tumors grew much more rapidly in $TF^{\Delta CT}$ mice relative to control animals and demonstrated increased vascular density, implying that TF-mediated signaling events within stromal cells support tumor angiogenesis. More detailed studies in these mice suggested that stromal cell–expressed TF exerts a negative regulation on angiogenesis through signaling events dependent on protease activated receptor-2 (PAR-2) (25). Deletion of the TF cytoplasmic domain in stromal cells apparently uncouples this negative regulatory pathway resulting in exuberant angiogenesis and more rapid tumor growth. A more detailed understanding of the importance of tumor cell– and stromal cell–derived TF in tumor growth will require experimental systems whereby both TF and potential TF-coupled signal transducers (e.g., PAR-1 and PAR-2) can be selectively eliminated from each component cell of the tumor microenvironment, including malignant, stromal, and inflammatory cells.

Circulating hemostatic factors have also been implicated in tumor growth and stroma formation. This relationship was first suggested by animal studies showing that tumor growth could be significantly altered by treatment with pharmacological anticoagulants, such as low molecular weight heparins (26). While these findings suggested a role for thrombin generation in tumor growth, the possibility of secondary pharmacological issues demanded some caution in interpreting these results. Furthermore, these early studies provided no insights into which of the many known thrombin substrates might be important to tumor biology. Thrombin could influence tumor growth and angiogenesis through a plethora of proteolytic targets. Based on the ability of provisional fibrin matrices to support cell adhesion, migration, and proliferation, one attractive hypothesis is that fibrin matrices within solid tumors support the formation of tumor stroma (8). Indeed, fibrin and fibrin degradation products are prominent components of the stroma of many human and murine tumors and may be biologically significant (8). Thrombin could also influence tumor stroma formation through local platelet activation. Platelet granules carry a remarkable array of chemokines, cytokines, and growth factors that have been shown to have angiogenic, inflammatory, and mitogenic properties in other contexts (27,28). Finally, thrombin-mediated signaling through PARs expressed on supporting cells, such as endothelium or mesenchymal cells, as well as tumor cell–associated PARs, could promote tumor growth and stroma formation. Depending on the context, thrombin generation, platelet activation, and fibrin deposition could also have a negative impact on tumor growth potential. For example, the growth of tumors anatomically located in an area prone to mechanical stress could be diminished by the development of intravascular microthrombi, resulting in diminished blood flow to tumor tissue (29). Indeed, targeting of procoagulants to tumor vasculature has been shown to be very effective in controlling tumor growth in mice (30).

Given the variety of potential mechanisms through which thrombin generation could influence tumor growth and stroma formation, the results of tumor growth studies in gene-targeted mice with defects in prothrombin, fibrinogen, and platelet function have been highly illuminating and often surprising. Outside of exceptional contexts (see the next section), each of these key hemostatic factors does not appear to be a critical determinant of tumor growth or stroma formation. For example, comparative analyses of the growth of several transplanted tumor cell lines in fibrinogen-deficient and control mice revealed that circulating fibrinogen is entirely dispensable for tumor growth and angiogenesis (31,32). The genetic imposition of a severe defect in platelet function (i.e., $G\alpha q^{-/-}$) also had no influence on the growth of subcutaneous tumors (33). Until recently, direct analyses of the role of prothrombin in cancer progression using transgenic mice were impossible because complete prothrombin deficiency results in either embryonic or perinatal mortality. However, the generation of transgenic mice rescued by low level expression of a human prothrombin transgene (~7–10% of normal) (34) has provided an opportunity to explore the role of this factor in disease. Initial cancer studies in these mice have likewise not revealed a general impediment in tumor growth (24). However, it is possible that genetically imposed defects resulting in even lower levels of prothrombin expression could reveal an important role for thrombin generation in tumor growth. In this regard, the potential role of thrombin-mediated PAR signaling in tumor stroma formation has not yet been fully explored.

Plasminogen Activation and Tumor Progression

Arguably, the element of the hemostatic system that has been most extensively studied with regard to tumor growth and dissemination is the plasminogen activation system. Multiple human and experimental tumor lines have been shown to express PA, PA receptor, and/or PA inhibitor, suggesting that the conversion of plasminogen to plasmin could play a role in tumor biology (35,36). A mechanistic link between plasminogen activation and tumor progression has been suggested by multiple animal studies showing that agents that impede plasminogen activation diminish tumor growth and/or metastatic potential (35,36). Plasmin has been shown to have a key role in matrix remodeling in the context of wound healing, suggesting it could support cell migration and proliferation in tumor stroma formation (37). Here, plasmin might support the remodeling of tumor stroma through the cleavage of both fibrin and nonfibrin substrates (e.g., metalloproteases, extracellular matrix glycoproteins, latent growth factors) (35–37).

Studies of tumor progression in gene-targeted mice with specific defects in plasminogen as well as components of the plasminogen activation system have generally supported the conclusion that plasminogen activation is a determinant of tumor biology. However, detailed studies of mutant mice lines have also yielded seemingly conflicting findings that, taken together, suggest that the contribution of the PA system to tumor biology is likely to be highly context dependent. For example, some studies have concluded that either plasminogen activation inhibitor-1 (PAI-1) deficiency or PAI-1 overexpression results in diminished tumor growth and angiogenesis (38–42), whereas other studies concluded that neither PAI-1 deficiency nor overexpression has any impact on tumor growth (43). These seemingly conflicting results may be explained, at least in part, by observations that PAI-1 may have a biological role in cell adhesion/migration separate from its role as a protease inhibitor (44). Studies of tumor growth and dissemination in mice with genetic deficits in plasminogen or PAs have also been seemingly inconsistent. For example, genetic elimination of either urokinase-type PA (45) or plasminogen (46) had no effect on the incidence or growth rate of primary tumors in an oncogene-driven mammary cancer model. Plasminogen deficiency likewise had no appreciable influence on primary tumor growth using the Lewis lung carcinoma model (47). In contrast, loss of plasminogen significantly diminished the growth of subcutaneously transplanted T241 fibrosarcoma cells (48). Notably, T241 fibrosarcoma tumors derived from plasminogen-deficient mice in these studies had an apparent diminution in macrophages infiltrating the tumor stroma, suggesting that loss of inflammatory cell–mediated events could explain the genotype-dependent differences in tumor growth (48). Taken together, these studies would suggest that the contribution of plasminogen activation to tumor growth is likely to be dependent on the precise tumor type.

Comprehensive studies of transplantable tumor cell lines in control and plasminogen-deficient mice have provided strong support for the notion that the importance of plasmin to tumor growth may depend not only on tumor type but also on tumor location. In these studies, plasminogen was shown not to be a major determinant of the growth of either Lewis lung carcinoma or T241 fibrosarcoma tumors when transplanted into the dorsal subcutis (29). However, the growth of both tumor types was dramatically diminished in plasminogen-deficient mice relative to control animals when transplanted into the footpad. Based on the presence of occlusive microthrombi within the vasculature of footpad tumors collected from plasminogen-deficient mice, but not tumors established in the dorsal subcutis, it was concluded that the major impediment to tumor growth in the footpad of plasminogen-deficient mice was a location-dependent disruption of vascular patency. This view was supported by the finding that both the plasminogen-dependent diminution in footpad tumor growth and the presence of occlusive microthrombi were entirely reversed by the concomitant genetic elimination of fibrinogen (29). Hence, the role of plasminogen activation in tumor growth may be dependent on multiple factors, including the precise tumor type and tumor location/microenvironment. Furthermore, these studies suggest that plasminogen and other hemostatic system components are likely to be a significant determinant of tumor growth in any location subject to repeated mechanical trauma, such as the footpad of ambulatory mice.

HEMOSTATIC FACTORS AND METASTASIS

Tumor Cell–Associated TF Expression Is Crucial for Metastasis

Although the data regarding the role of the hemostatic system components in tumor growth have been somewhat mixed, an important contribution of procoagulants to tumor cell metastasis has been a consistent finding. The expression of TF by malignant cells is commonplace in aggressively metastatic cancers (49) and this property appears to be critical to the metastatic phenotype. Multiple studies in rodents have shown that tumor cells lacking functional TF expression are nearly incapable of forming metastases, whereas comparable TF-expressing tumor cells are robustly metastatic (23,50–54). The expression of mutated Ras or other transforming oncogenes has been shown to lead to increased TF expression by tumor cells, suggesting that TF expression is fundamentally coupled to the malignant phenotype (3,55). TF expression could support metastasis through several mechanisms. Given that TF is effectively the "firing pin" leading to proteolytic conversion of prothrombin to thrombin, local thrombin generation could be coupled to the metastatic phenotype. However, several studies have suggested that TF may support metastasis by mechanism(s) uncoupled from its "traditional" role in initiating coagulation. In this regard, significant attention has focused on potential intracellular signaling events linked to the cytoplasmic domain of TF (23,51,54). This interest was driven in part by early studies indicating that tumor cells expressing mutant forms of TF with either altered or truncated cytoplasmic domains were far less metastatic than tumor cells expressing wild-type TF (23,51,54). Signaling events mediated by the TF cytoplasmic domain have been proposed to influence multiple cellular processes capable of affecting metastatic potential, including cytoskeletal organization, cell adhesion/migration, and apoptosis (56–61).

While signaling events mediated by the TF cytoplasmic tail may contribute to metastasis in certain contexts, it is increasingly clear that tumor cell–associated TF can support metastasis independent of the TF cytoplasmic domain. Recent comparative analyses of murine fibrosarcoma cell lines either expressing wild-type murine TF, a mutant form of TF lacking the cytoplasmic domain, or entirely devoid of TF strongly suggest that the extracellular domain of TF, rather than the cytoplasmic element, is the critical functional element that drives metastasis (24). Specifically, fibrosarcoma cells genetically incapable of TF expression were found to be nearly incapable of forming metastases, whereas TF-expressing cells were aggressively metastatic regardless of the presence or absence of the cytoplasmic domain (24).

The interaction of tumor cell–associated TF with its extracellular ligands, fVII and fX, could promote metastasis through several mechanisms. TF/fVIIa has been shown to support cell adhesion in vitro through interactions with matrix-immobilized Tissue Factor Pathway Inhibitor-1 (62), suggesting that tumor cell–associated TF/fVII could support tumor cell adhesion/migration. Alternatively, TF/fVIIa- or TF/fVIIa/fXa-mediated activation of either PAR-1 or PAR-2 (63,64) could influence metastatic potential. Here, it should be noted that a contribution of tumor cell–associated PAR activation to metastatic potential is an attractive possibility despite the finding that the genetic elimination of either PAR-1 or PAR-2 within all nontumor tissues in mice may have little impact on metastatic potential (65). Finally, TF may increase metastatic potential by supporting tumor cell–associated thrombin generation and platelet/fibrin deposition. This view is supported by comparative studies of TF-expressing and TF-deficient tumor cells transplanted into mice with and without selected genetic defects in prothrombin, fibrinogen, and platelet function (24). These studies showed that metastasis is exquisitely dependent on the combined availability of tumor cell–associated TF and circulating hemostatic factors (24). A working model consistent with these findings is that TF supports metastatic potential in large part, although not necessarily exclusively, through thrombin generation and ultimately thrombin-mediated proteolysis.

Circulating Hemostatic System Components and Metastasis

A potential link between thrombin and tumor cell metastatic potential has been appreciated for decades through studies of pharmacological or immunological inhibitors of thrombin or thrombin generation. Agents such as heparins, warfarin, and antibodies or inhibitors of fIIa and fXa have been repeatedly shown to inhibit metastatic potential in experimental animals (26). More recent studies using gene-targeted mice expressing low levels of human prothrombin have confirmed the view that thrombin is a major determinant of metastatic potential (24). These results have been further affirmed using mice that express diminished levels of murine prothrombin as a consequence of heterozygosity for a prothrombin null mutation ($fII^{+/-}$ mice) or due to the introduction of a conditional prothrombin knockout allele (fII^{flox} mice) (Fig. 1). One remarkable and somewhat surprising aspect of these studies is that even a relatively modest diminution in prothrombin levels (i.e., just 50% of normal) results in a dramatic diminution in metastatic success (Fig. 1). These results underscore the fundamental importance of thrombin-mediated proteolysis to tumor cell metastasis and suggest that even incremental changes in thrombin substrate conversion are biologically meaningful with regard to metastatic potential.

Any detailed understanding of the contribution of thrombin to cancer biology will require a firm understanding of which of the many known thrombin substrates are important in metastasis. In addition to directly controlling fibrin/platelet deposition, thrombin proteolysis activates coagulation factors XI, VIII, and V and protein C. Other thrombin substrates that might contribute to metastasis include factor XIII (transglutaminase), thrombin-activated fibrinolysis inhibitor, and at least three G protein-coupled PAR-1, -3, and -4. Viable mouse lines have been generated with specific defects in many of these proteins, permitting detailed analyses of their role in tumor dissemination. One of the first thrombin

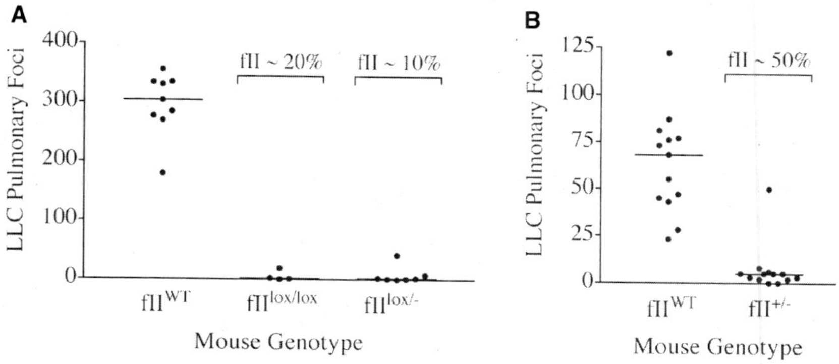

Figure 1 Prothrombin (fII) expression is a crucial determinant of metastatic potential. (**A**) Comparative analysis of pulmonary metastasis in wild-type mice and mutant animals carrying low levels of circulating prothrombin as a consequence of the introduction of a conditional (floxed) fII allele. Surface metastases were counted 14 days after intravenous injection of 5 x 10^5 LLC cells. Each point indicates the pulmonary metastases observed in individual mice ($P < 0.003$ for each comparison). (**B**) Comparative analysis of pulmonary metastasis in control and heterozygous mice carrying one null prothrombin allele formed 14 days after intravenous injection of 3.5 x 10^5 LLC cells. Note that even a relatively modest (i.e., 50%) reduction in circulating prothrombin levels results in a major reduction in pulmonary metastases ($P < 0.0001$). The horizontal bars represent median values. All P values were generated with the Mann Whitney U test. *Abbreviation*: LLC, Lewis lung carcinoma.

substrates to be extensively studied using gene-targeted mice was fibrinogen. The genetic deletion of fibrinogen resulted in a 5- to 10-fold diminution in the number of pulmonary metastases formed after intravenous injection of tumor cells (31). Furthermore, analyses of the more complex process of spontaneous metastases showed that loss of fibrinogen significantly diminished both hematogenous pulmonary metastases and lymphatic metastases (32). However, fibrinogen was not required for the growth of established tumors. Furthermore, tumor cell fate studies using radiolabeled tumor cells showed that fibrinogen was not required for the initial adhesion of circulating tumor cells in the lungs. Rather, fibrinogen dramatically improved the early survival of newly formed pulmonary micrometastases (31). While these results demonstrate that fibrinogen is an important determinant of metastatic potential, it is clearly not the only thrombin substrate important in metastasis. This conclusion was initially suggested by the finding that the already low metastatic potential observed in fibrinogen-deficient mice could be further diminished by the concomitant administration of the potent thrombin inhibitor, hirudin (31).

Considering the dual role of thrombin in fibrin deposition and platelet activation, an obvious second target of thrombin that might contribute to metastatic potential is platelets. This concept is supported by studies with platelet antagonists as well as recent studies showing reduced metastatic potential in mice lacking PAR-4, the primary thrombin-activated receptor directing platelet activation in mice (65). Furthermore, genetic alterations in mice resulting in more profound quantitative and qualitative platelet defects have been shown to dramatically diminish metastatic potential. Nuclear Factor Erythroid-Derived2-deficient mice, which lack circulating platelets, were found to have almost no capacity to support tumor cell metastasis (65). Loss of platelet function secondary to genetic elimination of Gαq, a G-protein signaling molecule critical for platelet activation, dramatically diminished metastasis in both experimental and spontaneous metastasis models (33). Other studies focused on specific proteins known to be important in platelet function, including $\alpha_{IIb}\beta_3$ (66–69) and P-selectin (70), also support the conclusion that platelets are an important determinant of metastatic potential.

Platelets and fibrinogen are undoubtedly not the only thrombin targets coupled to the metastatic phenotype. Preliminary studies of Lewis lung carcinoma metastasis in mice lacking the transglutaminase, fXIII, suggest that this thrombin target also supports metastasis (our unpublished results). Considering the importance of activated protein C both as a modulator of hemostatic function and innate immunity, this thrombin target is also a likely candidate to influence tumor progression. Lastly, thrombin-mediated PAR signaling on cells other than platelets, including tumor cells themselves, may be instrumental in supporting the metastatic phenotype. This concept is supported by studies showing that exposure of tumor cells to either thrombin or thrombin receptor agonists ex vivo prior to inoculation into mice increased metastatic potential (71,72). Considering the broad range of potential mechanisms through which thrombin could influence tumor dissemination, a detailed understanding of the role of this central hemostatic protease in cancer could provide multiple novel targets for treating metastatic disease.

The Platelet/Fibrinogen Axis and Innate Immune Surveillance

The compelling evidence linking the platelet/fibrinogen axis to metastasis raises the fundamental question of mechanism. Three major theories have been suggested to explain how platelets/fibrinogen support metastatic potential. First, platelets and fibrin associated with a newly embolized micrometastatic lesion could protect and stabilize tumor cells against mechanical sheer forces within the vasculature. This notion is supported by microscopic analyses showing that recently embolized tumor cells are associated with appreciable amounts of platelets and fibrin. However, tumor cell fate studies have indicated that neither platelet function nor fibrin(ogen) is a significant determinant of the initial localization of circulating tumor cells within the lung (31,33). Nevertheless, platelet/fibrin microthrombi could support the sustained adhesion of tumor cells within target tissues. A second theory is that the signals derived from the local release of platelet-derived products (e.g., growth factors, chemokines, cytokines) and/or fibrin matrices could support the safe exit of tumor cells into perivascular space or the formation of a supportive tumor stroma (27). A final, and increasingly attractive, hypothesis is that tumor cell–associated platelet/fibrin microthrombi could protect tumor cell emboli from innate immune surveillance mechanisms, particularly natural killer (NK) cells. Of course, these possibilities are not mutually exclusive and a combination of several distinct mechanisms may contribute to overall metastatic potential.

The concept that one advantage to tumors afforded by platelets and fibrinogen is protection from NK cell–mediated immune surveillance is supported by a number of compelling observations (24) (33,73). Several studies have shown that the dramatic diminution in metastatic potential conferred by the elimination of circulating platelets, the loss of platelet function, or fibrinogen deficiency can be entirely abrogated by the concomitant genetic or immunological elimination of NK cells (24) (33,73). Furthermore, tumor cell fate studies indicate that platelets/fibrin offer a survival advantage against NK cell–mediated clearance within just hours of tumor cell entrance into the circulation (24) (33). Whatever the mechanistic transaction between tumor cell–associated platelets/fibrin and NK cells that translates into increased metastatic success, it appears to occur very early following initial tumor cell localization, presumably while tumor cells are still within the vessel lumen. Platelet activation and fibrin(ogen) could influence NK cell function through a variety of potential mechanisms. The most obvious hypothesis is that tumor cell–associated platelets and fibrin constitute a physical barrier limiting access of NK cells to target tumor cells. NK cells recognize and kill potential target cells using a complex repertoire of upregulatory and downregulatory receptors that ultimately determine if a potential target cell is "aberrant" (74). The summation of these cell–cell interactions ultimately determines whether or not an NK cell kills a potential target cell. The concept that tumor cell–associated platelets/fibrin physically impede contact between NK cells and target tumor cells remains viable, but it should be noted that many other cells that support innate immunity readily negotiate both provisional fibrin matrices and immobilized platelets (75). Furthermore, NK cells are capable of migration through several other types of tissue/matrix barriers both in vitro and in vivo (76,77). A second possibility is that platelet-related signaling events downmodulate NK cell elimination of associated tumor cells in vivo. A complex mixture of growth factors, cytokines, and chemokines is known to be released from activated platelets that can affect immune function. It is particularly notable that several platelet-derived soluble factors (e.g., transforming growth factor-β_1 and prostaglandin E_2) have been shown to inhibit NK cell function in other contexts (78,79). An attractive related theory is that platelet activation could result in the appearance of surface proteins which, when engaged by NK cells, would result in their quiescence. Finally, fibrin(ogen) is known to possess a variety of integrin and nonintegrin binding motifs that might regulate NK cell function and limit tumor cell clearance. Of course, none of these potential mechanisms are mutually exclusive and it is possible that platelets/fibrin(ogen) could diminish NK cell–mediated killing through several mechanisms.

While there is a growing body of evidence suggesting that tumor cells can capitalize on the engagement of hemostatic system components as a means of protection from innate immune surveillance mechanisms, it is clearly not the only mechanism linking hemostasis to tumor progression. Recent analyses of TF-expressing fibrosarcoma cells revealed that TF-mediated thrombin generation could support early micrometastatic success by an additional mechanism independent of NK cell function (24). This thrombin-dependent but NK cell–independent mechanism has yet to be defined, but one simple hypothesis is that tumor cell–mediated activation of the full combination of thrombin substrates (e.g., fXI, fVIII, fV, fibrinogen, fXIII, and platelet and endothelial cell–associated PARs) results in increased resistance to shear forces within the vasculature that could disrupt or dissociate tumor cells newly localized within distant organs. Real-time microscopic analyses of circulating tumor cells and NK cells within the vasculature of mice with defects in prothrombin expression and individual thrombin targets may help better define the NK cell–coupled and NK cell–independent mechanisms that contribute to metastasis.

CONCLUSIONS AND FUTURE PROSPECTS

A substantial body of evidence has emerged supporting the view that hemostatic system components are major determinants of tumor dissemination. Hemostatic system components have been shown to influence multiple aspects of malignant disease, including tumor growth, stroma formation, metastasis, and evasion of innate immune surveillance. Consistent with the broad importance of hemostasis in tumor biology, recent clinical trials have shown that treatment with anticoagulants, such as low molecular weight heparin, can prevent cancer progression and improve survival (80,81). Notably, the patients that benefited most from anticoagulant therapy were those with minimal residual disease, consistent with the conclusion that procoagulants strongly influence micrometastases. While these findings are very exciting, they represent only the first steps toward targeting the hemostatic system as a means of treating cancer. As the precise mechanisms linking the hemostatic system to cancer progression become better understood, it is likely that novel therapies will become available which prevent or treat micrometastatic disease while maintaining hemostatic function.

REFERENCES

1. Korte W. Changes of the coagulation and fibrinolysis system in malignancy: their possible impact on future diagnostic and therapeutic procedures. Clin Chem Lab Med 2000; 8:679–692.
2. Laufs S, Schumacher J, Allgayer H. Urokinase-receptor (u-PAR): an essential player in multiple games of cancer: a review on its role in tumor progression, invasion, metastasis, proliferation/dormancy, clinical outcome and minimal residual disease. Cell Cycle 2006; 5(16):1760–1771.
3. Rak J, Yu JL, Luyendyk J, Mackman N. Oncogenes, trousseau syndrome, and cancer-related changes in the coagulome of mice and humans. Cancer Res 2006; 66(22):10643–10646.
4. Vrana JA, Stang MT, Grande JP, Getz MJ. Expression of tissue factor in tumor stroma correlates with progression to invasive human breast cancer: paracrine regulation by carcinoma cell-derived members of the transforming growth factor beta family. Cancer Res 1996; 56(21):5063–5070.
5. Pyke C, Kristensen P, Ralfkiaer E, et al. Urokinase-type plasminogen activator is expressed in stromal cells and its receptor in cancer cells at invasive foci in human colon adenocarcinomas. Am J Pathol 1991; 138(5):1059–1067.
6. Dvorak HF. Tumors: wounds that do not heal. Similarities between tumor stroma generation and wound healing. N Engl J Med 1986; 315(26):1650–1659.
7. Brown LF, Van de Water L, Harvey VS, Dvorak HF. Fibrinogen influx and accumulation of cross-linked fibrin in healing wounds and in tumor stroma. Am J Pathol 1988; 130(3):455–465.
8. Dvorak HF, Nagy JA, Berse B, et al. Vascular permeability factor, fibrin, and the pathogenesis of tumor stroma formation. Ann NY Acad Sci 1992; 667:101–111.
9. Degen JL, Drew AF, Palumbo JS, et al. Genetic manipulation of fibrinogen and fibrinolysis in mice. Ann NY Acad Sci 2001; 936:276–290.
10. Laurens N, Koolwijk P, de Maat MP. Fibrin structure and wound healing. J Thromb Haemost 2006; 4(5):932–939.
11. Li WY, Chong SS, Huang EY, Tuan TL. Plasminogen activator/plasmin system: a major player in wound healing? Wound Repair Regen 2003; 11(4):239–47.
12. Esmon CT. The interactions between inflammation and coagulation. Br J Haematol 2005; 131(4):417–430.
13. Coughlin SR. Protease-activated receptors in hemostasis, thrombosis and vascular biology. J Thromb Haemost 2005; 3(8):1800–1814.
14. von Hundelshausen P, Weber C. Platelets as immune cells: bridging inflammation and cardiovascular disease. Circ Res 2007; 100(1):27–40.
15. Toomey JR, Kratzer KE, Lasky NM, Broze GJ Jr. Effect of tissue factor deficiency on mouse and tumor development. Proc Natl Acad Sci U S A 1997; 94(13):6922–6926.
16. Carmeliet P, Mackman N, Moons L, et al. Role of tissue factor in embryonic blood vessel development. Nature 1996; 383(6595):73–75.
17. Bugge TH, Xiao Q, Kombrinck KW, et al. Fatal embryonic bleeding events in mice lacking tissue factor, the cell-associated initiator of blood coagulation. Proc Natl Acad Sci U S A 1996; 93(13):6258–6263.
18. Camerer E, Duong DN, Hamilton JR, Coughlin SR. Combined deficiency of protease-activated receptor-4 and fibrinogen recapitulates the hemostatic defect but not the embryonic lethality of prothrombin deficiency. Blood 2004; 103(1):152–154.
19. Griffin CT, Srinivasan Y, Zheng YW, Huang W, Coughlin SR. A role for thrombin receptor signaling in endothelial cells during embryonic development. Science 2001; 293(5535):1666–1670.

20. Palumbo JS, Zogg M, Talmage KE, Degen JL, Weiler H, Isermann BH. Role of fibrinogen- and platelet-mediated hemostasis in mouse embryogenesis and reproduction. J Thromb Haemost 2004; 2(8):1368–1379.
21. Sun WY, Witte DP, Degen JL, et al. Prothrombin deficiency results in embryonic and neonatal lethality in mice. Proc Natl Acad Sci U S A 1998; 95(13):7597–7602.
22. Abe K, Shoji M, Chen J, et al. Regulation of vascular endothelial growth factor production and angiogenesis by the cytoplasmic tail of tissue factor. Proc Natl Acad Sci U S A 1999; 96(15):8663–8668.
23. Bromberg ME, Sundaram R, Homer RJ, Garen A, Konigsberg WH. Role of tissue factor in metastasis: functions of the cytoplasmic and extracellular domains of the molecule. Thromb Haemost 1999; 82(1):88–92.
24. Palumbo JS, Talmage KE, Massari JV, et al. Tumor cell-associated tissue factor and circulating hemostatic factors cooperate to increase metastatic potential through natural killer cell-dependent and -independent mechanisms. Blood 2007; 110(1):133–141.
25. Belting M, Dorrell MI, Sandgren S, et al. Regulation of angiogenesis by tissue factor cytoplasmic domain signaling. Nat Med 2004; 10(5):502–509.
26. Bobek V, Kovarik J. Antitumor and antimetastatic effect of warfarin and heparins. Biomed Pharmacother 2004; 58(4):213–219.
27. Sierko E, Wojtukiewicz MZ. Platelets and angiogenesis in malignancy. Semin Thromb Hemost 2004; 30(1):95–108.
28. Weyrich AS, Zimmerman GA. Platelets: signaling cells in the immune continuum. Trends Immunol 2004; 25(9):489–495.
29. Palumbo JS, Talmage KE, Liu H, La Jeunesse CM, Witte DP, Degen JL. Plasminogen supports tumor growth through a fibrinogen-dependent mechanism linked to vascular patency. Blood 2003; 102(8):2819–2827.
30. Nilsson F, Kosmehl H, Zardi L, Neri D. Targeted delivery of tissue factor to the ED-B domain of fibronectin, a marker of angiogenesis, mediates the infarction of solid tumors in mice. Cancer Res 2001; 61(2):711–716.
31. Palumbo JS, Kombrinck KW, Drew AF, et al. Fibrinogen is an important determinant of the metastatic potential of circulating tumor cells. Blood 2000; 96(10):3302–3309.
32. Palumbo JS, Potter JM, Kaplan LS, Talmage K, Jackson DG, Degen JL. Spontaneous hematogenous and lymphatic metastasis, but not primary tumor growth or angiogenesis, is diminished in fibrinogen-deficient mice. Cancer Res 2002; 62(23):6966–6972.
33. Palumbo JS, Talmage KE, Massari JV, et al. Platelets and fibrin(ogen) increase metastatic potential by impeding natural killer cell-mediated elimination of tumor cells. Blood 2005; 105(1):178–185.
34. Sun WY, Coleman MJ, Witte DP, Degen SJ. Rescue of prothrombin-deficiency by transgene expression in mice. Thromb Haemost 2002; 88(6):984–991.
35. Sidenius N, Blasi F. The urokinase plasminogen activator system in cancer: recent advances and implication for prognosis and therapy. Cancer Metastasis Rev 2003; 22(2–3):205–222.
36. Dano K, Behrendt N, Hoyer-Hansen G, et al. Plasminogen activation and cancer. Thromb Haemost 2005; 93(4):676–681.
37. Castellino FJ, Ploplis VA. Structure and function of the plasminogen/plasmin system. Thromb Haemost 2005; 93(4):647–654.
38. Bajou K, Noel A, Gerard RD, et al. Absence of host plasminogen activator inhibitor 1 prevents cancer invasion and vascularization. Nat Med 1998; 4(8):923–928.
39. Bajou K, Masson V, Gerard RD, et al. The plasminogen activator inhibitor PAI-1 controls in vivo tumor vascularization by interaction with proteases, not vitronectin. Implications for antiangiogenic strategies. J Cell Biol 2001; 152(4):777–784.
40. Gutierrez LS, Schulman A, Brito-Robinson T, Noria F, Ploplis VA, Castellino FJ. Tumor development is retarded in mice lacking the gene for urokinase-type plasminogen activator or its inhibitor, plasminogen activator inhibitor-1. Cancer Res 2000; 60(20):5839–5847.
41. McMahon GA, Petitclerc E, Stefansson S, et al. Plasminogen activator inhibitor-1 regulates tumor growth and angiogenesis. J Biol Chem 2001; 276(36):33964–33968.

42. Swiercz R, Keck RW, Skrzypczak-Jankun E, Selman SH, Jankun J. Recombinant PAI-1 inhibits angiogenesis and reduces size of LNCaP prostate cancer xenografts in SCID mice. Oncol Rep 2001; 8(3):463–470.
43. Eitzman DT, Krauss JC, Shen T, Cui J, Ginsburg. Lack of plasminogen activator inhibitor-1 effect in a transgenic mouse model of metastatic melanoma. Blood 1996; 87(11):4718–4722.
44. Dellas C, Loskutoff DJ. Historical analysis of PAI-1 from its discovery to its potential role in cell motility and disease. Thromb Haemost 2005; 93(4):631–640.
45. Almholt K, Lund LR, Rygaard J, et al. Reduced metastasis of transgenic mammary cancer in urokinase-deficient mice. Int J Cancer 2005; 113(4):525–532.
46. Bugge TH, Lund LR, Kombrinck KK, et al. Reduced metastasis of Polyoma virus middle T antigen-induced mammary cancer in plasminogen-deficient mice. Oncogene 1998; 16(24):3097–3104.
47. Bugge TH, Kombrinck KW, Xiao Q, et al. Growth and dissemination of Lewis lung carcinoma in plasminogen-deficient mice. Blood 1997; 90(11):4522–4531.
48. Curino A, Mitola DJ, Aaronson H, et al. Plasminogen promotes sarcoma growth and suppresses the accumulation of tumor-infiltrating macrophages. Oncogene 2002; 21(57):8830–8842.
49. Ruf W, Mueller BM. Thrombin generation and the pathogenesis of cancer. Semin Thromb Hemost 2006; 32(suppl 1):61–68.
50. Bromberg ME, Bailly MA, Konigsberg WH. Role of protease-activated receptor 1 in tumor metastasis promoted by tissue factor. Thromb Haemost 2001; 86(5):1210–1214.
51. Bromberg ME, Konigsberg WH, Madison JF, Pawashe A, Garen A. Tissue factor promotes melanoma metastasis by a pathway independent of blood coagulation. Proc Natl Acad Sci U S A 1995; 92(18):8205–8209.
52. Hembrough TA, Swartz GM, Papathanassiu A, et al. Tissue factor/factor VIIa inhibitors block angiogenesis and tumor growth through a nonhemostatic mechanism. Cancer Res 2003; 63(11):2997–3000.
53. Mueller BM, Reisfeld RA, Edgington TS, Ruf W. Expression of tissue factor by melanoma cells promotes efficient hematogenous metastasis. Proc Natl Acad Sci U S A 1992; 89(24):11832–11836.
54. Mueller BM, Ruf W. Requirement for binding of catalytically active factor VIIa in tissue factor-dependent experimental metastasis. J Clin Invest 1998; 101(7):1372–1378.
55. Yu JL, May L, Klement P, Weitz JI, Rak J. Oncogenes as regulators of tissue factor expression in cancer: implications for tumor angiogenesis and anti-cancer therapy. Semin Thromb Hemost 2004; 30(1):21–30.
56. Ott I, Fischer EG, Miyagi Y, Mueller BM, Ruf W. A role for tissue factor in cell adhesion and migration mediated by interaction with actin-binding protein 280. J Cell Biol 1998; 140(5):1241–1253.
57. Ott I, Weigand B, Michl R, et al. Tissue factor cytoplasmic domain stimulates migration by activation of the GTPase Rac1 and the mitogen-activated protein kinase p38. Circulation 2005; 111(3):349–355.
58. Luther T, Dittert DD, Kotzsch M, et al. Functional implications of tissue factor localization to cell-cell contacts in myocardium. J Pathol 2000; 192(1):121–130.
59. Sharma L, Melis E, Hickey MJ, et al. The cytoplasmic domain of tissue factor contributes to leukocyte recruitment and death in endotoxemia. Am J Pathol 2004; 165(1):331–340.
60. Dorfleutner A, Hintermann E, Tarui T, Takada Y, Ruf W. Cross-talk of integrin alpha3beta1 and tissue factor in cell migration. Mol Biol Cell 2004; 15(10):4416–4425.
61. Jiang X, Guo YL, Bromberg ME. Formation of tissue factor-factor VIIa-factor Xa complex prevents apoptosis in human breast cancer cells. Thromb Haemost 2006; 96(2):196–201.
62. Fischer EG, Riewald M, Huang HY, et al. Tumor cell adhesion and migration supported by interaction of a receptor-protease complex with its inhibitor. J Clin Invest 1999; 104(9):1213–1221.
63. Camerer E, Huang W, Coughlin SR. Tissue factor- and factor X-dependent activation of protease-activated receptor 2 by factor VIIa. Proc Natl Acad Sci U S A 2000; 97(10):5255–5260.
64. Riewald M, Ruf W. Mechanistic coupling of protease signaling and initiation of coagulation by tissue factor. Proc Natl Acad Sci U S A 2001; 98(14):7742–7747.

65. Camerer E, Qazi AA, Duong DN, Cornelissen I, Advincula R, Coughlin SR. Platelets, protease-activated receptors, and fibrinogen in hematogenous metastasis. Blood 2004; 104(2):397–401.
66. Amirkhosravi A, Mousa SA, Amaya M, et al. Inhibition of tumor cell-induced platelet aggregation and lung metastasis by the oral GpIIb/IIIa antagonist XV454. Thromb Haemost 2003; 90(3):549–554.
67. Trikha M, Zhou Z, Timar J. Multiple roles for platelet GPIIb/IIIa and alphavbeta3 integrins in tumor growth, angiogenesis, and metastasis. Cancer Res 2002; 62(10):2824–2833.
68. Cohen SA, Trikha M, Mascelli MA. Potential future clinical applications for the GPIIb/IIIa antagonist, abciximab in thrombosis, vascular and oncological indications. Pathol Oncol Res 2000; 6(3):163–174.
69. Isoai A, Ueno Y, Giga-Hama Y, Goto H, Kumagai H. A novel Arg-Gly-Asp containing peptide specific for platelet aggregation and its effect on tumor metastasis: a possible mechanism of RGD peptide-mediated inhibition of tumor metastasis. Cancer Lett 1992; 65(3): 259–264.
70. Borsig L, Wong R, Feramisco J, Nadeau DR, Varki NM, Varki A. Heparin and cancer revisited: mechanistic connections involving platelets, P-selectin, carcinoma mucins, and tumor metastasis. Proc Natl Acad Sci U S A 2001; 98(6):3352–3357.
71. Nierodzik ML, Chen K, Takeshita K, et al. Protease-activated receptor 1 (PAR-1) is required and rate-limiting for thrombin-enhanced experimental pulmonary metastasis. Blood 1998; 92(10):3694–3700.
72. Nierodzik ML, Kajumo F, Karpatkin S. Effect of thrombin treatment of tumor cells on adhesion of tumor cells to platelets in vitro and tumor metastasis in vivo. Cancer Res 1992; 52(12):3267–3272.
73. Nieswandt B, Hafner M, Echtenacher B, Mannel DN. Lysis of tumor cells by natural killer cells in mice is impeded by platelets. Cancer Res 1999; 59(6):1295–1300.
74. Yokoyama WM. Natural killer cell immune responses. Immunol Res 2005; 32(1–3):317–325.
75. Diacovo TG, Roth SJ, Buccola JM, Bainton DF, Springer TA. Neutrophil rolling, arrest, and transmigration across activated, surface-adherent platelets via sequential action of P-selectin and the beta 2-integrin CD11b/CD18. Blood 1996; 88(1):146–157.
76. Allavena P, Bianchi G, Paganin C, Giardina G, Mantovani A. Regulation of adhesion and transendothelial migration of natural killer cells. Nat Immun 1996; 15(2–3):107–116.
77. Curtiss LK, Kubo N, Schiller NK, Boisvert WA. Participation of innate and acquired immunity in atherosclerosis. Immunol Res 2000; 21(2–3):167–176.
78. Bellone G, Aste-Amezaga M, Trinchieri G, Rodeck U. Regulation of NK cell functions by TGF-beta 1. J Immunol 1995; 155(3):1066–1073.
79. Yakar I, Melamed R, Shakhar G, et al. Prostaglandin e(2) suppresses NK activity in vivo and promotes postoperative tumor metastasis in rats. Ann Surg Oncol 2003; 10(4):469–479.
80. Kakkar AK, Levine MN, Kadziola Z, et al. Low molecular weight heparin, therapy with dalteparin, and survival in advanced cancer: the fragmin advanced malignancy outcome study (FAMOUS). J Clin Oncol 2004; 22(10):1944–1948.
81. Klerk CP, Smorenburg SM, Otten HM, et al. The effect of low molecular weight heparin on survival in patients with advanced malignancy. J Clin Oncol 2005; 23(10):2130–2135.

5

Chemotherapy-Induced Hemostatic Activation and Thrombosis in Cancer

Ilene Weitz and Howard A. Liebman

Division of Hematology, Department of Medicine, University of Southern California Keck School of Medicine and the Kenneth J. Norris, Jr. Comprehensive Cancer Center, Los Angeles, California, U.S.A.

- Patients with cancer receiving chemotherapy are more likely to develop venous thromboembolism (VTE) than cancer patients not receiving chemotherapy
- Preoperative chemotherapy-induced hemostatic activation may also increase the surgical VTE risk in the cancer patient
- Antiangiogenic and cytokine-modulating agents have been associated with a substantial increased risk for thrombosis when combined with chemotherapy
- Clinical studies have documented rapid chemotherapy-induced increases in plasma markers of thrombin generation
- The pathophysiology of this rapid chemotherapy-induced activation of the hemostatic system appears to be complex but may result from chemotherapy-induced tissue factor expression and endothelial activation
- An increase in basal thrombin generation is observed with repeated cycles of chemotherapy, which may account for the reported increased thrombotic risk with increasing cycles of chemotherapy

INTRODUCTION

The last 20 years have yielded significant advances in our understanding of the relationship between cancer biology, cancer-associated hemostatic activation, and the subsequent development of venous thromboembolism (VTE). Hemostatic activation can occur in patients with a variety of tumor types but may not translate into the development of clinically evident thrombosis due to the presence or absence of additional risk factors (1,2). Although arterial events can also occur in patients with malignancy, VTE is more frequently observed (1–3). Patients with cancer have at least a sevenfold increased risk of VTE compared to patients without cancer and the risk may be up to 20-fold in patients with metastatic disease (4). Various studies report the incidence of clinically significant VTE as 1% to 43% among cancer patients, depending on the type and stage of tumor, modality of cancer treatment, contributing risk factors, and comorbidities (5,6).

In addition to the type and stage of the malignancy, a number of classical risk factors such as surgery, intravenous catheters, infection, and bed rest further contribute to the cancer patient's thrombotic risk. However, a major thrombotic risk factor unique to the cancer patient results from the administration of systemic antineoplastic chemotherapy (1,2,4,5). Both population-based epidemiologic studies of VTE in cancer patients and the reported increased incidence of venous and arterial thrombosis observed in cancer treatment trials have shown that many chemotherapeutic drugs alone or in combination can significantly increase the thrombotic risk in cancer patients (7–30). In addition, newer targeted therapeutic agents and antiangiogenic drugs, while demonstrating a low thrombotic potential when given alone, can be associated with a markedly increased thrombotic risk when combined with other chemotherapeutic agents (31–47). Although a number of studies have demonstrated prothrombotic alterations in the hemostatic profile of cancer patients receiving chemotherapeutic agents, the precise mechanisms by which these drugs induce these pathogenic changes remains poorly understood.

In this chapter, we will review the evidence for an association between the systemic cancer chemotherapy and venous and arterial thrombosis and the proposed mechanisms by which these therapeutic agents contribute to the thromboembolic complications of cancer.

SYSTEMIC ANTINEOPLASTIC CHEMOTHERAPY AND VTE

A population-based, nested case-control study of VTE during a 15-year period in Olmstead County, Minnesota identified malignant neoplasm as a significant risk factor for VTE (7). For patients with cancer receiving chemotherapy the odds ratio for VTE was 6.5 [95% confidence interval (CI): 2.1–20.2] compared to an odds ratio of 4.1 (95% CI: 1.9–8.5) for cancer patients not receiving chemotherapy (7). A record linkage study of the Cancer Registry and the anticoagulation clinic databases in the Netherlands found that patients who received chemotherapy as initial treatment had an increased risk of VTE. The overall risk was 2.2 [relative risk (RR) 2.2, 95% CI: 1.8–2.6] when compared with that of patients who never received chemotherapy (8). The RR was even greater for patients receiving chemotherapy for metastatic disease (RR 2.4, 95% CI: 1.7–3.3).

A prospective observational multicenter study of 3003 patients with varied malignancies receiving chemotherapy reported an incidence of symptomatic VTE in 1.93% of patients (9). However, the incidence varied significantly by site of cancer (9). A retrospective single institution study of 206 consecutive cancer patients receiving chemotherapy reported objectively documented VTE in 7.3% of patients (10). The incidence of VTE was particularly increased in patients with colorectal cancer treated with fluorouracil (FU) and leucovorin chemotherapy (10). Since patients were not routinely screened for VTE in these studies, they most likely underestimated the incidence of VTE. Also, it cannot be determined from these studies whether the differences observed in VTE incidence for different cancers resulted from the specific malignancy or the chemotherapy used in treatment.

Levine et al. has analyzed the VTE incidence data from breast cancer treatment trials to show a relationship between antineoplastic therapy and VTE (2,5). In early-stage breast cancer in the absence of adjuvant therapy, the risk of VTE is reported between 0.2% and 0.8% (12,14,15). Although hormone therapy itself has been associated with an increased risk of VTE (11,12), when combined with chemotherapy, the risk significantly increases (12,13). In the International Breast Cancer Intervention Study on the effect of tamoxifen in a population of women with an elevated risk of developing breast cancer, the odds ratio for the development of VTE in women randomized to tamoxifen was 2.7 (95% CI: 1.6–4.6) (11). In women receiving adjuvant therapy for breast cancer, the incidence of VTE was fourfold higher among patients treated with both tamoxifen and chemotherapy compared with those who were treated with hormonal therapy alone (4.2–9.6% vs. 1.0–1.6%) (12,13). A retrospective study by the European Organization for Research and Treatment of Cancer, Breast Cancer Cooperative Group Study, showed that the incidence of VTE was increased in women receiving adjuvant chemotherapy within six weeks of surgery by 2.1% versus 0.8% for those patients who did not receive chemotherapy (14). A retrospective review of the records from Eastern Cooperative Oncology Group studies of adjuvant therapy reported an 8% incidence of VTE in postmenopausal women who received tamoxifen and chemotherapy compared to a 0.4% incidence ($p < 0.0001$) in women on the observation arms (15).

In a separate study by Levine, women receiving adjuvant chemotherapy for Stage II breast cancer were randomized to 12 weeks versus 36 weeks of chemotherapy, than prospectively followed for the development of VTE. There were 14 events in the 205 patients (6.8%), all occurring during the chemotherapy (16). All events occurred during 979 patient-months of chemotherapy, whereas none occurred during 2413 patient-months without treatment. A recent prospective study utilizing a routine ultrasound screening for VTE has found an objectively documented 4% incidence of VTE in women treated for Stage II breast cancer (Topic 1) (17). When chemotherapy is utilized in patients with advanced metastatic disease, the risk of VTE is significantly increased. A case series of women with Stage IV metastatic breast cancer receiving chemotherapy reported a 17% incidence of VTE (18). As observed in the Levine study, nearly all reported events occurred while patients were receiving systemic treatment for their malignancy.

A number of retrospective studies in other malignancies have also suggested a significant thrombotic risk associated with systemic chemotherapy, although these studies were less well controlled than the studies in breast cancer. However, they do lend support for a role for antineoplastic agents in contributing to the thrombotic risk in cancer patients. Table 1 presents the reported incidence of thrombotic events observed in various cancer treatment trials.

A single institution, retrospective study of patients with esophageal cancer receiving induction chemotherapy with cisplatinum, 5-FU infusion, with or without paclitaxel

Table 1 Incidence of VTE by Cancer Type and Treatment

Study	Cancer type	Cancer stage	Treatment	VTE (%)
Poplin et al. (20)	Colon	Stage II/III	FU/LV, levamisole	4.6
			Infusion FU/LV	6.9
Andre et al. (21)	Colon	Stage II/III	FU/LV; oxaliplatin	5.7
			FU/LV	6.5
Hurwitz et al. (22)	Colon	Stage IV	FU/LV	11.4
			FU/LV, bevacizamab	12.5
Cantwell et al. (23)	Lymphoma	Advanced	Various	10
Clarke et al. (24)	Lymphoma	Advanced	MACOP-B	27
Tateo et al. (27)	Ovarian	Stage III/IV	CDDP+—first line	6.4
			Follow-up treatment	4.8
Von Tempelhoff et al. (26)	Ovarian	Stage III/IV	CDDP, epirubicin, CTX	10.6
Lubiniecki et al. (28)	Prostate	Stage IV	Estramustine	6

Abbreviations: FU/LV, fluorouracil and leucovorin; CDDP+, cisplatinum alone or with additional chemotherapy; CTX, cyclophosphamide; MACOP-B, Methotrexate, Adriamycin, Cyclophospmide, Vincristin (Oncoin), Prednisone-Bleomycin; VTE, venous thromboembolism.

followed by radiation prior to surgical resection, reported an 8.4% incidence of symptomatic postsurgical VTE compared no thrombotic events observed in the patients who did not receive induction chemotherapy (19). This would suggest that preoperative chemotherapy-induced hemostatic activation might increase the surgical VTE risk in the cancer patient. Studies on the use of adjuvant chemotherapy in colon cancer report a 4% to 6% incidence of VTE (20,21). Up to a 12% incidence of VTE with combination chemotherapy for advanced colon cancer has been reported (Table 1) (22). The addition of the antiangiogenic agent, bevacizamab, to a standard chemotherapeutic regimen appeared to increase the risk of arterial thrombotic events (22). Other studies have suggested a causal role for systemic chemotherapy in the development of VTE in lymphoma (23,24), ovarian (25–27), prostate (28), glioma (29), and bladder cancers (Table 1) (30).

Antiangiogenic and cytokine-modulating agents such as SU5416 (31), thalidomide (32–45), and lenolinamide (46,47) have been associated with an increased risk for thrombosis, particularly when combined with chemotherapy. In 19 patients treated with *Cis*-platinum, gemcitabine, and SU5416, a molecule that inhibits autophosphorylation of the VEGF receptor, eight patients developed thrombotic events consisting of five arterial vascular events, two cerebral vascular accidents (CVAs), three transient ischemic attack, and four venous thromboembolic events (31). Although rare thromboembolic events had been observed with SU5416 alone, the combination appeared to significantly increase the thrombotic risk. In three patients on this study, plasma thrombin–antithrombin complexes (TAT) and prothrombin fragment 1+2 (F1+2), both sensitive markers of hemostatic activation, were measured prior to therapy, on day 8 and day 18 of a 21-day treatment cycle (31). Plasma TAT and F1+2 markedly increased by day 8 in all patients for each of the first and second treatment cycles. In all three patients, TAT and F1+2 remained elevated through day 18. Two of the three patients developed thromboembolic complications.

Thalidomide therapy, alone or in combination therapy, has been associated with the development of VTE (32–45). When given as a single agent in the treatment of multiple myeloma (MM), the reported incidence of VTE with thalidomide was 3% to 4% (32,33). When thalidomide is combined with dexamethasone alone or with other chemotherapeutic drugs for treatment of MM, the reported incidence of VTE ranges from 9% to 58% (Table 2) (34–41).

A similar high incidence of VTE has been reported for other trials combining thalidomide with other chemotherapeutic agents and/or biologics for the treatment of other malignancies and myelodysplasia (Table 2) (42–45). Lenolinamide, a potent analog of thalidomide, has also been reported to be associated with an increased risk of VTE, despite reduction in other thalidomide treatment–associated toxicities. The reported VTE incidence with lenolinamide and dexamethasone combination therapy is 19%, compared to 4% with lenolinamide alone (46,47).

Although the clinical trial data strongly support a causal role for systemic chemotherapy in the development of venous and arterial thrombosis in cancer patients, it does not provide any insights into the mechanism(s) by which antineoplastic treatment increases the thrombotic risk in these patients. In addition, the thrombotic risk related to systemic chemotherapy may depend upon the specific treatment regimen, the type of malignancy, cancer stage, and other contributing risk factors and comorbidities.

PATHOPHYSIOLOGY MARKERS OF HEMOSTATIC ACTIVATION

Several studies have documented chemotherapy-induced increases in plasma markers of thrombin generation such as TAT, prothrombin F1+2, fibrinopeptide A (FpA), and

Table 2 Incidence of VTE in Patients Treated with Thalidomide Alone or with Chemotherapy

Study	Cancer type	Patients	Treatment	VTE (%)
Glasmacher et al.[a] (32)	MM	1674	Th	3
Weber et al. (33)	MM	28	Th	4
			Th/D	15
Rajkumar et al. (34)	MM	102	D	3
		102	D/Th	17
Cavo et al. (35)	MM	61	D/Th	16
Palumbo et al. (36)	MM	164	M/P	2
		65	M/P/Th	17
		64	M/P/Th + enoxaparin	3
Hussein et al. (37);	MM	103	D/Th/VCR/LpDox (All)	
25				
Baz et al. (38)		19	D/Th/VCR/LpDox	58
		84	D/Th/VCR/LpDox + ASA	18
Offidani et al. (39)	MM	50	D/Th/LpDox	12
Dimopoulos et al. (40)	MM	50	D/Th/M	9
Lee et al. (41)	MM	236	D/Th/Dox/C/E	15
Desai et al. (42)	Renal CA	21	Th/FU/Gem	43
Dahut et al. (43)	Prostate	49	Th/Dtax	18
		25	Dtax	0
Fine et al. (44)	Glioma	40	Th/BCNU	30
Steurer et al. (45)	MDS	7	Th/darbopoietin	43

[a]A systematic review of phase II trials.

Abbreviations: Th, thalidomide; D, dexamethasone; M, mephalan; P, prednisone; VCR, vincristine; LpDox, liposomal doxorubicin; Dox, doxorubicin; E, etoposide; C, cyclophosphamide; P, cisplatinum; FU, fluorouracil; Gem, gemcitabine, Dtax, docetaxel; BCNU, carmustine; MM, multiple myeloma; MDS, myelodysplasia.

D-dimers. Edwards et al. measured plasma FpA levels in 16 cancer patients of various tumor types with metastatic disease before and after receiving infusions of an antineoplastic drug (48). Chemotherapeutic drugs given in the study included doxorubicin, methotrexate, FU, vincristine, and trimetrexate. Statistically significant elevations in FpA were documented within 45 minutes of receiving chemotherapy, although there were significant variations in responses for the different patients (48). This increase could be blocked by the concurrent administration of 5000 units of unfractionated heparin (48). A study of hemostatic activation during a single four-day continuous infusion of FU in 10 patients observed a significant increase in plasma FpA after 24 hours of infusion (49). Plasma levels of FpA returned to pretreatment levels at the end of the 24-hour infusion (49).

A study evaluating hemostatic activation in patients with non-Hodgkin's lymphoma compared an intensive COP-BLAM (cyclophosphamide, vincristine, prednisone, bleomycin, doxorubicin, and procarbazine) protocol with a less intensive COP regime (50). Markers of thrombin generation, plasma TAT, and prothrombin F1+2 were significantly elevated four hours after infusion of the intensive regimen (50). Although the less-intensive COP regimen also resulted in an increase in markers of thrombin generation, this did not reach statistical significance. Weitz et al. (51) studied the hemostatic alterations associated with chemotherapy in patients receiving treatment for breast and lung cancer. They demonstrated statistically significant increases in plasma TAT and D-Dimers within one hour of infusion of the systemic chemotherapy when compared to pretreatment levels. Plasma TAT and D-dimers remained significantly elevated 24 and 48 hours after treatment (51). Similar to the study of Edwards et al., hemostatic activation could be blocked by a single pretreatment dose of a low molecular weight heparin, dalteparin. In the patients with breast cancer, there was a statistically significant increase in basal pretreatment thrombin generation, as defined by increased plasma TAT, which appeared cumulative over the four months of treatment (51). Only one of the 10 patients with breast cancer had evidence of active cancer while receiving treatment.

The pathophysiology of this rapid chemotherapy-induced activation of the hemostatic system appears to be complex but strongly suggests a rapid increase in systemic functional tissue factor expression. Endothelial activation, due to the direct effects of chemotherapy, has been proposed as one cause of increased hemostatic activation (52). In vitro studies of human endothelial cell have demonstrated enhanced thrombin-induced tissue factor expression by paclitaxel (53). This enhanced expression appears to result from paclitaxel activation of c-Jun terminal NH_2 kinase (53). Direct endothelial cell toxicity has been described with exposure to bleomycin. Vacuolization and necrosis of murine endothelial cells have been described in histologic sections of lung after bleomycin exposure (54). In vitro exposure of endothelial cells to various cancer drugs has been reported to induce retraction from its subendothelial matrix, resulting in platelet adherence to the exposed matrix (55). Exposure of the subendothelial matrix would also expose blood to subendothelial tissue factor, leading to hemostatic activation. Exposure of cultured human endothelial cells to postchemotherapy plasma from breast cancer patients resulted in increased platelet–endothelial interaction (56). These changes were correlated with increased plasma interleukin (IL)-1 (56), a cytokine known to induce endothelial and monocytes tissue factor expression (57).

Direct or indirect chemotherapy-induced endothelial perturbation may result in increases in plasma levels of von Willebrand factor (vWF) and Factor VIII coagulant protein (58–62). CVAs, reported following bleomycin, or vindesine and cisplatinum chemotherapy for head and neck cancer, have been associated with markedly elevated levels of vWF. The patients who developed CVA had elevated baseline vWF levels, which increased with chemotherapy (58). In 65 patients with testicular cancer treated with cisplatin and bleomycin chemotherapy, plasma von Willebrand levels increased significantly by completion of their chemotherapy (59). Venous thrombotic events occurred in five (7.7%) patients and arterial events occurred in two (3%) patients (59). Although increases in vWF levels in the plasma of cancer patients receiving chemotherapy could result directly from drug-induced endothelial activation, indirect endothelial activation mediated by either chemotherapy-induced inflammatory cytokines or by thrombin-mediated endothelial release is also possible. Patients receiving chemotherapy for breast and lung cancer had increases in plasma levels of IL-6 compared to pretreatment levels (60).

Microangiopathic thrombocytopenia has been noted as a consequence of exposure to mitomycin C and gemcitabine. The role of ultralarge vWF multimers in chemotherapy-associated thrombotic thrombocytopenic purpura (TTP)/hemolytic uremic syndrome (HUS) is unclear. The presence of ultralarge multimers of vWF was noted in five of six cancer patients who had received chemotherapy and/or cyclosporine who subsequently developed thrombotic microangiopathy (61). Other investigators have failed to detect similar abnormalities in von Willebrand multimer patterns associated with mitomycin C–related TTP/HUS (62). Unlike classical TTP, decreased cleavage of vWF was not observed in patients developing a TTP-like picture following bone marrow transplant (63). In these patients, A Disintegin And Metalloproteinase with ThromboSondin like Motif- number 13 activity appears to be normal, unlike classical TTP where ADAMTS13 activity is significantly reduced (63). This may explain why chemotherapy-induced TTP/HUS responds poorly to plasma exchange.

The increase in basal levels of thrombin generation observed with repeated cycles of chemotherapy may result from cumulative prothrombotic changes in patient plasma. Alterations in protein C plasma levels have been described during breast cancer chemotherapy with several studies reporting decreases in protein C levels as a consequence of chemotherapy (64,65). In a study of 15 patients receiving cyclophosphamide, FU, and methotrexate for breast cancer, statistically significant decreases in protein C activity and antigen and protein S antigen developed by day 8 of treatment (64). Concomitant with the decrease in proteins C and S was a statistically significant decrease in Factor VII activity, suggesting that the coagulation inhibitor decreases could have resulted from consumption secondary to hemostatic activation (64). A prospective analysis of nine patients receiving cyclophosphamide, methotrexate, and 5-FU for breast cancer treatment demonstrated a statistically significant reduction in protein C activity ($p < 0.001$) in all patients after two months of treatment (65). Protein C levels returned to baseline after completion of the chemotherapy (65). Of interest, eight of nine patients had midtherapy elevations of Factor VIII, an independent risk factor for thrombosis (65). Ten patients receiving 5-FU alone or in combination with cisplatinum, cyclophosphamide, methotrexate, or doxorubicin developed statistically significant increases in FpA with a simultaneous decrease in protein C activity (47). The question remains in regard to these studies as to whether the depressions reported in protein C activity and antigen result from enhanced consumption via increased tissue factor–mediated thrombin generation or whether drug-induced suppression of this natural anticoagulant results in an enhanced malignancy-related hemostatic activation.

L-asparginase is an important antineoplastic drug used in the treatment of acute lymphoblastic leukemia. Its unique biologic effect results from depletion of plasma L-asparagine, an essential amino acid required for protein synthesis and, therefore, inhibiting leukemic cell growth. L-asparginase also suppresses hepatic protein synthesis, resulting in decreases in multiple plasma hemostatic and anticoagulant proteins including fibrinogen, plasminogen, antithrombin, proteins C and S, and other coagulation factors (66–76). The combined effects of the underlying malignancy and an apparent disproportionate suppression of natural anticoagulant levels have resulted in a significant incidence of thrombosis in children and adults treated with the agent (77–79). Most events occur within one to two weeks after initiation of asparaginase treatment, which coincides with greatest depression in the levels of the natural anticoagulants. Depressions in antithrombin plasma levels have been correlated with elevations in markers of hemostatic activation including FpA, TAT, and prothrombin F1 + 2 (70,71,74). However, the levels of antithrombin or other natural anticoagulants such as protein C or S do not consistently correlate with thrombotic events or predict for the development of thrombosis (67,71,75).

SUMMARY

Clinical studies strongly support a role for antineoplastic chemotherapy in increasing the thrombotic risk in cancer patients. Experimental data suggests that chemotherapeutic agents can directly or indirectly increase tissue factor expression in endothelial cells and monocytes and macrophages. Treatment with a number of chemotherapeutic agents can result in changes in patients' plasma that are prothrombotic, by lowering the levels of natural anticoagulants such as antithrombin, proteins C and S, while simultaneously increasing the prothrombotic levels of fibrinogen, vWF and Factor VIII coagulant protein. Despite these well-documented effects of chemotherapy, there is no evidence at present that supports a predictive value for any marker of hemostatic activation or plasma natural anticoagulant or coagulation factor for the risk of thrombosis cancer patients receiving systemic chemotherapy.

An important observation from recent clinical studies is that the use of targeted therapeutic agents and antiangiogenic medications may not result in a decrease in the treatment related thrombotic risk in cancer patients, particularly when combined with classical cytotoxic chemotherapy. Future clinical trials of newer therapeutic agents should carefully consider the thrombotic risks associated with their use as single agents or in combination therapy.

REFERENCES

1. Rickles FR, Levine MN, Dvorak HB. Abnormalities of hemostasis in malignancy. In: Coleman RW, Hirsch J, Marder VJ, et al., eds. Hemostasis and Thrombosis. Philadelphia, PA: Lippincott, Williams & Watkins, 2001:1132–1152.
2. Rickles FR, Levine MN. Epidemiology of thrombosis in cancer. Acta Haematol 2001; 106:6–12.
3. Sack GH, Levin J, Bell W. Trousseau's syndrome and other manifestations of chronic disseminated coagulopathy in patients with neoplasms: clinical, pathophysiologic and therapeutic features. Medicine (Baltimore) 1977; 56:1–37.
4. Blom JW, Doggen CJ, Osanto S, et al. Malignancies, prothrombotic mutations, and the risk of venous thrombosis. JAMA 2005; 293:715–722.
5. Lee AYY, Levine MN. The thrombophilic state induced by therapeutic agents in the cancer patient. Semin Thrombo Hemost 1999; 25(2):137–146.
6. Sallah S, Wan JY, Nguyen NP. Venous thrombosis in patients with solid tumors: determination of frequency and characteristic. Thromb Haemost 2002; 87:575–579.
7. Heit JA, Silverstein MD, Mohr DN, et al. Risk factors for deep vein thrombosis and pulmonary embolism: a population-based case-control study. Arch Intern Med 2000; 160:809–815.
8. Blom JW, Vanderschoot JPM, Oostindier MJ, et al. Incidence of venous thrombosis in a large cohort of 66,329 cancer patients: results of a record linkage study. J Thromb Haemost 2006; 4:529–535.
9. Khorana AA, Francis CW, Culakova E, Lyman GH. Risk factors for chemotherapy-associated venous thromboembolism in a prospective observational study. Cancer 2005; 104:2822–2829.
10. Otten H-M, Mathijssen J, ten Cate H, et al. Symptomatic venous thromboembolism in cancer patients treated with chemotherapy. Arch Intern Med 2004; 164:190–194.
11. Duggan C, Marriott K, Edwards R, Cuzick J. Inherited and acquired risk factors for venous thromboembolic disease among women taking Tamoxifen to prevent breast cancer. J Clin Oncol 2003; 21:3588–3593.
12. Fisher B, Constantino J, Redmond C, et al. A randomized clinical trial evaluating tamoxifen in the treatment of patients with node-negative breast cancer who have estrogen receptor-positive breast cancer. N Engl J Med 1989; 320:479–484.
13. Fisher B, Dignma J, Wolmark N, et al. Tamoxifen and chemotherapy for lymph node-negative, estrogen receptor-positive breast cancer. J Natl Cancer Inst 1997; 89:1673–1682.
14. Clahsen PE, van de Velde CJH, Julien JP, et al. Thromboembolic complications after perioperative chemotherapy in women with early breast cancer: a European Organization for research and treatment of Cancer Breast cancer Cooperative Group Study. J Clin Oncol 1994; 12:1266–1271.
15. Saphner T, Tormey DC, Gray R. Venous and arterial thrombosis in patients who receive adjuvant therapy for breast cancer. J Clin Oncol 1991; 9:286–294.
16. Levine MN, Gent M, Hirsch J, et al. The thrombogenic effects of anticancer drug therapy in women with stage II breast cancer. New Eng J Med 1988; 297:179–180.
17. Haas SK, Kakkar AK, Kemkes-Matthes B, et al. Prevention of thromboembolism with low-molecular weight heparin in patients with metastatic breast or lung cancer-results of the TOPIC studies (abstract). J Thromb Haemost 2005; 3(suppl 1):OR059.
18. Goodnough LT, Saito H, Manni A, et al. Increased incidence of thromboembolism in stage IV breast cancer patients treated with a five-drug chemotherapy regimen. A study of 159 patients. Cancer 1984; 54:1264–1268.
19. Berger AC, Scott WJ, Freedman G, et al. Morbidity and mortality are not increased after induction chemoradiotherapy followed by esophagectomy in patients with esophageal cancer. Semin Oncol 2005; 32(suppl 9):16–20.

20. Poplin EA, Benedetti JK, Estes NC, et al. Phase III southwest oncology group 9415/intergroup randomized trial of fluorouracil, leucovorin and levamisole for adjuvant treatment of stage III and high-risk stage II colon cancer. J Clin Oncol 2005; 23:1819–1825.
21. Andre T, Boni C, Mounedji-Boudiaf L, et al. Oxaliplatin, fluorouracil, and leucovorin as adjuvant treatment for colon cancer. N Engl J Med 2004; 350:2343–2351.
22. Hurwitz H, Fehrenbacher L, Novotny W, et al. Bevacizumab plus irinotecan, fluorouracil, and leucovorin for metastatic colorectal cancer. N Engl J Med 2004; 350:2335–2342.
23. Cantwell BM, Carmichael J, Ghani SE, Harris AL. Thromboses and thromboemboli in patients with lymphoma during cytotoxic chemotherapy. BMJ 1998; 297:179–180.
24. Clarke CS, Otridge BW, Carney DN. Thromboembolism: a complication of weekly chemotherapy in the treatment of non-Hodgkin's lymphoma. Cancer 1990; 66:2027–2030.
25. Shlebak AA, Smith DB. Incidence of objectively diagnosed thromboembolic disease in cancer patients undergoing cytotoxic chemotherapy and/or hormonal therapy. Cancer Chemother Pharmacol 1997; 39:462–466.
26. Von Tempelhoff GF, Dietrich M, Niemann F, et al. Blood coagulation and thrombosis with ovarian malignancy. Thromb Haemost 1997; 77:456–461.
27. Tateo S, Mereu L, Salamano S, et al. Ovarian cancer and venous thromboembolic risk. Gynecol Oncol 2005; 99:119–125.
28. Lubiniecki GM, Berlin JA, Weinstein RB, Vaughn DJ. Thromboembolic events with estramustine phosphate-based chemotherapy in patients with hormone-refractory prostate carcinoma. Results of a meta-analysis. Cancer 2004; 101:2755–2759.
29. Quevado JF, Buckner JC, Schmidt JL, et al. Thromboembolism in patients with high-grade glioma. Mayo Clin Proc 1994; 69:329–332.
30. Czaykowski PM, Moore M, Tannock IF. High risk of vascular events in patients with urothelial transitional cell carcinoma treated with cis-platin based chemotherapy. J Urol 1998; 160:2021–2024.
31. Kuenen BC, Rosen L, Smit EF, et al. Dose-finding and pharmacokinetic study of cisplatin, gemcitabine and SU5416 in patients with solid tumors. J Clin Oncol 2002; 20:1657–1667.
32. Glasmacher A, Hahn C, Hoffmann F, et al. A systematic review of phase-II trials of monotherapy in patients with relapsed or refractory multiple myeloma. Br J Haematol 2005; 132:584–593.
33. Weber D, Rankin K, Gavino M, Delasalle K, Alexanian R. Thalidomide alone or with dexamethasone for previously untreated multiple myeloma. J Clin Oncol 2003; 21:16–19.
34. Rajkumar SV, Blood E, Vesole D, et al. Phase III clinical trial of thalidomide plus dexamethasone compared with dexamethasone alone in newly diagnosed multiple myeloma: a clinical trial coordinated by the Eastern Cooperative Oncology Group. J Clin Oncol 2006; 24:431–436.
35. Cavo M, Zamagni E, Tose P, et al. First-line therapy with thalidomide and dexamethasone in preparation for autologous stem cell transplant for multiple myeloma. Haematologica 2004; 89:826–831.
36. Palumbo A, Bringhen S, Caravita T, et al. Oral melphalan and prednisone plus thalidomide compared with melphalan and prednisone alone in elderly patients with multiple myeloma: randomized controlled trial. Lancet 2006; 367:825–831.
37. Hussein MA, Baz R, Srkalovic G, et al. Phase 2 study of pegylated liposomal doxorubicin, vincristine, decreased frequency dexamethasone, and thalidomide in newly diagnosed and relapsed-refractory multiple myeloma. Mayo Clin Proc 2006; 81:889–895.
38. Baz R, Li L, Kottke-Marchant K, et al. The role of aspirin in the prevention of thrombotic complications of thalidomide and anthracycline-based chemotherapy for multiple myeloma. Mayo Clin Proc 2005; 80:1568–1574.
39. Offidani M, Corvatta L, Marconi M, et al. Low-dose thalidomide with pegylated liposomal doxorubicin and high-dose dexamethasone for relapsed/refractory multiple myeloma: a prospective, phase II study. Haematologica 2006; 91:133–136.
40. Dimopoulos M, Anagnostopoulos A, Terpos E, et al. Primary treatment with pulsed melphalan, dexamethasone and thalidomide for elderly symptomatic patients with multiple myeloma. Haematologica 2006; 91:252–254.

41. Lee C-K, Barlogie B, Munshi N, et al. DTPACE: an effective, novel combination chemotherapy with thalidomide for previously treated patients with myeloma. J Clin Oncol 2003; 21:12732–12739.
42. Desai AA, Vogelzang NJ, Rini BI, et al. A high rate of venous thromboembolism in a multi-institutional phase II trial of weekly intravenous gemcitabine with continuous infusional flurouracil and daily thalidomide in patients with metastatic renal cell carcinoma. Cancer 2002; 95:1629–1636.
43. Dahut WL, Gulley JL, Arlen PM, et al. Randomized phase II trial of doxetaxel plus thalidomide in androgen-independent prostate cancer. J Clin Oncol 2004; 22:2532–2539.
44. Fine HA, Wen PY, Maher EA, et al. Phase II trial of thalidomide and carmustine for patients with recurrent high-grade gliomas. J Clin Oncol 2003; 21:2299–2304.
45. Steurer M, Sudmeier I, Stauder R, Gastl G. Thromboembolic events in patients with myelodysplastic syndrome receiving thalidomide in combination with darbepoietin. Br J Haematol 2003; 121:101–103.
46. Dimopoulos M, Weber D, Chen C, et al. Evaluating oral lenalinomide (Revlimid) and dexamethasone versus placebo and dexamethasone in patients with relapsed or refractory multiple myeloma [abstr. 0402]. Haematologica 2005; 90(suppl 2):160.
47. Rajkumar SV, Hayman SR, Lacy MQ, et al. Combination therapy with lenalinomide plus dexamethasone (Rev/Dex) for newly diagnosed myeloma. Blood 2005; 106:4050–4053.
48. Edwards RL, Klaus M, Mathews E, et al. Heparin abolishes the chemotherapy-induced increase in plasma fibrinopeptide A levels. Am J Med 1990; 89:25–28.
49. Kuzel T, Esparaz B, Green D, Kies M. Thrombogenicity of intravenous 5-flurouracil alone or in combination with cisplatin. Cancer 1990; 65:885–889.
50. Zurborn KH, Granm J Glander K, et al. Influence of cytostatic treatment on the coagulation system and fibrinolysis in patients with non-Hodgkin's lymphomas and acute leukemias. Eur J Haematol 1991; 47:55–59.
51. Weitz IC, Israel VK, Waisman JR, et al. Chemotherapy-induced activation of hemostasis: effect of a low molecular weight heparin (dalteparin sodium) on plasma markers of hemostatic activation. Thromb Haemost 2002; 88:213–220.
52. Lazo JS. Endothelial injury caused by antineoplastic agents. Biochem Pharmacol 1986; 35:1912–1923.
53. Stahli BE, Camici GG, Steffel J, et al. Paclitaxel enhances thrombin-induced endothelial tissue factor expression via c-Jun terminal NH_2 kinase activation. Circ Res 2006; 99:149–155.
54. Adamson IYR, Bowden DH. The pathogenesis of bleomycin-induced pulmonary fibrosis in mice. Am J Pathol 1974; 77:185–198.
55. Nicolson GL, Custead S. Effect of chemotherapeutic drugs on platelets and metatastic tumor cell-endothelial cell interactions as a model for assessing vascular endothelial integrity. Cancer Res 1985; 45:331–336.
56. Bertomeu MC, Gallo S, Lauri D, et al. Chemotherapy enhances endothelial reactivity to platelets. Clin Expl Metast 1990; 8:511–518.
57. Bevilacqua MP, Pober JS, Majeau GR, et al. Interleukin 1 (IL-1) induces biosynthesis and cell surface expression of procoagulant activity in human vascular endothelial cells. J Exp Med 1984; 160:618–623.
58. Licciardello JT, Moake JL, Rudy CK, Karp DD, Hong WK. Elevated plasma von Willebrand factor levels and arterial occlusive complications associated with cisplatin based chemotherapy. Oncology 1985; 42:296–300.
59. Nuver J, Smit AJ, van der Meer J, et al. Acute chemotherapy-induced cardiovascular changes in patients with testicular cancer. J Clin Oncol 2005; 23:9130–9137.
60. Weitz IC, Liebman HA. Chemotherapy-induced activation of hemostasis: dalteparin suppresses both thrombin and interleukin-6 expression in breast cancer patients receiving adjuvant chemotherapy. Blood 2004; 104(suppl):956a.
61. Charba D, Moake JL, Harris MA, Hester JP. Abnormalities of von Willebrand factor multimers in drug associated thrombotic microangiopathies. Am J Hematol 1993; 42:268–277.
62. Monteaguado J, Pereira A, Roig S, et al. Investigation of plasma von Willebrand factor and circulating platelet aggregating activity in mitomycin C-related hemolytic-uremic syndrome. Am J Hematol 1990; 33:46–49.

63. van der Plas RM, Schiphorst ME, Huizinga EG, et al. von Willebrand factor proteolysis is deficient in classic, but not in the bone marrow transplantation-associated, thrombotic thrombocytopenic purpura. Blood 1999; 93:3798–3802.
64. Rogers JS, Murgo AJ, Fontana JA, Raich PC. Chemotherapy for breast cancer decreases plasma protein C and protein S. J Clin Oncol 1988; 6:276–281.
65. Feffer SE, Carmosino LS, Fox RL. Acquired protein C deficiency in patients with breast cancer receiving cyclophosphamide, methotrexate and 5-fluorouracil. Cancer 1989; 63:1303–1307.
66. Liebman HA, Wada JK, Patch MJ, McGehee W. Depression of functional and antigenic plasma antithrombin III (ATIII) due to therapy with L-asparaginase. Cancer 1982; 50:451–456.
67. Priest JR, Ramsay NKC, Bennett AJ, Krivit W, Edson JR. The effect of l-asparaginase on antithrombin, plasminogen and plasma coagulation during treatment for acute lymphoblastic leukemia. J Pediatr 1982; 100:990–995.
68. Barbui T, Rodeghiero F, Meli S, Dini E. Fatal pulmonary embolism and antithrombin III deficiency in acute lymphoblastic leukemia during l-asparaginase therapy. Acta Haematol 1983; 69:188–191.
69. Conrard J, Horellou MH, van Dreden P, et al. Decrease in protein C in l-asparaginase-treated patients. Br J Haematol 1985; 59:725–727.
70. Gugliotta L, D'Angelo A, Mattioli Belmonte M, et al. Hypercoaguability during l-asparaginase treatment: the effect of antithrombin III supplementation in vivo. Br J Haematol 1990; 74:465–470.
71. Leone G, Gugliotta L, Mazzucconi MG, et al. Evidence of a hypercoagulable state in patients with acute lymphoblastic leukemia treated with low dose of *E. coli* l-asparaginase. A GIMEMA study. Thromb Haemost 1993; 69:12–15.
72. Castaman G, Rodeghiero F. Erwinia- and *E. coli*-derived l-asparaginase have similar effects on hemostasis. Pilot study of 10 patients with acute lymphoblastic leukemia. Haematologica 1993; 78(suppl 2):57–60.
73. Rodeghiero F, Castaman G, Dini E. Fibrinopeptide A changes during remission induction treatment with l-asparaginase in acute lymphoblastic leukemia. Evidence for activation of blood coagulation. Thromb Res 1990; 57:31–38.
74. Pui CH, Chesney CM, Bergum PW, Jackson CW, Rapaport SI. Lack of pathogenic role of protein C and S in thrombosis associated with asparaginase-prednisone-vincristine therapy for leukemia. Br J Haematol 1986; 64:283–290.
75. Pogliani EM, Parma M, Bargetti I, et al. L-asparaginase in acute lymphoblastic leukemia treatment: the role of human antithrombin III concentrates in regulating the prothrombotic state induced by therapy. Acta Haematol 1995; 93:5–8.
76. Pui CH, Jackson CW, Chesney CM, Abildgaard CF. Involvement of von Willebrand factor in thrombosis following asparaginase-prednisone-vincristine therapy for leukemia. Am J Hematol 1978; 25:291–298.
77. Kucuk O, Kwaan HC, Gunnar W, Vazquez RM. Thromboembolic complications associated with l-asparaginase. Cancer 1985; 55:702–706.

6

Angiogenesis Inhibitors, Cancer-Associated Thrombosis, and Bleeding

H. M. W. Verheul
Department of Medical Oncology, University Medical Center Utrecht, Utrecht, The Netherlands, and Department of Medical Oncology, Johns Hopkins Medical Institutions, Baltimore, Maryland, U.S.A.
M. E. Belderbos and R. Pili
Department of Medical Oncology, Johns Hopkins Medical Institutions, Baltimore, Maryland, U.S.A.
H. M. Pinedo
Department of Medical Oncology, VU Medical Center, Amsterdam, The Netherlands

- Angiogenesis inhibitors disturb vascular homeostasis, leading to arterial and venous thrombosis, bleeding, and hypertension.
- The risk of arterial thrombotic events with bevacizumab is estimated to be around 5%.
- Arterial and venous thrombosis have been observed with other angiogenesis inhibitors that are still in development, suggesting that this may be a class effect; however, rates vary widely between specific agents and among various clinical trials.
- The close linkage between coagulation, angiogenesis, and platelet activation is likely responsible for the vascular complications of angiogenesis inhibitors but the mechanisms are not completely understood.
- Aspirin may reduce arterial thrombosis associated with bevacizumab, but this has not been well studied.
- More research is needed to identify patients at high risk for vascular complications during angiogenesis-inhibitor therapy.

INTRODUCTION

The development of cancer is dependent on new blood vessel formation, the process of angiogenesis (1). This process is stimulated by tumors through the release of angiogenic growth factors. Angiogenesis is required not only for tumor growth, but also for wound healing, growth, and the menstrual cycle (2). The coagulation cascade plays an important role in the angiogenic process (3,4). A clear correlation between tissue factor (TF), the main initiator of coagulation, and vascular endothelial growth factor (VEGF) has been recognized in both preclinical and clinical studies (5–7). In addition, platelets are transporters of angiogenesis factors, and activation of platelets stimulates new vessel formation (8–10). Taking these findings together, the observation that angiogenesis inhibitors also affect coagulation could have been expected. In several clinical trials, various angiogenesis inhibitors caused venous and arterial thrombotic complications as well as delayed wound healing and bleeding complications. The first severe thrombotic complications occurred in a dose-finding early clinical trial with SU5416, an antiangiogenic receptor tyrosine kinase inhibitor (RTKI), in combination with chemotherapy (11). This study contributed to the early termination of the clinical development of SU5416. In this chapter, we summarize the clinically observed coagulation abnormalities during antiangiogenic therapy.

ANGIOGENESIS INHIBITORS

The stimulation and inhibition of angiogenesis is strictly regulated in the human body. Many endogenous stimulators and inhibitors of angiogenesis have been discovered. Well known are the stimulators basic fibroblast growth factor and VEGF, while thrombospondin and endostatin are examples of endogenous inhibitors (12,13).

The interaction of growth factors and their receptors regulates the process of new vessel formation. The receptors are mostly of the tyrosine kinase type that signal intracellularly. Many growth factors and more than 50 receptor tyrosine kinases have been identified. Altogether, approximately 20 families of growth factor and receptor pathways have been recognized (14,15). Growth factor binding results in dimerization of the receptor tyrosine kinase, causing autophosphorylation of the cytoplasmic domains and activation of tyrosine kinase activity. Subsequently, intracellular signaling pathways become activated. These include the phosphatidylinositol 3'-kinase (PI3K)/Akt (protein kinase B) pathway, the Ras/Raf mitogen-activated protein kinase (MAPK) pathway, and the protein kinase C pathway, among others. Activated signaling pathways induce cell growth, proliferation, and migration as well as differentiation and prevention of the death of endothelial cells and other cells (16–18).

Inhibition of angiogenesis was proposed as a therapeutic strategy against cancer by Judah Folkman in 1971 (19). This hypothesis was based on preclinical findings that tumors remain dormant when they are unable to recruit new vessels. Like any organ that is growing, a tumor needs nutrients and oxygen. New vessel formation contributes to these needs. On the other hand, tumor dormancy has been described as the state in which tumors are unable to stimulate angiogenesis. Microscopically small tumor nests have been found in preclinical studies as well as in tumor specimens of patients at autopsy (20,21).

Since 1990, several angiogenesis inhibitors have been developed for clinical use. This development was stimulated by promising preclinical experiments showing that inhibition of angiogenesis reduced tumor growth and metastasis formation. In 2004, the first angiogenesis inhibitor was approved by the Food and Drug Administration (FDA) for clinical use. This humanized antibody against VEGF, bevacizumab, in combination with chemotherapy, prolonged the survival of patients with advanced colorectal cancer by five months (22). Recently, it has also been approved for lung and ovarian cancer in combination with chemotherapy (23). In addition, two antiangiogenic RTKIs, sorafenib and sunitinib, have been approved by the FDA for patients with advanced renal cell cancer based on a significant doubling of disease-free survival compared to either placebo or interferon-alpha, respectively. Further clinical trials are ongoing in other cancer types and in combination with chemotherapy with these agents

(24). Currently, many antibody-based angiogenesis inhibitors as well as antiangiogenic tyrosine kinase inhibitors are in clinical development. For example, VEGF-Trap is an antibody-based fusion product of the Fc region of immunoglobulin G1 (IgG1) and the high-affinity domains of VEGF receptor-1 (VEGFR1) and VEGF receptor-2 (VEGFR2). In preclinical in vivo experiments, VEGF-Trap treatment resulted in potent tumor growth inhibition, including inhibition of ascites formation in ovarian cancer (25,26). New antiangiogenic RTKIs include ZD6474, an inhibitor of all VEGFRs as well as epidermal growth factor receptor and fibroblast growth factor receptor. This agent is very potent in preclinical tumor models, but its clinical activity remains to be determined (27,28). In patients with heavily pretreated breast cancer, no responses to this agent were seen (29). AG013736, an RTKI of VEGFR1/2 and Platelet Derived Growth Factor Receptor-β, and AZD2171, an RTKI of VEGFR1–3, are also in clinical development and have shown promising results in preliminary reports. Thus, antiangiogenic agents have begun to impact on cancer care, but more effective inhibitors and improved treatment strategies with these agents are eagerly awaited. Multiple angiogenesis inhibitors are currently in clinical development as monotherapy as well as in combination strategies with chemotherapy or radiotherapy for various cancer types.

ANGIOGENESIS AND THE COAGULATION CASCADE

Up to 40% of patients with a malignancy develop clinical symptoms due to a coagulation abnormality such as deep venous thrombosis or pulmonary embolism (PE), while in up to 90% of patients, clinical and laboratory-based coagulation abnormalities are observed (30). Systemic markers of an activated coagulation cascade in cancer patients have been detected, including elevated concentrations of thrombin–antithrombin complexes (TAT-complexes) and prothrombin fragments (31). Also, in tumor fluids from patients with soft tissue sarcomas, high levels of TAT-complexes, TF, and extremely high VEGF levels were present (32). In the past two decades, it has become clear that the coagulation cascade plays an important role in tumor development, especially in tumor-induced angiogenesis and metastasis formation. Preclinical studies showed, for example, in a transgenic mouse model of dermal fibrosarcoma that tumors occurred predominantly in areas prone to wounding and that high tumor TF-expression induced enhanced tumor growth and metastasis formation (33,34). In addition, the MET oncogene generates tumor formation (hepatocellular carcinomas) by activation of the coagulation cascade (35). A direct biological interaction between VEGF and TF expression has been identified. These factors act in parallel, reciprocally stimulating endothelial cells (5,36). TF knockout mice die because of inappropriate vascular development causing loss of vascular integrity (37). A strong correlation between TF and VEGF expression in breast cancer tissues from patients has been reported (6). In addition, increased TF expression has been detected at the angiogenic sites of invasive breast carcinomas (38). TF expression in tumor specimens of patients with non–small cell lung cancer correlated significantly with microvessel density and VEGF expression (36).

Stimulation of angiogenesis by activation of the coagulation cascade includes release of growth factors by platelets upon their activation. Platelets are circulating depots of pro-angiogenic growth factors including VEGF (8). Both in vitro as well as in vivo studies have shown that platelets stimulate angiogenesis (10,39). In patients, release of angiogenic factors by platelets in wound-healing areas has been detected, which could be inhibited by anticoagulants (40). In addition, platelet–tumor interactions have been widely recognized since the studies of Gasic et al. in 1968 (41). These investigators showed that thrombocytopenia inhibits tumor metastasis formation and growth.

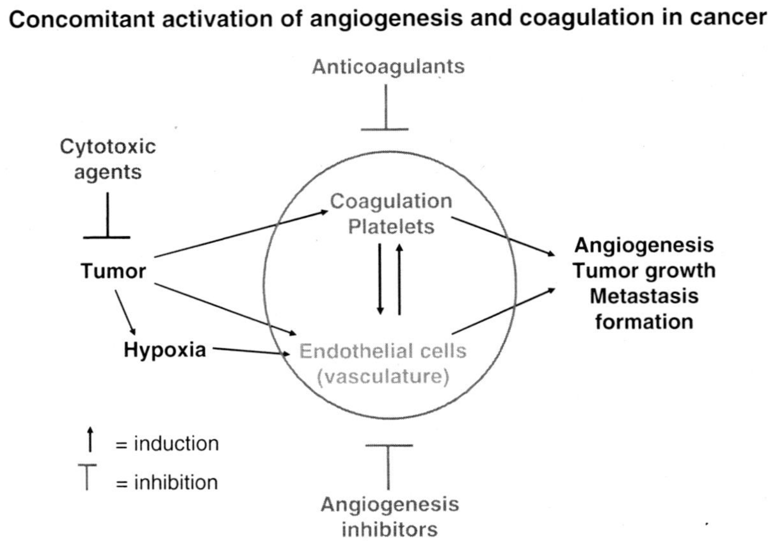

Figure 1 Tumors secrete many angiogenic factors, including VEGF. The secretion of angiogenic factors is enhanced by the hypoxic tumor microenvironment. In addition, tumors secrete procoagulants and most tumor cells express TF. TF is the main activator of the coagulation cascade. Upon binding of factor VIIa and factor X to TF, factor Xa is generated and subsequent thrombin is formed from prothrombin. Thrombin converts fibrinogen into fibrin, activates platelets with subsequent VEGF release, and stimulates endothelial cell proliferation. TF expression is also induced on endothelial cells through tumor-released VEGF. By activation of the vasculature, endothelial cells lose their natural anticoagulatory phenotype and promote coagulation as well, mainly through TF. The coagulation cascade is directly activated by tumors or procoagulatory endothelial cells provide the endothelium with an ideal angiogenic matrix compound, fibrin, to form new vessels. In conclusion, concomitant activation of angiogenesis and coagulation occurs in tumor growth. TF and VEGF play key roles in the interactions between both pathways. Inhibition of angiogenesis or coagulation impairs tumor growth and metastasis formation in a variety of preclinical in vivo tumor models. *Abbreviations*: VEGF, vascular endothelial growth factor; TF, tissue factor.

Other coagulation factors have also been shown to stimulate angiogenesis, including thrombin and fibrin (ogen), while some of the endogenous anticoagulants inhibit the angiogenic process, for example antithrombin III (42).

Taken together, it is clear that both intra- and extravascular activation of the coagulation cascade occurs in the tumor microenvironment including the extracellular matrix (ECM) and that this activation is important for tumor development including angiogenesis and metastasis formation. Figure 1 depicts the close interaction between angiogenesis and coagulation cascade in tumor growth and metastasis.

OVERVIEW OF ANGIOGENESIS-INHIBITOR RELATED THROMBOTIC CLINICAL ADVERSE EVENTS

Table 1 provides an overview of angiogenesis-related thrombotic events or other coagulation-dependent events in phase I or higher clinical trials of agents that are approved or in

Table 1 Thromboembolic Complications in Clinical Studies with Angiogenesis Inhibitors That Are Currently in Phase II or III Development or Already Approved

Drug	Phase	Treatment	Diagnosis	*n*	SAE	Ref.
Bevacizumab: mAb against VEGF-A	I	0.1–10 mg/kg; days 0, 28, 35, and 42	Various	25	Bleeding 4 pts, hypertension 10 pts	43
	II	Control 40 pts, 3 mg/kg 37 pts, 10 mg/kg 39 pts	Adv renal	116	Epistaxis 1, 5, and 8 pts respectively, hypertension 2, 1, and 14 pts respectively, 1 PE in control arm	44
	II	Carboplatin (C)/paclitaxel (P) ($n = 32$); C/P/bevacizumab 7.5 mg/kg ($n = 32$); C/P/bevacizumab 15 mg/kg ($n = 35$)	Adv lung	99	6× hemoptysis (5 in low dose group), hypertension	45
	II	Bevacizumab 3–10 mg/kg	Adv breast	35	2× severe hypertension	46
	II	5FU/LV ($n = 35$); 5FU/LV/bevacizumab 5 mg/kg ($n = 36$); 5FU/LV/bevacizumab 10 mg/kg ($n = 33$)	Adv colorectal	104	3× gastrointestinal hemorrhage (hd); 11× Hypertension (3 ld, 8 hd); 8 thromb events (5 ld, 2 hd)	47
	II	5FU/LV/placebo ($n = 105$); 5FU/LV/bevacizumab 5 mg/kg ($n = 104$)	Adv colorectal	209	2× gastrointestinal perforation; 15 48 arterial event (5 in control arm)	
	III	Irinotecan (I)/5FU/LV ($n = 397$); I/5FU/LV/bevacizumab 10 mg/kg ($n = 393$)	Adv colorectal	790	Grade 3 hypertension (2.3% vs. 11.0%); any thrombotic event (16.2% vs. 19.4%); PE (3.6% vs. 5.1%); GI perforation (1.5% vs. 0%)	22 49
	III	Capacetabine (Cap)/placebo ($n = 230$); Cap/bevacizumab (15 mg/kg) ($n = 232$)	Adv breast	462	Hypertension (2.4% vs. 33.5%); any thrombotic event (5.6% vs. 7.3%); grade I–III bleeding (11.2% vs. 28.8%)	

(Continued)

Table 1 Thromboembolic Complications in Clinical Studies with Angiogenesis Inhibitors That Are Currently in Phase II or III Development or Already Approved (*Continued*)

Drug	Phase	Treatment	Diagnosis	*n*	SAE	Ref.
VEGF-Trap: IgG-based decoy receptor for VEGF A, and B	I	0.3–3.0 mg/kg i.v. 1st injection followed by 4 wk rest, followed by 3× every 2 wk	Macular degeration	19	—	50
	I	0.3–3.0 mg/kg i.v./2 wk	Various	16	—	51
	I	VEGF-Trap 2 and 4 mg/kg plus I/5FU/LV	Various	10	Hypertension 1 pt	52
	I	VEGF-Trap 2 and 4 mg/kg plus FOLFOX4	Various	6	Hypertension 2 pts	53
PTK787/ZK222584: RTKI of VEGFR1/2/3, c-KIT, and Platelet Derived Growth Factor Receptor	I	FOLFIRI/PTK787 500–1500 mg/day	Adv colorectal	21	1× grade 3 hypertension (1000 mg/day)	54
	II	FOLFOX-4/PTK787 500–2000 mg/day	Adv colorectal	35	1× grade 3 thrombocytopenia (1250 mg)	55
	III	FOLFOX (n = 583); FOLFOX+PTK787 1250 mg qd (n = 583)	Adv colorectal	1168	Hypertension 5.9% vs. 20.6%; DVT 3.0% vs. 4.7%; PE 1.4% vs. 6.0%; art thromb 1.7% vs. 3.6%	56
SU5416: Small molecule inhibitor of VEGFR2	I	Cisplatin (CIS)/gemcitabine (GEM); GEM/SU5416 85 mg/m^2 (n = 13); CIS/GEM/SU5416 145 mg/m^2 (n = 6)	Various	19	3× transient ischemic attack; 2× cerebrovascular accident; 4× DVT; 1× hemorrhage	11
	I	IFL/SU5416 85 mg/m^2 (n = 5); IFL/SU5416 145 mg/m^2 (n = 6)	Adv colorectal	11	—	57
	I	I/SU5416 85 mg/m^2 (n = 3); I/SU5416 110 mg/m^2 (n = 4); I/SU5416 145 mg/m^2 (n = 3)	Adv colorectal	10	—	58
	IB	P 70 mg/m^2/SU5416 110 mg/m^2 (n = 6); P 55 mg/m^2/SU5416 110 mg/m^2 (n = 6)	Adv head and neck	12	2× DVT; 1× transient ischemic attack	59

	II	SU5416 145 mg/m^2 (all patients received prophylactic anticoagulation)	Adv soft tissue sarcomas	13	1× thrombosis	60
	II	Dexamethasone/SU5416 145 mg/m^2	Hormone-refractory prostate	16	—	61
	II	SU5416 145 mg/m^2	Adv renal	30	1× cardiac ischemia/infarction; 2× VTE	62
	II	145 mg/m^2	Adv renal, melanoma and soft tissue sarcoma	80	1× MI; 4× thromboembolic event	63
SU11248/Sunitinib: RTKI of VEGFR-1/2/3, c-Fms, Flt-3, c- KIT and PDGFR	I	50–75 mg/day; 4 wk on, 2 wk off	AML	16	2 fatal bleeding (brain and lung)	64
	I	50–150 mg/day, 4 wk on, 2 wk off	Various	28	1 PE, 5 pts thrombocytopenia, 2 pts hypertension	65
	II	50 mg; 4 wk on, 2 wk off	Adv renal	168	Thrombocytopenia 21 pts, hypertension 17 pts	66, 67
	II	50 mg; 4 wk on, 2 wk off	Imatinib-refractory GIST	202	Epistaxis 14 pts, hypertension 17 pts	68
	III	50 mg 4 wk on; 2 wk off	Adv renal	375	Thrombocytopenia 65% (8% grade III–IV), HT 24% (8% grade III–IV)	69
BAY43-9006/sorafenib: (R)TKI of VEGFR 2/3, Flt-3, c-KIT, PDGR, Raf kinase	I	Sorafenib 100–800 mg bid	Various	22	–	70

(*Continued*)

Table 1 Thromboembolic Complications in Clinical Studies with Angiogenesis Inhibitors That Are Currently in Phase II or III Development or Already Approved (*Continued*)

Drug	Phase	Treatment	Diagnosis	*n*	SAE	Ref.
	I	50–800 mg bid 21 days, 7 days off	Various	44	–	71
	II	400 mg bid	Melanoma	37	Hypertension 6 pts	72
	II	400 mg bid	Hepatocellular carcinoma	137	Only grade III and IV toxicities reported not related to coagulation	73
	II	400 mg bid	Adv renal cell carcinoma	202	Hypertension 43%, hemorrhage 22%; no thrombotic events reported	74
ZD6474 Vandetanib: (R)TKI of VEGFR-1/2/3, EGFR, FGFR, and RET	I	50–600 mg/day	Various	77	1× thrombocytopenia (600 mg); 1× DVT (100 mg); 1× PE (100 mg); 1× intestinal ischemia (600 mg)	75
	II	100 mg/day ($n = 22$); 300 mg/day ($n = 24$)	Adv breast cancer	46	No thromboembolic complications	29
AG013736: RTKI of VEGFR-1/2, PDGFR-β	I	5–30 mg bid	Various	36	Hypertension 22 pts, fatal lung bleeding 2 pts, gr 1 rectal bleeding 1 pt, DVT 1 pt	76
VEGF-AS: antisense against VEGF	I	15–250 mg/m^2 i.v. every other week for 5 days	Various	51	PE 1 pt, thrombocytopenia 6 pts	77
AZD2171: RTKI of VEGFR1/2/3	I	0.5–60 mg/day oral	Various	36	Fatal cerebral hemorrhage 1 pt, hypertension 3pts	78
	I	1–30 mg/day oral	Adv prostate cancer	18	Transient ischemic attack 1 pt, hematuria 1 pt	79
	I	30–45 mg/day oral	Non-Small Cell Lung Cancer	20	Hypertension 6 pts	80

Abbreviations: Adv, advanced; pt, patient; 5FU/LV, 5-fluorouracil and leucovorin; PE, pulmonary embolism; VEGF, vascular endothelial growth factor; RTKI, receptor tyrosine kinase inhibitor; DVT, deep vein thrombosis.

current clinical development. These agents can be categorized broadly into antiangiogenic monoclonal antibodies and antiangiogenic small molecule RTKIs. Thrombotic events occur frequently in patients treated with angiogenesis inhibitors, especially when these agents are given in combination with chemotherapy (11,22,60).

Bevacizumab, an IgG1-based antibody against VEGF, has been studied as monotherapy and in combination with chemotherapy. As monotherapy, no thrombotic events were diagnosed in patients with kidney cancer in a phase I clinical trial (43,44). However, in combination studies of bevacizumab and chemotherapy, the number of thrombotic events was greater compared to chemotherapy alone (22,47). These thrombotic events are mostly of arterial origin. In a phase III trial comparing irinotecan, 5-fluorouracil (5FU), and leucovorin (LV) with or without bevacizumab, an increase in the number of thrombotic events from 16.2% to 19.4% occurred in the bevacizumab arm (22). In a phase II study with 5FU/LV in combination with bevacizumab in patients with colorectal cancer, 15 arterial thrombotic events were observed (48). Although these studies suggest that bevacizumab induces thrombosis, this effect was not observed in all clinical studies. These thrombotic events can be explained partially by the fact that cancer patients are prone to develop thrombosis. For example, when three phase II trials with the combination of 5FU/LV plus bevacizumab in colorectal cancer were analyzed together, no differences in thrombotic complications between chemotherapy plus bevacizumab versus no bevacizumab were observed (81). Still, arterial thrombotic events rarely occur with chemotherapy alone, and the data from the clinical trials with bevacizumab clearly indicate that bevacizumab treatment is related to these events. It was concluded that bevacizumab is responsible for a twofold increase in the risk of any thrombotic event (82). Recently, Roncalli et al. described the rare appearance of a thrombotic event related to bevacizumab treatment (83). They found an intracardiac thrombus during 5FU/LV plus bevacizumab treatment in a patient with colorectal cancer, which disappeared completely with anticoagulation. With other chemotherapy schedules or in other cancer types, thrombotic events were also observed in relation to bevacizumab. For example, in a group of patients with metastatic breast cancer, when capacetabine plus bevacizumab was given after at least two previous chemotherapy regimens, a trend to an increased incidence of thrombotic events was observed (from 6.6% to 7.3%) (49). In conclusion, the manufacturer estimates that the risk of developing any thrombotic event related to bevacizumab treatment is about 5% (84). Whether patients should be treated prophylactically with an anticoagulant to reduce this risk is controversial, because there is also an increased bleeding risk due to bevacizumab therapy. We propose that low-dose anticoagulation may be of benefit for selected patients (such as those not at risk for pulmonary hemorrhage) treated with bevacizumab-containing regimens in the advanced cancer setting.

As mentioned, other coagulation abnormalities also occur. Especially, bleeding complications of bevacizumab have been observed in clinical studies. These are mostly confined to epistaxis or other insignificant bleeding events (grade I or II). However, in some cases, bevacizumab-induced bleeding complications can be fatal. In particular, in patients with lung cancer, such fatal complications have been observed (23). In addition, wound-healing problems of surgery have been observed for bevacizumab treatment if given close to the procedure. Surgery in patients with colorectal cancer before or during bevacizumab-containing combination treatment with chemotherapy compared to the same chemotherapy regimens without bevacizumab increased wound-healing problems from 0.5% to 1.3% and 3.4% to 13%, respectively (85). Overall, bleeding toxicities of all grades including epistaxis have been reported in up to 44% of patients treated with bevacizumab (86). Therefore, antiangiogenic agents should be given with caution perioperatively. Especially, bevacizumab should be halted for a prolonged period, because of its long half-life time.

Another vascular side effect observed with bevacizumab therapy is hypertension. In some studies, up to 35% of patients had hypertension due to bevacizumab, which, however, is generally easily managed (87).

For VEGF-Trap, an IgG-based decoy receptor against VEGF, not enough data are available to make firm conclusions about its effects on coagulation at this point, but thus far, no serious problems regarding thrombosis or bleeding have been reported (52,53). Hypertension has been observed in a few patients.

RTKIs are less frequently associated with thrombotic events. However, the first serious indication that angiogenesis inhibitors affect the coagulation system in cancer patients came from a study with the RTKI SU5416 (11). This was the first agent of a range of Sugen compounds that inhibit RTKs. In combination with chemotherapy, severe thrombotic complications were observed that ultimately led to the early termination of the clinical development of SU5416. As was shown later in a preclinical study by the group of Kerbel, SU5416 in combination with gemcitabine and/or cisplatin induced TF expression and activity on endothelial cells (88). TF leads to thrombin formation, and thrombin directly activates platelets and will convert fibrinogen into fibrin, both potentially leading to thrombosis. PTK787 has also been shown to induce thrombotic complications in combination with chemotherapy (FOLFOX) in patients with colorectal cancer. The difference between the percentage of patients diagnosed with PE in this study of 1158 patients is especially striking between FOLFOX alone compared to FOLFOX plus PTK787, 1.4% versus 6%, respectively (89). However, more recent studies with newer RTKIs have not shown such significant thrombotic complications. Of note is the fact that these studies have been mainly performed as monotherapy. Combination studies with chemotherapy are ongoing, and little data on the incidence of thrombotic complications are available yet. However, preliminary reports indicate that thrombotic events occur less frequently compared to studies with SU5416 and PTK787. In monotherapy as well as combination studies with these agents, bleeding complications are of general concern. Up to 25% or 22% of patients who are treated with sunitinib or sorafenib, respectively, experience low-grade bleeding complications (90,91). Bleeding events ranging from minor subungual splinter bleedings up to fatal lung bleedings in patients have been reported in clinical trials with angiogenesis inhibitors, especially RTKIs (92,93).

Furthermore, hypertension is a major concern in patients treated with these agents. Hypertension is very well manageable with standard antihypertensive agents, but in some patients, malignant hypertension can present. Preexisting hypertension is not an absolute contraindication for starting treatment.

ANGIOGENESIS INHIBITOR–RELATED THROMBOSIS

Under physiological circumstances, endothelial cells play a major role in preventing blood cells from adhering to the vascular wall leading to coagulation activation. Endothelial cells produce and secrete numerous factors to prevent the activation and propagation of coagulation. These include endothelium-derived relaxing factor/nitric oxide (NO), endothelial membrane-associated ecto-ADPase, thrombomodulin (TM), prostacyclin (PGI2), glycosaminoglycans, TF pathway inhibitor (TFPI), and tissue type plasminogen activator (tPA) (94). NO, ecto-APDase, and PGI2 prevent platelet aggregation and activation. TM and TFPI inhibit the TF-mediated activation of thrombin, and tPA converts plasminogen into plasmin for the immediate breakdown of fibrin that may be formed despite endothelial antithrombotic activity. In addition, endothelial cells express binding sites for antithrombotic proteins such as TM, TFPI, protein C, and heparan sulfates, and these also contribute to the anticoagulant cell surface. Heparan sulfate promotes the binding of antithrombin III, an anticoagulant that inhibits thrombin activity. When the vessel wall or antithrombotic homeostasis is disturbed, endothelial cells undergo a programmed phenotypic change and become prothrombotic (95). The key factor in this change is increased expression of TF. Therefore, one may expect that an inhibitor of VEGF would reduce the prothrombotic state. However, this effect of VEGF seems dose dependent. At high concentrations, VEGF stimulates coagulation by inducing TF activity, vascular permeability, and endothelial cell proliferation and migration, whereas at low concentrations, VEGF is a survival and maintenance factor for the endothelial cells. Inhibition of VEGF can decrease TF activity of endothelial cells (88). However, single-agent SU5416 treatment increased the amount of circulating soluble TF and increased potential thrombin generation (96). These contradictory results from in vitro experiments and clinical observations may be explained by SU5416 inhibition at a relatively high dose (nanograms/mL) of VEGF stimulation of the endothelial cells in vitro. When used in patients, SU5416 inhibits endothelial cells that are mostly quiescent and only stimulated with a very low dose of VEGF (picograms/mL) as a survival factor. SU5416 may induce apoptosis of quiescent endothelial cells in vivo by interfering with the survival activity of VEGF rather than inhibiting the angiogenesis activity (97). Not only proliferating endothelial cells, but also apoptotic endothelial cells become procoagulant (98). Under physiological circumstances, platelets may act as providers of these growth (maintenance) factors for the endothelium by delivering growth factors in low amounts. When this growth factor–signaling pathway is disturbed by treatment, the platelet–endothelial cell maintenance interaction is disturbed (96). Due to the disturbed endothelial cell homeostasis and the initiation of apoptosis, the endothelial cell anticoagulant phenotype will disappear, cells will become procoagulant, and thrombotic events can occur (99). Another related explanation for the increased risk of thrombosis is that the renewal capacity of endothelial cells in response to trauma is disturbed by inhibition of the VEGF pathway. This may cause increased exposure of the underlying ECM containing collagen (100). The incidence of drug-related thrombotic events vary significantly with RTKIs, and most of these complications were not as impressive as observed with SU5416. However, most of these RTKIs have not been tested in combination treatment with similar chemotherapy regimens as SU5416.

Bevacizumab-induced thrombosis occurs mainly in arteries, and this may be due to a disturbed platelet function in these patients. Recently, we found that platelets take up bevacizumab (101), and this uptake reduces the stimulatory activity of platelets on endothelial cells. Within eight hours after treatment, more than 97% of platelet VEGF is neutralized. Consequently, platelets cannot provide the endothelial cells with VEGF, and thereby the close interaction between platelets and the endothelial cell lining is disturbed. We hypothesize that additional aspirin treatment, standard treatment for patients at risk for arterial thrombosis, may reduce arterial thrombotic events during treatment with bevacizumab. However, the risk of major bleeding will be increased with aspirin. Therefore, a method to identify patients at risk for thrombosis or for bleeding is needed. If that were available, it would be possible to determine whether a patient should also be treated with an anticoagulant during treatment with bevacizumab.

Another factor that may increase the risk of venous versus arterial thrombosis may be differences in endothelial cell signaling. The PI3K pathway is involved in the formation of the venous vascular system, while the RAF–ERK pathway is involved in arteries (102). One may hypothesize that bevacizumab preferentially acts on the RAF–ERK pathway rather than the PI3K pathway, causing more arterial than venous thrombotic complications.

In conclusion, thrombotic events due to antiangiogenic therapy can be fatal. Neutralization of platelet VEGF due to uptake of bevacizumab may be responsible for bevacizumab-related arterial thrombotic and, to a lesser extent, venous thrombotic events.

RTKI-related thrombotic events differ so much between the various agents that it is hard to determine whether this is a class effect of these clinical agents or is actually dependent on specific formulations.

ANGIOGENESIS INHIBITOR–RELATED BLEEDING

Angiogenesis is essential for wound healing. Under normal conditions, endothelial cells are quiescent. They do not proliferate or migrate, but survive, presumably due to stimulation by small amounts of survival factors. VEGF plays a major role in this survival (12). As described above, one source of survival factors for endothelial cells is platelets (39), and another source may be perivascular cells (103). An old observation is that isolated organs can be kept alive for a few days when perfused with platelet-rich, but not platelet-poor, plasma (104). These experiments suggested that platelet-derived growth factors are essential for homeostasis of the endothelium. Serum, which is used in vitro to grow cells, contains most of these platelet-derived angiogenic growth factors. Platelets help maintain vascular integrity in patients (105,106), and low platelet counts are associated with edema and extravasation of blood plasma and cells.

When vascular signaling pathways in endothelial and vascular supporting cells are inhibited by an angiogenesis inhibitor, normal endothelial cell homeostasis is also disturbed (96), and wound healing is inhibited (107,108). Platelets secrete VEGF in wound-healing areas, and inhibition of platelet activation results in a decrease of VEGF in wounds (40). The angiogenesis-promoting activity of platelets has been demonstrated in both in vitro and in vivo assays (9,10,109). As mentioned above, we demonstrated that platelets take up the therapeutic antibody bevacizumab, and bevacizumab blocks the angiogenic activity of platelets (101). Upon activation (for example, during wound healing), platelets release their contents, primarily growth factors. This release may neutralize VEGF derived from other sources during wound healing due to the large excess amount of bevacizumab that is taken up by platelets over the amount of VEGF contained by platelets (Verheul et al., unpublished). We propose that uptake of bevacizumab by platelets may be related to bleeding and wound-healing complications. The interaction of platelets and endothelial cells seems well balanced, and interference by bevacizumab may increase the risk of thrombosis, because platelets are unable to adequately support endothelial cells. On the other hand, this may increase the risk for bleeding because platelet stimulation of endothelial cells during wound healing is disturbed by bevacizumab uptake. In the case of severe bleeding complications, platelet transfusions may be used to restore proper platelet function for a short period of time.

Whether RTKIs also influence platelet release of VEGF or primarily affect endothelial cells has to be determined. Interestingly, platelets express VEGF receptors, and thrombin-induced platelet activation is enhanced by VEGF, suggesting that RTKIs may inhibit platelet activation (110). In addition, RTKIs induce thrombocytopenia (65). In one patient, severe complications of thrombocytopenia with peripheral signs of microangiopathy were observed. In this patient, normal maturating megakaryocytes were present in the bone marrow, and indications of hemolytic anemia were found. The disturbance of the platelet–endothelial cell interactions by angiogenesis inhibitors may be potentiated by chemotherapy-induced thrombocytopenia (11). Interactions between VEGF and TF, the principal physiologic initiator of coagulation, may be of importance as well (111). Both in vitro and in vivo, increased endothelial TF expression in relation to VEGF stimulation has been demonstrated (6,36). In wound healing or other organ damage, endothelial cell–induced coagulation promotes wound healing and presumably angiogenesis. Therefore, inhibition of this pathway by blocking either VEGF or its receptor or other growth factor receptors might be responsible for inadequate wound healing. Thus far, no studies have been performed to determine the effect of angiogenesis inhibitors on TF expression other than preclinical and clinical studies with SU5416. Monotherapy with SU5416 reduced VEGF-induced TF activity of endothelial cells in vitro (88). The effects of RTKIs on wound healing are minimal in preclinical studies (112,113). In summary, bleeding complications and disturbed wound healing are most likely caused by disturbance of the tight endothelial cell–platelet interaction that maintains vascular integrity.

ANGIOGENESIS INHIBITOR–RELATED HYPERTENSION

The underlying mechanism of VEGF-mediated regulation of blood pressure has been extensively studied. Endothelial cells promote vasodilation by secretion of NO and PGI2 (114), and VEGF induces the release of these factors by endothelial cells. Downstream of the VEGF receptor on endothelial cells, the PI3K and MAPK signaling cascades are responsible for endothelial nitric oxide synthetase induction (115). Blockade of this VEGF pathway will lead to a decreased production of these vasodilators and therefore to vascular resistance. Inhibition of the MAPK and Akt pathways by angiogenesis inhibitors leading to respectively downregulation of PGI2 and NO release of vascular or perivascular cells may also directly be involved in treatment-induced hypertension (116).

CONCLUSION

In conclusion, both antiangiogenic antibodies as well as RTKIs disturb vascular homeostasis, causing thrombosis, bleeding, and hypertension. The underlying mechanisms are not completely understood. Because antiangiogenic agents have become the standard of care for many cancer types, determining the risk factors for these complications and managing them are of major importance. For example, one possibility in the case of a serious bleeding complication during bevacizumab therapy might be simple platelet transfusion. On the other hand, it has to be determined if anticoagulants should be used for patients with increased thrombotic risk factors. Therefore, the challenge in coming years is not only to improve the efficacy of antiangiogenic therapy with or without combination chemotherapy, but also to develop new clinical guidelines to manage these new kind of toxicities.

REFERENCES

1. Kerbel R, Folkman J. Clinical translation of angiogenesis inhibitors. Nat Rev Cancer 2002; 2(10):727–739.
2. Carmeliet P. Angiogenesis in life, disease and medicine. Nature 2005; 438(7070):932–936.
3. Rickles FR, Patierno S, Fernandez PM. Tissue factor, thrombin, and cancer. Chest 2003; 124(suppl 3):58S–68S.
4. Daly ME, Makris A, Reed M, Lewis CE. Hemostatic regulators of tumor angiogenesis: a source of antiangiogenic agents for cancer treatment? J Natl Cancer Inst 2003; 95(22):1660–1673.
5. Zucker S, Mirza H, Conner CE, et al. Vascular endothelial growth factor induces tissue factor and matrix metalloproteinase production in endothelial cells: conversion of prothrombin to thrombin results in progelatinase A activation and cell proliferation. Int J Cancer 1998; 75(5):780–786.

6. Shoji M, Hancock WW, Abe K, et al. Activation of coagulation and angiogenesis in cancer: immunohistochemical localization in situ of clotting proteins and vascular endothelial growth factor in human cancer. Am J Pathol 1998; 152(2):399–411.
7. Yu JL, May L, Lhotak V, et al. Oncogenic events regulate tissue factor expression in colorectal cancer cells: implications for tumor progression and angiogenesis. Blood 2005; 105(4):1734–1741.
8. Pinedo HM, Verheul HM, D'Amato RJ, Folkman J. Involvement of platelets in tumour angiogenesis? Lancet 1998; 352(9142):1775–1777.
9. Verheul HM, Jorna AS, Hoekman K, Broxterman HJ, Gebbink MF, Pinedo HM. Vascular endothelial growth factor-stimulated endothelial cells promote adhesion and activation of platelets. Blood 2000; 96(13):4216–4221.
10. Kisucka J, Butterfield CE, Duda DG, et al. Platelets and platelet adhesion support angiogenesis while preventing excessive hemorrhage. Proc Natl Acad Sci USA 2006; 103(4):855–860.
11. Kuenen BC, Rosen L, Smit EF, et al. Dose-finding and pharmacokinetic study of cisplatin, gemcitabine, and SU5416 in patients with solid tumors. J Clin Oncol 2002; 20(6):1657–1667.
12. Ferrara N. Vascular endothelial growth factor: basic science and clinical progress. Endocr Rev 2004; 25(4):581–611.
13. Folkman J. Endogenous angiogenesis inhibitors. Apmis 2004; 112(7–8):496–507.
14. Pawson T. Regulation and targets of receptor tyrosine kinases. Eur J Cancer 2002; 38 (suppl 5):S3–S10.
15. Gschwind A, Fischer OM, Ullrich A. The discovery of receptor tyrosine kinases: targets for cancer therapy. Nat Rev Cancer 2004; 4(5):361–370.
16. Schlessinger J. Cell signaling by receptor tyrosine kinases. Cell 2000; 103(2):211–225.
17. Bogdan S, Klambt C. Epidermal growth factor receptor signaling. Curr Biol 2001; 11(8): R292–R295.
18. Blume-Jensen P, Hunter T. Oncogenic kinase signalling. Nature 2001; 411(6835):355–365.
19. Folkman J. Tumor angiogenesis: therapeutic implications. N Engl J Med 1971; 285(21):1182–1186.
20. Hanahan D, Folkman J. Patterns and emerging mechanisms of the angiogenic switch during tumorigenesis. Cell 1996; 86(3):353–364.
21. Folkman J, Kalluri R. Cancer without disease. Nature 2004; 427(6977):787.
22. Hurwitz H, Fehrenbacher L, Novotny W, et al. Bevacizumab plus irinotecan, fluorouracil, and leucovorin for metastatic colorectal cancer. N Engl J Med 2004; 350(23):2335–2342.
23. Jain RK, Duda DG, Clark JW, Loeffler JS. Lessons from phase III clinical trials on anti-VEGF therapy for cancer. Nat Clin Pract Oncol 2006; 3(1):24–40.
24. Patel PH, Chaganti RS, Motzer RJ. Targeted therapy for metastatic renal cell carcinoma. Br J Cancer 2006; 94(5):614–619.
25. Lau SC, Rosa DD, Jayson G. Technology evaluation: VEGF Trap (cancer), Regeneron/sanofi-aventis. Curr Opin Mol Ther 2005; 7(5):493–501.
26. Byrne AT, Ross L, Holash J, et al. Vascular endothelial growth factor-trap decreases tumor burden, inhibits ascites, and causes dramatic vascular remodeling in an ovarian cancer model. Clin Cancer Res 2003; 9(15):5721–5728.
27. Drevs J, Konerding MA, Wolloscheck T, et al. The VEGF receptor tyrosine kinase inhibitor, ZD6474, inhibits angiogenesis and affects microvascular architecture within an orthotopically implanted renal cell carcinoma. Angiogenesis 2004; 7(4):347–354.
28. Beaudry P, Force J, Naumov GN, et al. Differential effects of vascular endothelial growth factor receptor-2 inhibitor ZD6474 on circulating endothelial progenitors and mature circulating endothelial cells: implications for use as a surrogate marker of antiangiogenic activity. Clin Cancer Res 2005; 11(9):3514–3522.
29. Miller KD, Trigo JM, Wheeler C, et al. A multicenter phase II trial of ZD6474, a vascular endothelial growth factor receptor-2 and epidermal growth factor receptor tyrosine kinase inhibitor, in patients with previously treated metastatic breast cancer. Clin Cancer Res 2005; 11(9):3369–3376.

30. Nash GF, Walsh DC, Kakkar AK. The role of the coagulation system in tumour angiogenesis. Lancet Oncol 2001; 2(10):608–613.
31. Goldenberg N, Kahn SR, Solymoss S. Markers of coagulation and angiogenesis in cancer-associated venous thromboembolism. J Clin Oncol 2003; 21(22):4194–4199.
32. Verheul HM, Hoekman K, Lupu F, et al. Platelet and coagulation activation with vascular endothelial growth factor generation in soft tissue sarcomas. Clin Cancer Res 2000; 6(1):166–171.
33. Lacey M, Alpert S, Hanahan D. Bovine papillomavirus genome elicits skin tumours in transgenic mice. Nature 1986; 322(6080):609–612.
34. Zhang Y, Deng Y, Luther T, et al. Tissue factor controls the balance of angiogenic and antiangiogenic properties of tumor cells in mice. J Clin Invest 1994; 94(3):1320–1327.
35. Boccaccio C, Sabatino G, Medico E, et al. The MET oncogene drives a genetic programme linking cancer to haemostasis. Nature 2005; 434(7031):396–400.
36. Koomagi R, Volm M. Tissue-factor expression in human non-small-cell lung carcinoma measured by immunohistochemistry: correlation between tissue factor and angiogenesis. Int J Cancer 1998; 79(1):19–22.
37. Carmeliet P, Mackman N, Moons L, et al. Role of tissue factor in embryonic blood vessel development. Nature 1996; 383(6595):73–75.
38. Contrino J, Hair G, Kreutzer DL, Rickles FR. In situ detection of tissue factor in vascular endothelial cells: correlation with the malignant phenotype of human breast disease. Nat Med 1996; 2(2):209–215.
39. Verheul HM, Hoekman K, Luykx-de Bakker S, et al. Platelet: transporter of vascular endothelial growth factor. Clin Cancer Res 1997; 3(12 Pt 1):2187–2190.
40. Weltermann A, Wolzt M, Petersmann K, et al. Large amounts of vascular endothelial growth factor at the site of hemostatic plug formation in vivo. Arterioscler Thromb Vasc Biol 1999; 19(7):1757–1760.
41. Gasic GJ, Gasic TB, Stewart CC. Antimetastatic effects associated with platelet reduction. Proc Natl Acad Sci USA 1968; 61(1):46–52.
42. van Hinsbergh VW, Koolwijk P, Hoekman K. The hemostatic system in angiogenesis. Exs 2005; 94:247–266.
43. Gordon MS, Margolin K, Talpaz M, et al. Phase I safety and pharmacokinetic study of recombinant human anti-vascular endothelial growth factor in patients with advanced cancer. J Clin Oncol 2001; 19(3):843–850.
44. Yang JC, Haworth L, Sherry RM, et al. A randomized trial of bevacizumab, an anti-vascular endothelial growth factor antibody, for metastatic renal cancer. N Engl J Med 2003; 349(5):427–434.
45. Johnson DH, Fehrenbacher L, Novotny WF, Herbst RS, Nemunaitis JJ, Jablons DM, Langer CJ, DeVore RF 3rd, Gaudreault J, Damieo LA, Holmgren E, Kabbinavar F. Randomized phase II trial comparing bevacizumab plus carboplatin and paclitaxel with carboplatin and paclitaxel alone in previously untreated locally advanced or metastatic non-small-cell lung cancer. J Clin Oncol, 2004 Jun 1;22(11):2184-91.
46. Sledge, G., Miller, K., Novotny, W., Gaudreault, J.,Ash, M., Cobleigh, M. A phase II trial of Single-Agent Rhumab VEGF (Recombinant Humanized Monoclonal Antibody to Vascular Endothelial cell Growth Factor) in Patients with Relapsed Metastatic Breast Cancer. Proc Am Soc Clin Oncol 19:2000 (abstr 5C)
47. Kabbinavar F, Hurwitz HI, Fehrenbacher L, et al. Phase II, randomized trial comparing bevacizumab plus fluorouracil (FU)/leucovorin (LV) with FU/LV alone in patients with metastatic colorectal cancer. J Clin Oncol 2003; 21(1):60–65.
48. Kabbinavar FF, Schulz J, McCleod M, et al. Addition of bevacizumab to bolus fluorouracil and leucovorin in first-line metastatic colorectal cancer: results of a randomized phase II trial. J Clin Oncol 2005; 23(16):3697–3705.
49. Miller KD, Chap LI, Holmes FA, et al. Randomized phase III trial of capecitabine compared with bevacizumab plus capecitabine in patients with previously treated metastatic breast cancer. J Clin Oncol 2005; 23(4):792–799.

50. Nguyen et al. Ophthalmology 2006; 113:1522.
51. Dupont J,Rothenberg ML, Spriggs DR, et al. Safety and pharmacokinetics of intravenous VFGF Trap in a phase I clinical trial of patients with advanced solid tumors. Abstract No:3029 Journal of clinical Oncology, 2005 ASCO Annual Meeting Proceedings.Vol 23, No.16s, Part I of II (June 1 Supplement), 2005:3029
52. Rixe O, Verslype C, Méric JB, et al. Safety and pharmacokinetics of intravenous VEGF Trap plus irinotecan, 5-fluorouracil, and leucovorin (I-LV5FU2) in a combination phase I clinical trial of patients with advanced solid tumors. Annual Meeting of ASCO 2006; Abstr Nr 13161.
53. Mulay M, Limentani SA, Carroll M, Furfine ES, Cohen DP, Rosen LS. Safety and pharmacokinetics of intravenous VEGF Trap plus FOLFOX4 in a combination phase I clinical trial of patients with advanced solid tumors. Annual Meeting ASCO 2006; Abstr Nr 13061.
54. Trarbach T, Schleucher N, Tewes M, et al. Phase I/II study of PTK787/ZK 222584 (PTK/ZK), a Novel, Oral Angiogenesis Inhibitor in Combination With FOLFIRI as First-line Treatment for Patients With Metastatic Colorectal Cancer (CRC) Abstract No: 3605. Journal of Clinical Oncology, 2005 ASCO Annual Meeting Proceedings. Vol 23, No.16S, Part I of II (June 1 Supplement), 2005:3605.
55. Steward WP, Thomas A, Morgan B, et al. Expanded phase I/II study of PTK787/ZK 222584 (PTK/ZK), a novel, oral angiogenesis inhibitor, in combination with FOLFOX-4 as first-line treatment for patients metastatic colorectal cancer. Abstract No: 3556 Journal of Clinical Oncology, 2004 ASCO Annual Meeting Proceedings (Post-Meeting Edition). Vol 22, No.14s (July 15 Supplement), 2004:3556.
56. Hecht JR, Trarbach T, Jaeger E, et al. A randomized, double-blind, placebo-controlled, phase III study in patients (Pts) with metastatic adenocarcinoma of the colon or rectum receiving first-line chemotherapy with oxaliplatin/5-fluorouracil/leucovorin and PTK787/ZK 222584 or placebo (CONFIRM-I) Abstract No: 3 Journal of Clinical Oncology, 2005 ASCO Annual Meeting Proceedings. Vol 23, No. 16s Part I of II (June 1 Supplement) 2005:3.
57. Lockhart AC, Cropp GF, Berlin JD, Donnelly E, Schumaker RD, Schaff IJ, Hande KR, Fleischer AC, Hannah AL, Rothenberg ML, Phase I/pilot study of SU5416 (semaxinib) in combination with irinotecan/bolus 5-FU/LV(IFL) in patients with metastatic colorectal cancer. Am J Clin Oncol. 2006 Apr;29(2):109-15.
58. Hoff PM, Wolff RA, Bogaard K, Waldrum S, Abbruzzese JL. A Phase I study of escalating doses the tyrosine kinase inhibitor semaxanib (SU5416) in combination with irinotecan in patients with advanced colorectal carcinoma. Jpn J Clin Oncol. 2006 Feb; 36(2):100-3. Epub 2006 Jan 31.
59. Cooney MM, Tsemg KY, Makar V, Mcpeak RJ, Ingalls ST, Dowlati A,Overmoyer B, MeCrae K, Ksenich P, Lavertu P, Ivy P, Hoppel CL, Remick S. A phase IB clinical and pharmacokinetic study of the angiogenesis inhibitor SU5416 and paclitaxel in recurrent or metastatic carcinoma of the head and neck. Cancer Chemother. Pharmacol, 2005 Mar;55(3):295-300. Epub 2004 Nov 6.
60. Heymach JV, Desai J, Manola J, et al. Phase II study of the antiangiogenic agent SU5416 in patients with advanced soft tissue sarcomas. Clin Cancer Res 2004; 10(17):5732–5740.
61. Stadler WM, Cao D, Vogelzang NJ, Ryan CW, Hoving K, Wright R, Karrison T, Vokes EE. A randomized phase II trial of the antiangiogenic agent SU5416 in hormone-refractory prostate cancer. Clin Cancer Res 2004 May 15;10(10):3365-70.
62. Lara PN, Quinn DI, Margolin K, Meyers FJ, Longmate J, Frankel P, Mack PC, Turrel C, Valk P, Rao J, Buckley P, Wun T, Gosselin R, Galvin I, Gumerlock PH, Lenz HJ, Doroshow JH, Gandara DR; SU5416 plus interferon alpha in advanced renal cell carcinoma; a phase II California Cancer Consorlium Study with biological and imaging correlates of angiogenesis inhibition. Clin. Cancer Res 2003 Oct 15;9(13):4772-81.
63. Kuenen BC, Tabernero J, Baselga J, Cavalli F, Pfanner E, Conte PF, Seeber S, Madhusudan S, Deplanque G, Huisman H, Scigalla P, Hoekman K, Harris AL Efficacy and toxicity of the angiogenesis inhibitor SU5416 as a single agent in patients with advanced renal cell carcinoma, melanoma,and soft tissue sarcoma. Clin Cancer Res 2003 May;9(5):1648-55.
64. Fielder W, Serve H, Da hner II, et al. A phase I study of SU11248 in the treatment of patients with refractory or resistant acute myeloid leukemia (AML) or not amenable to conventional therapy for the disease. Blood. 2005 Feb 1;105(3):986-93. Epub 2004 Sep 30.

65. Faivre S, Delbaldo C, Vera K, et al. Safety, pharmacokinetic, and antitumor activity of SU11248, a novel oral multitarget tyrosine kinase inhibitor, in patients with cancer. J Clin Oncol 2006; 24(1): 25–35.
66. Motzer RJ, Michaelson MD, Redman B G, et al. Activity of SU11248, a multitargeted inhibitor of vascular endothelial growth factor receptor and platlet-derived growth factor receptor, in patients with metastatic renal cell carcinoma. J Clin Oncol, 24:16-24, 2006.
67. Motzer RJ, Rini BI, Bukowski RM, et al. Sunitinib in patients with metastatic renal cell carcinoma. Jama, 295:2516-2524, 2006.
68. Demetri GD, van Oosterom AT, Garrett CR, et al. Efficacy and safety of sunitinib in patients with advanced gastrointestinal stromal tumor after failure of imatinib: a randomised controlled trail. Lancet, 368: 1329–1338, 2006.
69. Motzer RJ, Hutson T E, Tomezak P, et al. Sunitinib versus interferon alfa in metastatic renal-cell carcinoma. N Engl J Med, 356: 115–124, 2007.
70. Strumberg D, Richly H, Hilger R A, et al. Phase I clinical and Pharamacokinetic study of the Novel Raf kinase and vascular endothelial growth factor receptor inhibitor BAY 43-9006 in patients with advanced refractory solid tumors. J Clin Oncol, 23: 965–972, 2005.
71. Awada A, Hendlisz A, Gil T, et al. Phase I safety and pharmacokinetics of BAY 43-9006 administered for 21 days on/7 day off in patients with advanced, refractory solid tumors. Br J Cancer, 92: 1855–1861, 2005.
72. Eisen T, Ahmad T, Flaherty KT, et al. Sorafenib in advanced melanoma: a phase II randomized discontinuation trail analysis. Br J Cancer, 95: 581–586, 2006.
73. Abou-Alfa GK, Schwartz I, Ricci S, et al. (2006). Phase II study of sorafenib in patients with advanced hepatocellular carcinoma. J Clin Oncol 24, 4293–4300.
74. Ratain MJ, Eisen T, Stadler WM, et al. Phase II placebo-controlled randomized discontinuation trial of sorafenib in patients with metastatic renal cell carcinoma. J Clin Oncol, 24: 2505–2512, 2006.
75. Holden SN, Eckhardt SG, Basser R, et al. Clinical evaluation of ZD6474, and orally active inhibitor of VEGF and EGF receptor signaling, in patients with solid malignant tumors. Ann Oncol 16: 1391–1397, 2005.
76. Rugo HS, Herbst RS, Llu G, et al. Phase I trial of the oral antiangiogenesis agent AG-013736 in patients with advanced solid tumors: pharmacokinetic and clinical results. J Clin Oncol, 23: 5474–5483, 2005.
77. Levine AM, Tulpulc A, Quinn DI, et al. Phase I study of antisense oligonucleotide against vascular endothelial growth factor; decrease in plasma vascular endothelial growth factor with potential clinical efficacy. J Clin Oncol, 24: 1712-1719, 2006.
78. Drevs J, Medinger M, Mross K, et al. Phase I clinical evaluation of AZD2171, a highly potent VEGF receptor tyrosine kinase inhitor, in patients with advanced tumors Journal of Clinical Oncology, 2005 ASCO Annual Meeting Proccedings. Vol 23, No. 16S, Part I of (June 1 Supplement), 2005: 3002
79. Ryan C, Stadler WM, Roth BJ, et al. Safety and tolerability of AZD2171, a highly potent VEGFR inhibitor, in patients with advanced prostate adenocarcinoma Abstract No: 3049, Journal of Clinical Oncology, 2005 ASSCO Annual Meeting Proceeding. Vol 23, No. 16S, Part I of (June I Supplement), 2005: 3049
80. Laurie SA, Arnold A, Gauthier I, et al. Final results of a phase I study of daily oral AZD2171, an inhibitor of vascular endothelial growth factor receptors (VEGFR), in combination with carboplatin (C) + paclitaxel (T) in patients with advanced non-small cell lung cancer (NSCLC); A study of the National Cancer Institute of Canada Clinical Trials Group (NCIC VTG) Journal of Clinical Oncology, 2006 ASCO Annual Meeting Proceeding Part I. Vol 24, No. 18S (June 20 Supplement), 2006: 3054
81. Kabbinavar FF, Hambleton J, Mass RD, et al. Combined analysis of efficacy: the addition of bevacizumab to fluorouracil/leucovorin improves survival for patients with metastatic colorectal cancer. J Clin Oncol 2005; 23(16):3706–3712.
82. Motl S. Bevacizumab in combination chemotherapy for colorectal and other cancers. Am J Health Syst Pharm 2005; 62(10):1021–1032.

83. Roncalli J, Delord JP, Galinier M, et al. Bevacizumab in metastatic colorectal cancer: a left intracardiac thrombotic event. Ann Oncol 2006; 17(7):1177–1178.
84. Ratner M. Genentech discloses safety concerns over Avastin. Nat Biotechnol 2004; 22(10):1198.
85. Scappaticci FA, Fehrenbacher L, Cartwright T, et al. Surgical wound healing complications in metastatic colorectal cancer patients treated with bevacizumab. J Surg Oncol 2005; 91(3):173–180.
86. Sanborn RE, Sandler AB. The safety of bevacizumab. Expert Opin Drug Saf 2006; 5(2):289–301.
87. Dincer M, Altundag K. Angiotensin-converting enzyme inhibitors for bevacizumab-induced hypertension (December). Ann Pharmacother 2006.
88. Ma L, Francia G, Viloria-Petit A, et al. In vitro procoagulant activity induced in endothelial cells by chemotherapy and antiangiogenic drug combinations: modulation by lower-dose chemotherapy. Cancer Res 2005; 65(12):5365–5373.
89. Hecht JR, Trarbach T, Jaeger E, et al. A randomized, double-blind, placebo-controlled, phase III study in patients (Pts) with metastatic adenocarcinoma of the colon or rectum receiving first-line chemotherapy with oxaliplatin/5-fluorouracil/leucovorin and PTK787/ZK 222584 or placebo (CONFIRM-1). Annual Meeting ASCO; 2005:3.
90. Motzer RJ, Hudson TE, Tomczak P, et al. Phase III randomized trial of sunitinib malate (SU11248) versus interferon-alfa as first-line systemic therapy for patients with metastatic renal cell carcinoma. In: ASCO Annual Meeting; 2006:LBA3.
91. Escudier B, et al. Randomized Phase III trial of the Raf kinase and VEGFR inhibitor sorafenib (BAY 43–9006) in patients with advanced renal cell carcinoma (RCC) Anual meeting ASCO 2005; Abstr No LBA4510.
92. Robert C, Faivre S, Raymond E, et al. Subungual splinter hemorrhages: a clinical window to inhibition of vascular endothelial growth factor receptors? Ann Intern Med 2005; 143(4):313–314.
93. Herbst RS, Sandler AB. Non-small cell lung cancer and antiangiogenic therapy: what can be expected of bevacizumab? Oncologist 2004; 1 (suppl 9):19–26.
94. Pearson JD. Normal endothelial cell function. Lupus 2000; 9(3):183–188.
95. Cines DB, Pollak ES, Buck CA, et al. Endothelial cells in physiology and in the pathophysiology of vascular disorders. Blood 1998; 91(10):3527–3561.
96. Kuenen BC, Levi M, Meijers JC, et al. Analysis of coagulation cascade and endothelial cell activation during inhibition of vascular endothelial growth factor/vascular endothelial growth factor receptor pathway in cancer patients. Arterioscler Thromb Vasc Biol 2002; 22(9):1500–1555.
97. Taraseviciene-Stewart L, Kasahara Y, Alger L, et al. Inhibition of the VEGF receptor 2 combined with chronic hypoxia causes cell death-dependent pulmonary endothelial cell proliferation and severe pulmonary hypertension. Faseb J 2001; 15(2):427–438.
98. Bombeli T, Karsan A, Tait JF, Harlan JM. Apoptotic vascular endothelial cells become procoagulant. Blood 1997; 89(7):2429–2442.
99. Hathcock JJ. Flow effects on coagulation and thrombosis. Arterioscler Thromb Vasc Biol 2006; 26(8):1729–1737.
100. Kilickap S, Abali H, Celik I. Bevacizumab, bleeding, thrombosis, and warfarin. J Clin Oncol 2003; 21(18):3542; author reply 3543.
101. Verheul HM, Lolkema MP, Qian DZ, et al. Platelets take up the monoclonal antibody bevacizunab. Clin cancer Res (In press) 2007.
102. Hong CC, Peterson QP, Hong JY, et al. Artery/vein specification is governed by opposing phosphatidylinositol-3 kinase and MAP kinase/ERK signaling. Curr Biol 2006; 16(13):1366–1372.
103. Okuda Y, Tsurumaru K, Suzuki S, et al. Hypoxia and endothelin-1 induce VEGF production in human vascular smooth muscle cells. Life Sci 1998; 63(6):477–484.
104. Gimbrone MA Jr, Aster RH, Cotran RS, et al. Preservation of vascular integrity in organs perfused in vitro with a platelet-rich medium. Nature 1969; 222(188):33–36.
105. Hanson SR, Slichter SJ. Platelet kinetics in patients with bone marrow hypoplasia: evidence for a fixed platelet requirement. Blood 1985; 66(5):1105–1109.

106. Slichter SJ. Relationship between platelet count and bleeding risk in thrombocytopenic patients. Transfus Med Rev 2004; 18(3):153–167.
107. te Velde EA, Kusters B, Maass C, et al. Histological analysis of defective colonic healing as a result of angiostatin treatment. Exp Mol Pathol 2003; 75(2):119–123.
108. McCarty ME, Ellis LM. Mechanisms of anti-angiogenic tyrosine kinase inhibition on wound healing—the obvious and not so obvious. Cancer Biol Ther 2002; 1(2):127–129.
109. Rhee JS, Black M, Schubert U, et al. The functional role of blood platelet components in angiogenesis. Thromb Haemost 2004; 92(2):394–402.
110. Selheim F, Holmsen H, Vassbotn FS. Identification of functional VEGF receptors on human platelets. FEBS Lett 2002; 512(1–3):107–110.
111. Pawlinski R, Pedersen B, Erlich J, et al. Role of tissue factor in haemostasis, thrombosis, angiogenesis and inflammation: lessons from low tissue factor mice. Thromb Haemost 2004; 92(3):444–450.
112. Duan WR, Patyna S, Kuhlmann MA, et al. A multitargeted receptor tyrosine kinase inhibitor, SU6668, does not affect the healing of cutaneous full-thickness incisional wounds in SKH-1 mice. J Invest Surg 2006; 19(4):245–254.
113. Haroon ZA, Amin K, Saito W, et al. SU5416 delays wound healing through inhibition of TGF-beta 1 activation. Cancer Biol Ther 2002; 1(2):121–126.
114. Scotland RS, Madhani M, Chauhan S, et al. Investigation of vascular responses in endothelial nitric oxide synthase/cyclooxygenase-1 double-knockout mice: key role for endothelium-derived hyperpolarizing factor in the regulation of blood pressure in vivo. Circulation 2005; 111(6):796–803.
115. Gelinas DS, Bernatchez PN, Rollin S, et al. Immediate and delayed VEGF-mediated NO synthesis in endothelial cells: role of PI3K, PKC and PLC pathways. Br J Pharmacol 2002; 137(7):1021–1030.
116. Umemoto S, Kawahara S, Hashimoto R, et al. Different effects of amlodipine and enalapril on the mitogen-activated protein kinase/extracellular signal-regulated kinase kinase-extracellular signal-regulated kinase pathway for induction of vascular smooth muscle cell differentiation in vivo. Hypertens Res 2006; 29(3):179–186.

7

Heparin in Cancer: Role of Selectin Interactions

Lubor Borsig
University of Zürich, Zürich, Switzerland

Jennifer L. Stevenson
*University of California, San Diego, California, U.S.A.**

Ajit Varki
University of California, San Diego, California, U.S.A.

- Heparin therapy has potential benefits for cancer patients that extend beyond its anticoagulant activity.
- Experimental evidence from various systems consistently support the ability of heparin to attenuate metastasis.
- Clinical studies support a beneficial role for heparin in cancer, which is in contrast to the limited effects of other anticoagulants.
- P- and L-selectin are vascular cell adhesion molecules mediating initial steps of intravascular cell adhesion, and these interactions are efficiently inhibited by heparin.
- Carcinoma cells are common carriers of selectin ligands, and their high expression correlates with poor prognosis due to metastasis.
- Metastasis is facilitated by P- and L-selectin–mediated interaction of tumor cells with platelets, leukocytes, and endothelial cells.
- Heparin at clinically acceptable levels is a potent inhibitor of P- and L-selectin–mediated interactions.
- Heparin attenuates experimental metastasis largely via the inhibition of cell–cell interactions mediated by P- and L-selectin.

HEPARIN EFFECTS ON CANCER: CLINICAL EVIDENCE

The close relationship between hypercoagulability and cancer was first identified in 1865 (1), and has been extensively studied since (2). Heparin is a highly sulfated glycosaminoglycan that has been in clinical use as an anticoagulant for many years (3–5). Many retrospective

* Currently with AMGEN, Thousand Oaks, California, U.S.A.

analyses of clinical data implicate heparin in improving survival of cancer patients (6–10), as do studies using various mouse models of cancer (see below). In contrast, clinical trials using oral vitamin K antagonists, another type of anticoagulant, showed no significant improvement of survival in most cancers (11–14). This suggests that the anticoagulant effects of heparin are not primarily responsible for the antimetastatic effect. Based on encouraging observations with heparin treatment, several recent prospective clinical trials have been performed to evaluate this phenomenon (14–18). The CLOT clinical trial, in which patients with a solid tumor and venous thromboembolism were treated with dalteparin or a vitamin K antagonist, demonstrated no effect on survival (15). However, analysis of a subset of patients who were metastasis-free at the beginning of the trial demonstrated a significant increase in survival with dalteparin in that population (14). The Fragmin Advanced Malignancy Outcome Study (FAMOUS) trial evaluated the effect of the low-molecular-weight heparin (LMWH) dalteparin on the survival of patients with advanced carcinoma (16). No improvement in survival was seen in patients with an originally poor prognosis, but those with a better prognosis demonstrated a statistically significant increase in survival. A trial of patients with small cell lung cancer also demonstrated increased survival in patients who were given dalteparin in combination with traditional chemotherapy, compared to patients who received traditional chemotherapy alone, regardless of the initial stage of the patients (17). Finally, the Malignancy and Low-Molecular-Weight Heparin Therapy (MALT) trial of patients with advanced solid tumors demonstrated an improvement in survival in patients who received the LMWH nadroparin compared to those who received a placebo (18).

Given these promising results and the related animal data (see below), it seems likely that heparin treatment in cancer patients directly affects tumorigenesis and/or metastasis, rather than simply serving to prevent thromboembolism. Delineation of a mechanism is currently a topic of investigation in several laboratories. As will be addressed below, heparin has a variety of biological activities, one or many of which may be involved in reduction of metastasis and increase in survival (19,20). We summarize some of the work that has been done in this field and suggest conclusions that can be drawn from this work, which have implications for cancer treatment.

HEPARIN EFFECTS ON CANCER: EXPERIMENTAL EVIDENCE

A variety of animal models have been developed as preclinical models to evaluate potential cancer therapies. Of these, mice have proven to be particularly useful, as their genetics are easily manipulated (21). There are two main techniques by which metastasis can be studied in mouse models (22). The first is the spontaneous model of metastasis, in which a primary tumor is formed (either by injection of exogenous tumor cells or by genetic manipulation of endogenous cells) and allowed to metastasize spontaneously. This model provides an opportunity to recapitulate many of the steps of the metastatic cascade, including invasion of the basement membrane, intravasation, extravasation at a distant site, and growth of the metastatic foci. There are, however, many limitations to this model when evaluating the effect of a therapy, as the timing of the treatment with respect to the various stages of metastasis and the route of metastasis (hematogenous vs. lymphatic) cannot be fully understood. The second model is experimental metastasis, in which tumor cells are administered directly into the blood. This provides a means by which the effect of a treatment can be evaluated at specific time points, and narrows the number of interactions affected by the treatment.

Many mouse studies on the effect of heparin on metastasis have been reported. Table 1 summarizes reported metastasis studies in mice to evaluate the role of heparin since 1990. For a previous review that includes studies prior to 1990, see Ref. (40)

Table 1 Murine Experimental Metastasis Experiments with Heparin

Tumor type	Heparin[a]	Heparin dose[b]	Heparin timing[c]	Route[d]	Effect on metastasis	References
Mouse mammary carcinoma	UFH	40 IU/mouse	−1 day and −1 hr	i.p.	Decrease	Lee et al. (23)
Mouse melanoma	UFH	0.4 mg/mouse	−20 min	i.v.	Decrease	Vlodavsky et al. (24)
			−1 day		No effect	
	LMWH	0.4 mg/mouse	−20 min		Decrease	
			−1 day		No effect	
Mouse melanoma	LAC LMWH	10 mg/kg	−20 min and twice a week	i.v.	Decrease	Sciumbata et al. (25)
Mouse melanoma	UFH, modified	50 or 100 mg/kg	−1 hr and once daily for next 3 days	s.q.	Decrease	Lapierre et al. (26)[e]
		10 mg/kg			No effect	
Human colon carcinoma	UFH	100 U/mouse	−30 min	i.v.	Decrease	Borsig et al. (27)
Mouse colon carcinoma	UFH	100 U/mouse	−30 min	i.v.	Decrease	Borsig et al. (28)
Mouse melanoma	UFH	0.2–0.5 mg/mouse	Coinjected	i.v.	Decrease	Poggi et al. (29)
Mouse melanoma Mouse lung carcinoma	LAC or LMWH	1.0 mg/mouse	Once daily, days 1–7	i.v.	Decrease	Ono et al. (30)
Mouse melanoma	LMWH	10 mg/kg	−4 hr	s.q.	Decrease	Amirkhosravi et al. (31)
Mouse melanoma	UFH	12.5 or 60 IU/mouse	−30 min	Not specified	Decrease	Ludwig et al. (32)
		60 IU/mouse	+1 day and then every second day		no effect	
Mouse lung carcinoma	LAC	0.5–2.0 mg/mouse	−10 min	i.v.	Decrease	Yoshitomi et al. (33)
			−1 hour	s.q.	No effect	
Mouse colon carcinoma	UFH	6.6 U/mouse	−30 min	s.q.	Decrease	Stevenson et al. (34)
	LMWH	7.3 IU/mouse				
Mouse melanoma	UFH	6.6 U/mouse				
	LMWH	7.3 IU/mouse				

(Continued)

Table 1 Murine Experimental Metastasis Experiments with Heparin (*Continued*)

Tumor type	Heparin[a]	Heparin dose[b]	Heparin timing[c]	Route[d]	Effect on metastasis	References
Mouse melanoma	LMWH	50 mg/kg	–4 hr	s.q.	No effect	Kragh et al. (35)
Human melanoma	UFH & LMWH	200 IU/kg	–1 day and once daily for 3 days	i.p.	Decrease	Bereczky et al. (36)
Mouse colon carcinoma	UFH	100 IU/mouse	+6 hr and +12 hr	i.v.	Decrease	Laubli et al. (37)
Mouse lung carcinoma	UFH	100 IU/kg	+1 hr	s.q.	No effect	Szende et al. (38)
	LMWH	38 IU/kg			No effect	
		57 IU/kg			Decrease	
Mouse melanoma	UFH	10–60 IU/mouse	–30 min	i.v.	Decrease	Ludwig et al. (39)
	LMWH	60 IU/mouse				

[a]UFH, modified is 2,3- *O*-desulfated; LAC (obtained by chemical modification of the heparin); LMWH encompasses a variety of low-molecular-weight heparins.
[b]The doses provided here are those given in the corresponding references. Note that many of these doses can be directly compared by assuming an approximate average weight of 20 g/mouse. However, correlating heparin mass with activity depends upon the type of heparin being used and, while fairly consistent approximations can be found in the literature for UFH, much variation is observed in the literature for LMWH correlations. Therefore, it is left to the reader to perform these conversions, should it be desired.
[c]Timing of the heparin administration is given in reference to administration of tumor cells. A negative value indicates that heparin was administered prior to tumor cell injection.
[d]Route of heparin administration.
[e]This study was performed as a survival study; however, numerous visible lung metastases were confirmed in all animals that received the vehicle-alone control injection.
Abbreviations: UFH, unfractionated heparin; LAC, low anticoagulant; LMWH, low-molecular-weight heparin; i.v., intravenous; s.q., subcutaneous; i.p., intraperitoneal.

These involved a variety of heparins, including unfractionated heparin, various LMWHs, and heparins with various chemical modifications, including some that decrease the anticoagulant activity. Studies also have been performed using a variety of tumor cells, including human and mouse colon carcinoma and melanoma, mouse lung carcinoma, and mouse breast carcinoma, using a variety of heparin doses, routes, and timing of administration. A few recent ones are highlighted below, and further discussion will follow.

Studies of colon carcinoma metastasis models demonstrated that a single bolus of unfractionated heparin given just prior to tumor cell injection attenuates metastasis (27). A more recent study showed the same for melanoma cells (32). Experimental metastasis assays performed with heparin dosing at clinically relevant levels demonstrated a reduction in metastasis of both colon carcinoma and melanoma cells, in a manner that was dependent on the type of heparin administered (34). While unfractionated heparin and the LMWH tinzaparin reduced metastasis, the synthetic pentasaccharide fondaparinux had no effect. All of these were administered to achieve the same clinically relevant anticoagulant levels. Thus, a single clinically relevant dose of heparin is capable of dramatically reducing metastasis (34).

WHICH OF MANY BIOLOGICAL ACTIONS OF HEPARIN INTERDICT CANCER METASTASIS?

Heparin is a complex mixture of natural glycosaminoglycans extracted from porcine intestine (4,41). Although clinical preparations are enriched for the ability to inhibit the clotting, the mixtures also have a wide variety of biological effects other than anticoagulation. The anticoagulant activity of heparin is carried only by a subset of the preparations, and it is determined by a distinct pentasaccharide responsible for binding to antithrombin III (40,42). In addition to blockade of P- and L-selectin binding (43–47), heparin can alter interactions with integrins, affect the action of various growth factors and cytokines, inhibit angiogenesis and heparanases, and modulate the activity of some proteases and extracellular matrix components (40,42,48). Despite these many biological effects, the earliest actions in the metastatic cascade are likely to be the most important. In the experimental model of metastasis in which tumor cells are administered directly into the vasculature and immediately interact with blood cells, the selectins are likely one of the first steps in the metastatic cascade. Additionally, as the heparin administered in most animal studies is cleared within a few hours, many of the additional effects of heparin (e.g., heparanase and angiogenesis inhibition) are likely not relevant during this time frame.

ANIMAL STUDIES SHOWING BENEFITS OF OTHER ANTICOAGULANTS WERE DONE AT LEVELS FAR EXCEEDING CLINICALLY TOLERABLE DOSES

As discussed above, heparin has many potential antimetastatic effects, including anticoagulation. Some experimental studies have demonstrated that anticoagulation using the antithrombin agent hirudin can reduce metastasis. In one of these studies, 20 mg/kg of hirudin was given to mice immediately before, four hours after, and then every other day after intravenous injection of tumor cells, for 10 days (49). A significant decrease in metastatic foci was observed. Another group injected mice with hirudin at 10 mg/kg 20 minutes prior to tumor cell injection (50). Again, decreased pulmonary arrest of tumor cells with hirudin treatment was demonstrated. However, when anticoagulation by hirudin was measured at the time of tumor cell injection, the results were almost all above the limits of detection (clotting time >300 seconds in an activated partial thromboplastin time test). As this dose was about half that given in the first mentioned study, both results are very likely not to be clinically relevant, given the excessive anticoagulation achieved. In this regard, other groups have designed chemically modified, non-anticoagulant heparins, the use of which still showed a decrease in metastasis (26,51). Finally, we have recently compared unfractionated heparin with the synthetic pentasaccharide fondaparinux, which has no selectin inhibitory activity. We found that the pentasaccharide had no effect on hematogenous metastasis when given at similar clinically acceptable levels of anticoagulation (34).

SELECTINS: ADHESION MOLECULES FOR CELLS IN THE VASCULATURE

Selectins are vascular cell adhesion molecules involved in adhesive interactions of leukocytes and platelets within the circulation. The physiological functions of selectins are well described in processes of inflammation, immune response, wound repair, and hemostasis (52). The initial steps in leukocyte tethering and rolling on endothelium are supported by rapid and reversible interactions of selectins with their carbohydrate ligands. Selectins are membrane-anchored glycoproteins containing a lectin domain, which mediates binding to carbohydrates (53), This family of Ca^{2+}-dependent lectins consists of three members: E-, P-, and L-selectin (Fig. 1A).

P-selectin is present in the storage granules of endothelial cells (Weibel-Palade bodies) and platelets (α-granules), thus enabling rapid exteriorization on cell surfaces upon activation (53). In contrast, E-selectin requires de novo transcription and is found on activated endothelial cell surfaces several hours after exposure to the stimulus (53). Almost all leukocyte subpopulations carry L-selectin constitutively on their cell surfaces. The role of selectins has been elucidated in mouse models deficient in selectins to delineate important aspects of their function. The synergy of L- and P-selectin in the rolling of neutrophils was determined, where the rolling flux of leukocytes was higher in wild type (wt) mice with functional P- and L-selectins (54). Mice deficient in one or both selectins had a low proportion of leukocyte rolling (55). The distinct role of individual selectins in leukocyte rolling was found to be due to differences in the rolling velocities characteristic for each selectin in vivo (53,56). While L-selectin mediates fast rolling of leukocytes on endothelium, P- and E-selectin support rolling at lower velocities. Thus, partially overlapping, yet specific contributions of selectins have been identified (Fig. 1A). Selectin expression is tightly regulated during homeostasis, thereby ensuring leukocyte adhesion/recruitment only at the proper time and location. While cell surface expression of P- and E-selectin is temporal in nature and lasts only a short time, L-selectin on leukocytes is proteolytically shed after a cell–cell interaction leading to activation (57). Aberrant selectin action can also lead to excessive accumulation of leukocytes, contributing to the pathogenesis of inflammatory disorders such as ischemia-reperfusion injury.

The natural ligands for selectins consist of distinct glycan structures that are usually carried on a protein backbone. The ability of selectins to bind to various classes of molecules (mucins, sulfated glycolipids, glycosaminoglycans, and negatively charged polysaccharides) in vitro made the identification of biologically relevant selectin ligands critically dependent on the assay conditions (58). Only the use of mouse models enabled the understanding of which ligands facilitate selectin-mediated interactions also in vivo. In addition, the presence of the selectin ligands at the right place (accessible to the selectins) at the right time (when selectins are present) determines the identification of "the real selectin ligand" (59). Over the years, several molecules have been described to be biologically relevant selectin ligands. In general, most selectin ligands carry sialylated, fucosylated lactosamine oligosaccharide structures containing the terminal tetrasaccharide sialyl Lewis^x (sLe^x) (53,60). Depending on the selectin, additional sulfation of the glycan itself or of the protein backbone in close proximity to the oligosaccharide is a prerequisite for selectin recognition (61).

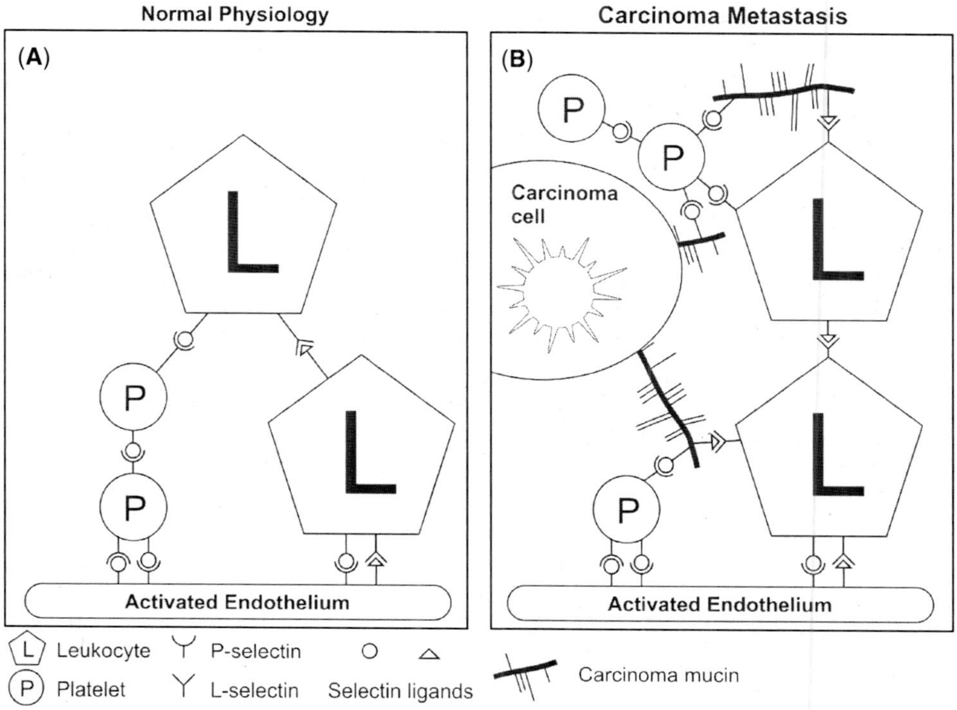

Figure 1 Selectin-mediated interactions during homeostasis and carcinoma metastasis. (**A**) The physiological roles of selectins include the mediation of leukocyte–endothelial cell interactions leading to leukocyte extravasation. Activation of endothelial cells by certain stimuli leads to translocation of P-selectin from endothelial Weibel-Palade bodies and platelet α-granules to the cell surface, thereby enabling loose binding to leukocytes. (**B**) Possible selectin-mediated tumor cell interactions in the bloodstream. Blood-borne carcinoma cells, carrying selectin ligands on cell surface mucins or other glycoconjugates, can induce interactions with platelets, leukocytes, and endothelium. Although all these interactions were shown to take place in mouse models in vivo, their temporal and spatial occurrence in the process of metastasis requires further investigation. E-selectin participation during homeostasis is well described. Due to delayed cell-surfce expression of E-selectin and the inability of heparin to block E-selectin mediated interactions, possible E-selectin contacts are not depicted in this figure.

The best characterized selectin ligand is the P-selectin glycoprotein ligand-1 (PSGL-1), which is concentrated on the tips of microvilli on leukocyte cell surfaces. In the absence of PSGL-1, leukocyte rolling on activated endothelium is virtually eliminated, emphasizing the crucial role of selectin-mediated interactions by leukocyte recruitment (62). Finally, PSGL-1 mediates not only P-selectin but also E-selectin–dependent leukocyte rolling, as demonstrated in small-to-medium blood vessels (63). Selectin–selectin ligand interactions between activated platelets, leukocytes, and activated endothelium in normal physiology are depicted in Figure 1A. As detailed previously, these interactions have all been demonstrated through numerous in vitro and in vivo studies.

CARCINOMA CELLS ARE CARRIERS OF SELECTIN LIGANDS

Hematogenous metastasis is the most common route of cancer spread for carcinomas. Epithelial cells covered with mucins normally line the lumen of hollow organs, and soluble mucins are also secreted to the apical surfaces of the epithelium. Mucins are high-molecular-weight molecules containing a protein core substituted with a large number of *O*-linked glycan structures. The glycan component accounts for 30% to 70% of the total molecular weight (64). The emergence of neoplasia is associated with the loss of epithelial cell polarity and alterations of surface glycosylation. The major carriers of altered glycosylation are mucins in most carcinomas, carrying enhanced expression of sLe^x or sialyl Lewis^a (its isomer), or Tn and sialyl-Tn antigen structures (65). Levels of carcinoma mucins (e.g., CA-125, CA19-9) are routinely used as markers in the diagnosis of cancer and are useful in following the response to treatment. Furthermore, experimental evidence of efficient recombinant soluble selectin binding to primary carcinoma tumors has been documented (66).

It was found that patients with sLe^x-positive colorectal carcinoma had a survival of only 58.3%, while patients whose tumors did not express sLe^x had an improved survival of 93.0% (67). This and other studies of colorectal carcinoma demonstrated that sLe^x expression also correlated with the stage of the disease, disease recurrence, and the presence of lymph node metastases (67,68). Studies of patients with non–small cell lung cancer also correlated sLe^x expression with decreased disease free survival (69). Further studies demonstrated that expression of an enzyme involved in the synthesis of sLe^x also correlated with poor prognosis in lung carcinoma (70). The relationship between sLe^x expression and decreased survival and increased disease severity has been shown for a variety of additional cancers, including gastric (71,72), prostate (73,74), and breast cancer (75,76), cutaneous squamous cell carcinoma (77), melanoma (78), renal cell carcinoma (79), Hodgkin's disease (80), and pancreatic ductal adenocarcinoma (81). From all of this information, it can be seen that there is frequent association between sLe^x expression and increased disease severity among various cancers (82), which is consistent with the idea that selectins facilitate metastasis.

P- AND L-SELECTIN ARE FACILITATORS OF THE EARLY PHASES OF HEMATOGENOUS METASTASIS

Most tumor cells that enter the vasculature do not survive and form metastatic foci (83). Hematogenous metastasis consists of a cascade of events in which the metastatic tumor cells enter the bloodstream, evade innate immune surveillance, adhere to endothelial cells of distant organs, and extravasate. Of these events, cell–cell interactions with the endothelium of a seeding organ, and with platelets and leukocytes appear to be critical for metastatic progression. The entrance of invasive carcinomas carrying selectin ligands into the blood makes these cells potential candidates for interactions with endothelium, platelets, and leukocytes through selectin interactions. This hypothesis has been explored by several laboratories, and recent evidence confirmed P- and L-selectin contributions to metastasis (27,32,34,37). Carcinomas generally carry selectin ligands, and all three selectin members (P-, L-, and E-selectin) are known "initiating" cell adhesion molecules in the vasculature, making selectin-mediated interactions with blood-borne carcinomas likely (Fig. 1B). In the context of metastasis initiation, the rapid nature of P-selectin expression upon activation of endothelia or platelets, together with the constant presence of L-selectin on leukocytes, makes these selectins possible contributors to metastasis. Consequently, the presence of early-response receptors P- and L-selectin in the circulation suggests a role not only of the endothelium, but also of platelets and leukocytes in the process of metastasis. Figure 1B depicts the potential interactions of intravascular carcinoma cells via mucinous ligands to P- and L-selectin. Direct interactions between tumor cells and activated platelets, leukocytes, and activated endothelium can all be mediated by P- and L-selectin.

PLATELETS, LEUKOCYTES, AND THEIR ROLE DURING METASTASIS

Platelets are involved in many physiological and pathological processes including hemostasis, thrombosis, and inflammation. Tumor cell emboli, consisting of platelets and leukocytes, may also potentiate tumor metastasis (84–86). Formation of platelet–tumor cell thrombi may help evade host responses and contribute to colonizing distant organs (27,84–87). Indeed, experimentally induced thrombocytopenia led to attenuation of metastasis in mice (88). Intravenous injection of tumor cells in mice is mostly associated with platelet–fibrin aggregates, which seem to help tumor cell retention in the lung vasculature due to their size. In the absence of platelet–tumor cell interactions, tumor cells are cleared also by natural killer (NK) cells (87,89). Although an exact molecular mechanism of platelet–tumor cell complex formation has not been identified, considerable evidence suggests that P-selectin is one of the mediators in this process (27,90). P-selectin deficiency leads to reduced platelet–tumor cell interactions and tumor cell seeding to the lung vasculature (27,37). Enhanced association of monocytes with tumor cells has also been detected (27,89), and the "platelet cloak" may protect against NK cells (87). The reduction of selectin ligands on tumor cells also caused the inhibition of platelet–tumor cell emboli formation, which led to attenuation of metastasis (27,28,89). In addition, platelet aggregates were detected around tumor cells not expressing selectin ligands (50). Thus, it is possible that while P-selectin–mediated platelet aggregation facilitates interactions among platelets, contact of platelets with tumor cells could be of a different nature.

P-selectin–mediated interactions apart from platelets were also reported (32). Lethal irradiation of mice followed by bone marrow rescue was used to address the contribution of endothelial P-selectin to metastasis. When P-selectin–deficient mice were rescued with wt bone marrow, a significant reduction of metastasis was observed. Such chimeric mice had P-selectin on platelets only. This study indicates that early activation of endothelium and concomitant expression of P-selectin contributes to metastasis.

Patients with occult or overt cancer often develop thromboemboli (the so-called Trousseau's syndrome) and are in a sustained hypercoagulable state (91). Clinical manifestations of this hypercoagulable state in cancer vary from deep venous thrombosis to disseminated intravascular coagulation. In particular, mucin-producing carcinomas are frequently associated with microvascular thromboembolism in cancer patients. The hypercoagulation is due to alterations in hemostasis and the activation of fluid phase coagulation modulated by tissue factor (91). In this regard, it is also interesting to note that platelet-rich microthrombi formation can be associated with cancer cell–platelet interactions, which are at least partially mediated by P-selectin. Recent evidence supports the notion that carcinoma mucins are implicated in thrombus formation (92). Purified human carcinoma mucin triggered selectin-dependent platelet aggregation upon intravenous injection in mice (92). These findings provided evidence for a direct association of carcinoma mucins with platelet aggregation, which is typically associated with the Trousseau syndrome.

Participation of leukocytes in tumor cell emboli is already part of the textbook descriptions of hematogenous metastasis. However, their contribution to this process remained somewhat unclear until recently. While there is a large amount of evidence about the primary tumor environment being populated largely by leukocytes, there is limited knowledge about the role of leukocytes during metastasis (93). The potential of leukocytes to modulate metastasis was tested in an L-selectin–deficient mouse model (37,28). Metastatic progression was dependent on L-selectin, because its genetic absence in mice led to attenuation of metastasis, implicating leukocytes in the process. L-selectin mediated recruitment of leukocytes to the tumor emboli subsequent to P-selectin–mediated platelet–tumor cell complex formation. This suggests that L-selectin mediates the interaction of leukocytes with the tumor cell microenvironment, either with the thrombus itself or with the surrounding endothelium. Indeed, an increase in the presence of leukocytes near vascular tumor cells correlated with enhanced expression of L-selectin ligands around the tumor cell embolus, indicative of locally activated endothelium (37). Leukocytes associated with tumor cells in the vasculature were found to be neutrophils and monocytes (37). One possible explanation for the leukocyte contribution to metastasis comes from the capacity of L-selectin–positive leukocytes to transmigrate through L-selectin ligand–positive endothelium (94,95). Thus, leukocytes may assist tumor cells breaching the endothelial barrier at sites of intravascular embolization, thereby facilitating metastasis (96,97).

Figure 2A summarizes the potential interactions of intravascular carcinoma cells with platelets, leukocytes, or endothelial cells.

Direct P- and L-selectin–mediated interactions between the tumor cell and the vascular environment can contribute to tumor cell adhesion, platelet aggregation, and leukocyte activation.

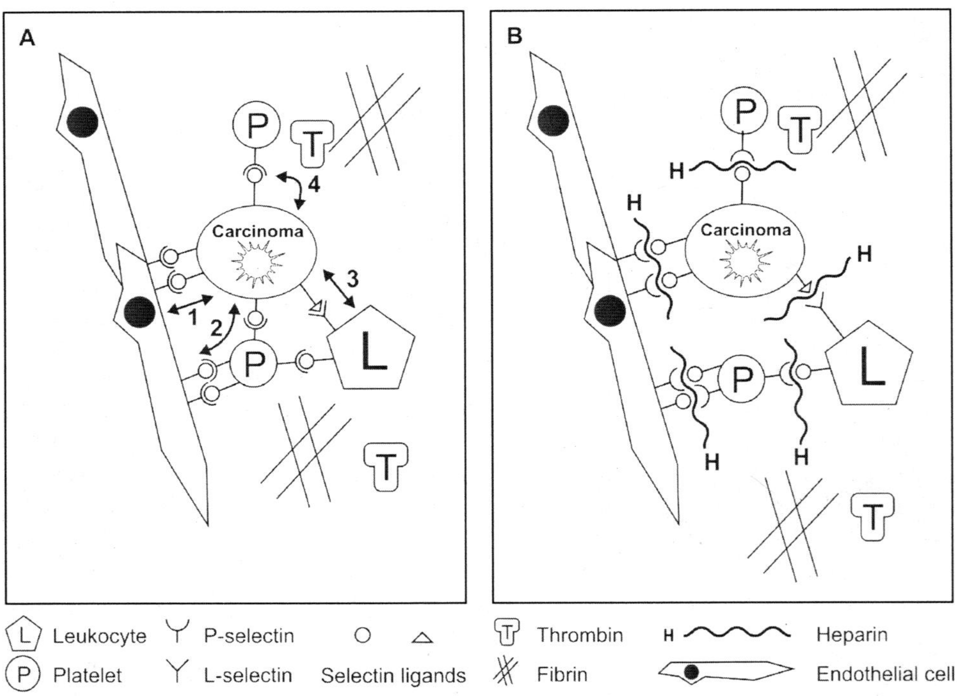

Figure 2 Selectin-mediated interactions during malignancy and the potential of heparin to inhibit metastasis. (**A**) Multiple interactions among leukocytes, activated platelets, endothelium, and tumor cells are possible. The carcinoma mucins serve as selectin ligands for activated endothelium associated with P-selectin expression (1); platelet-mediated carcinoma adhesion to the endothelium is P-selectin dependent (2); direct L-selectin–meditated interactions between leukocytes and cancer cells could further contribute to platelet activation and thrombi formation (3); and direct cancer cell–mediated platelet activation, associated also with thrombin generation, could lead to thrombi formation tightened by fibrin deposits (4). (**B**) Heparin, with its potential to bind to P- and L-selectin, could interfere with early interactions amongst cancer cells and platelets, leukocytes, and endothelium. Although interactions among the metastatic cancer cells and blood constituents can be mediated by many processes, the early role of selectins in the initiation of such interactions suggests a crucial role in the metastatic cascade.

HEPARINS ARE POTENT INHIBITORS OF P- AND L-SELECTIN BINDING AT CLINICALLY TOLERABLE LEVELS

Due to its biological origin and heterogeneous structure, heparin has biological activities distinct from anticoagulation associated with subsets of molecules (40,42,48). As discussed previously, heparin binds to growth factors, inhibits the activity of the extracellular hydrolase heparanase, and inhibits P- and L-selectin–mediated interactions. Although any of these biological activities could potentially modulate cancer progression, results from metastasis experiments suggest that inhibition of selectins is one of the earliest processes affected (Fig. 2). Heparin efficiently binds to P- and L-selectin despite having no obvious structural similarities to the natural selectin ligands (43,45). This activity of heparin is likely explained by the dense cluster of multiple negatively charged sulfates and carboxylates, but the exact structure recognized is unknown. However, heparin efficiently inhibited P- and L-selectin–mediated interactions with cancer cells in in vitro and in vivo experiments (27,32,37,45,98,99). Unfractionated heparin was first shown to inhibit P- and L-selectin binding to sLe^x structures at concentrations currently used for anticoagulation (45). Incubation of human mucin producing carcinoma cells with platelets resulted in a strong P-selectin–dependent platelet aggregation around tumor cells (27). These interactions were carcinoma mucin dependent and were blocked by unfractionated heparin. Injection of heparins (unfractionated or LMWH) also attenuated metastasis in experimental mouse models (Table 1).

The contribution of P- and L-selectins in the facilitation of metastasis was studied in mice deficient either in individual P- or L-selectin or in double P/L-selectin (27,28,32,37). While the absence of P- or L-selectin significantly attenuated metastasis of carcinoma cells, there was virtually no metastasis observed in the P/L double deficient mice (P/L-sel–/–), suggesting a synergistic effect of both selectins (28). Heparin injection 30 minutes before tumor cell injection attenuated metastasis in wt mice to levels similar to that observed in P-selectin–deficient mice (P-sel–/–) (27,28,32). In L-selectin–deficient mice (L-sel–/–), injection of heparin 30 minutes prior to tumor cells further attenuated metastasis (28). Additional effects of heparin administration prior to tumor cells in L-sel–/– mice suggest that the involvement of leukocytes, through L-selectin, is subsequent to the initial P-selectin–mediated platelet aggregation. No further reduction of metastasis in PL-sel–/– indicated that no other biological activity of heparin was contributing to the attenuation of metastasis (unpublished observations) (28). The recent finding of L-selectin participation in metastasis indicated that leukocytes contribute to this process in a time period subsequent to P-selectin–dependent platelet interactions (37). Heparin injection several hours after the tumor cells led to attenuation of metastasis, primarily due to L-selectin inhibition. These results are clinically relevant since the tumor cells were already in circulation at the time of heparin treatment, similar to clinical situations in cancer patients at an advanced stage.

Taken together, it can be inferred that the effect of heparin on metastasis in mice is time dependent. Heparin pharmacokinetics in mouse circulation after intravenous injection showed rapid clearance, with the biological effect determined by inhibition of P-selectin–mediated platelet–tumor cell interactions lasting for about six to eight hours (27). The short presence of heparin in circulation, together with the strong attenuation of metastasis, emphasizes the significant role of this short-term interaction. Such interactions were shown to be at least in part P- and L-selectin dependent, thus implicating platelets, endothelium, and leukocytes in metastasis progression (27,28,90).

A summary of mouse metastasis studies using various cancer cells and treatment with heparin, LMWH, or low-anticoagulant heparin (LAC heparin) is presented in Table 1. Studies performed before 1990 are reviewed by Smorenburg and Van (40). Despite the large variation in the heparin or LMWH dose used in various laboratories, injection of heparin in a time period around the tumor cell injection (shortly before or after) was associated with reduction of metastasis. However, treatment with heparin either one day before or one day after tumor cell injection did not affect metastasis (24,32). The exception to this is the study of Bereczky et al. (36), in which heparin injected one day prior to tumor cells reduced metastasis. Unfortunately, the time of repeated heparin injection in this study could not be identified.

In general, the doses of heparin and LMWH used in these studies were several times higher than the currently acceptable doses in humans. Inhibition of human P-selectin has previously been reported to occur at concentrations lower than those required to inhibit mouse P-selectin (27). Therefore, assuming that inhibition of selectins is the main mechanism for heparin attenuation of metastasis, the potential for a heparin effect on metastasis is even greater than that in mice. Nevertheless, two recent studies have shown that heparin and LMWH used at clinically relevant doses (generally targeting 1 anti-Xa unit/mL) are as efficient at inhibiting metastasis as higher doses (34,39). Based on these observations, it can be concluded that heparin or LMWH are efficient inhibitors of metastasis and their efficiency correlates with the time of administration. In principle, all observations of metastasis attenuation by heparin in mice (Table 1) are in agreement with the possible inhibition of P- and/or L-selectin. While other biological effects of heparin on angiogenesis and heparanase inhibition are possible, the time-limited presence of heparin in the mouse circulation limits their potential to be the leading mechanisms for the effect on metastasis. In addition, the attenuation of metastasis observed even with LAC heparin excludes the anticoagulant activity of heparin as its biological activity in this process (Table 1). Taken together, experimental evidence from various mouse models supports the role of heparin as an effective inhibitor of metastasis. Based on observations in selectin-deficient mice, heparins seem to affect early processes (within the first 24 hours) during metastasis, which are mediated predominantly by P- and L-selectin (Fig. 2B).

HEPARINS AND LMWHs: POTENTIAL FOR ANTIMETASTATIC TREATMENTS

Hematogenous metastasis is a very important field of research, because with many types of cancer, it is the metastatic foci that prove to be fatal for the patient, not the primary tumor itself (100). Tumor cells have been shown to survive for up to several days within the vasculature (101). It is also known that most of the tumor cells that enter the vasculature do not go on to form metastatic foci (83). Thus, it is clear that the period of time that the tumor cells are in the vasculature is when the tumor cells are susceptible, either to killing by the immune system or to potential therapies.

As many types of cancers are diagnosed well after the tumor is established, it is impossible to treat patients for the entire duration of time in which they have cancer. It has been suggested that heparin inhibition of P- and L-selectin be used immediately following initial cancer diagnosis until a period of time (e.g., a few weeks) after surgical removal of the primary tumor (102). This is a particularly crucial window of opportunity, as it is known that when a patient is undergoing surgery for removal of a primary tumor, the tumor cells are often introduced into the vasculature during the surgical process (103). Therefore, the pre-, peri-, and postoperative administration of heparin is most likely to be beneficial to a cancer patient. There are many patient years of experience with heparin anticoagulation; therefore, the mechanism of managing heparin treatment and the potential side effects are well known.

Preclinical analyses clearly show significant variation among LMWH in their potential to inhibit metastasis, correlating with the mechanisms discussed above. Thus, selectin-blocking ability can vary between preparations of the same formulation of heparin.

Work performed previously has shown that one of the three formulations of unfractionated heparin that was tested had no selectin-inhibitory activity (47). Therefore, while previous testing has demonstrated that specific heparins (unfractionated heparin and tinzaparin) are superior in inhibiting P- and L-selectin (34), it should not be assumed that this is independent of the specific lot, and testing should be performed to determine selectin inhibition for each lot of heparin. However, taken together, the available evidence from preclinical studies and clinical trials discussed strongly argue for the further study of heparins as antimetastatic therapy.

REFERENCES

1. Plegmasia alba dolens. In: Trousseau A, ed. Lectures on Clinical Medicine, Delivered at the Hotel-Dieu, Paris. London: New Sydenham Society, 1865; 5:281–332.
2. Rickles FR, Falanga A. Molecular basis for the relationship between thrombosis and cancer. Thromb Res 2001; 102:V215–V224.
3. Rosenberg RD, Lam L. Correlation between structure and function of heparin. Proc Natl Acad Sci USA 1979; 76:1218–1222.
4. Rosenberg RD. Biochemistry and pharmacology of low molecular weight heparin. Semin Hematol 1997; 34(suppl 4):2–8.
5. Hirsh J, Raschke R. Heparin and low-molecular-weight heparin: the Seventh ACCP Conference on Antithrombotic and Thrombolytic Therapy. Chest 2004; 126:188S-203S.
6. Kakkar AK, Hedges RA, Williamson RCN, Kakkar VV. Perioperative heparin therapy inhibits late death from metastatic cancer. Int J Oncol 1995; 6:885–888.
7. Hettiarachchi RJK, Smorenburg SM, Ginsberg J, Levine M, Prins MH, Büller HR. Do heparins do more than just treat thrombosis? The influence of heparins on cancer spread. Thromb Haemost 1999; 82:947–952.
8. Ornstein DL, Zacharski LR. The use of heparin for treating human malignancies. Haemostasis 1999; 29(suppl 1):48–60.
9. Smorenburg SM, Hettiarachchi RJK, Vink R, Büller HR. The effects of unfractionated heparin on survival in patients with malignancy—a systematic review. Thromb Haemost 1999; 82:1600–1604.
10. Zacharski LR, Ornstein DL, Mamourian AC. Low-molecular-weight heparin and cancer. Semin Thromb Hemost 2000; 26(suppl 1):69–77.
11. Zacharski LR, Henderson WG, Rickles FR, et al. Effect of warfarin anticoagulation on survival in carcinoma of the lung, colon, head and neck, and prostate. Final report of VA Cooperative Study #75. Cancer 1984; 53:2046–2052.
12. Levine M, Hirsh J, Gent M, et al. Double-blind randomised trial of a very-low-dose warfarin for prevention of thromboembolism in stage IV breast cancer. Lancet 1994; 343:886–889.
13. Hejna M, Raderer M, Zielinski CC. Inhibition of metastases by anticoagulants. J Nat Cancer Inst 1999; 91:22–36.
14. Lee AY, Rickles FR, Julian JA, et al. Randomized comparison of low molecular weight heparin and coumarin derivatives on the survival of patients with cancer and venous thromboembolism. J Clin Oncol 2005; 23:2123–2129.
15. Lee AY, Levine MN, Baker RI, et al. Low-molecular-weight heparin versus a coumarin for the prevention of recurrent venous thromboembolism in patients with cancer. N Engl J Med 2003; 349:146–153.
16. Kakkar AK, Levine MN, Kadziola Z, et al. Low molecular weight heparin, therapy with dalteparin, and survival in advanced cancer: the fragmin advanced malignancy outcome study (FAMOUS). J Clin Oncol 2004; 22:1944–1948.
17. Altinbas M, Coskun HS, Er O, et al. A randomized clinical trial of combination chemotherapy with and without low-molecular-weight heparin in small cell lung cancer. J Thromb Haemost 2004; 2:1266–1271.

18. Klerk CP, Smorenburg SM, Otten HM, et al. The effect of low molecular weight heparin on survival in patients with advanced malignancy. J Clin Oncol 2005; 23:2130–2135.
19. Lever R, Page CP. Novel drug development opportunities for heparin. Nat Rev Drug Discov 2002; 1:140–148.
20. Castelli R, Porro F, Tarsia P. The heparins and cancer: review of clinical trials and biological properties. Vasc Med 2004; 9:205–213.
21. Sharpless NE, Depinho RA. The mighty mouse: genetically engineered mouse models in cancer drug development. Nat Rev Drug Discov 2006; 5:741–754.
22. Fidler IJ. New developments in in vivo models of neoplasia. Cancer Metast Rev 1991; 10:191–192.
23. Lee AE, Rogers LA, Longcroft JM, Jeffery RE. Reduction of metastasis in a murine mammary tumour model by heparin and polyinosinic-polycytidylic acid. Clin Exp Metast 1990; 8:165–171.
24. Vlodavsky I, Mohsen M, Lider O, et al. Inhibition of tumor metastasis by heparanase inhibiting species of heparin. Invasion Metast 1994; 14:290–302.
25. Sciumbata T, Caretto P, Pirovano P, et al. Treatment with modified heparins inhibits experimental metastasis formation and leads, in some animals, to long-term survival. Invasion Metast 1996; 16:132–143.
26. Lapierre F, Holme K, Lam L, et al. Chemical modifications of heparin that diminish its anticoagulant but preserve its heparanase-inhibitory, angiostatic, anti-tumor and anti-metastatic properties. Glycobiology 1996; 6:355–366.
27. Borsig L, Wong R, Feramisco J, Nadeau DR, Varki NM, Varki A. Heparin and cancer revisited: mechanistic connections involving platelets, P-selectin, carcinoma mucins, and tumor metastasis. Proc Natl Acad Sci USA 2001; 98:3352–3357.
28. Borsig L, Wong R, Hynes RO, Varki NM, Varki A. Synergistic effects of L- and P-selectin in facilitating tumor metastasis can involve non-mucin ligands and implicate leukocytes as enhancers of metastasis. Proc Natl Acad Sci USA 2002; 99:2193–2198.
29. Poggi A, Rossi C, Casella N, et al. Inhibition of B16-BL6 melanoma lung colonies by semisynthetic sulfaminoheparosan sulfates from *E. coli* K5 polysaccharide. Semin Thromb Hemost 2002; 28:383–391.
30. Ono K, Ishihara M, Ishikawa K, et al. Periodate-treated, non-anticoagulant heparin-carrying polystyrene (NAC-HCPS) affects angiogenesis and inhibits subcutaneous induced tumour growth and metastasis to the lung. Br J Cancer 2002; 86:1803–1812.
31. Amirkhosravi A, Mousa SA, Amaya M, Francis JL. Antimetastatic effect of tinzaparin, a low-molecular-weight heparin. J Thromb Haemost 2003; 1:1972–1976.
32. Ludwig RJ, Boehme B, Podda M, et al. Endothelial P-selectin as a target of heparin action in experimental melanoma lung metastasis. Cancer Res 2004; 64:2743–2750.
33. Yoshitomi Y, Nakanishi H, Kusano Y, et al. Inhibition of experimental lung metastases of Lewis lung carcinoma cells by chemically modified heparin with reduced anticoagulant activity. Cancer Lett 2004; 207:165–174.
34. Stevenson JL, Choi SH, Varki A. Differential metastasis inhibition by clinically relevant levels of heparins--correlation with selectin inhibition, not antithrombotic activity. Clin Cancer Res 2005; 11:7003–7011.
35. Kragh M, Binderup L, Vig Hjarnaa PJ, Bramm E, Johansen KB, Frimundt Petersen C. Non-anti-coagulant heparin inhibits metastasis but not primary tumor growth. Oncol Rep 2005; 14:99–104.
36. Bereczky B, Gilly R, Raso E, Vago A, Timar J, Tovari J. Selective antimetastatic effect of heparins in preclinical human melanoma models is based on inhibition of migration and microvascular arrest. Clin Exp Metast 2005; 22:69–76.
37. Laubli H, Stevenson JL, Varki A, Varki NM, Borsig L. L-selectin facilitation of metastasis involves temporal induction of Fut7–dependent ligands at sites of tumor cell arrest. Cancer Res 2006; 66:1536–1542.
38. Szende B, Paku S, Racz G, Kopper L. Effect of Fraxiparine and heparin on experimental tumor metastasis in mice. Anticancer Res 2005; 25:2869–2872.

39. Ludwig RJ, Alban S, Bistrian R, et al. The ability of different forms of heparins to suppress P-selectin function in vitro correlates to their inhibitory capacity on bloodborne metastasis in vivo. Thromb Haemost 2006; 95:535–540.
40. Smorenburg SM, Van NCJF. The complex effects of heparins on cancer progression and metastasis in experimental studies. Pharmacol Rev 2001; 53:93–105.
41. Lindahl U, Kjellén L. Heparin or heparan sulfate--what is the difference? Thromb Haemost 1991; 66:44–48.
42. Engelberg H. Actions of heparin that may affect the malignant process. Cancer 1999; 85:257–272.
43. Nelson RM, Cecconi O, Roberts WG, Aruffo A, Linhardt RJ, Bevilacqua MP. Heparin oligosaccharides bind L- and P-selectin and inhibit acute inflammation. Blood 1993; 82:3253–3258.
44. Norgard-Sumnicht KE, Varki NM, Varki A. Calcium-dependent heparin-like ligands for L-selectin in nonlymphoid endothelial cells. Science 1993; 261:480–483.
45. Koenig A, Norgard-Sumnicht KE, Linhardt R, Varki A. Differential interactions of heparin and heparan sulfate glycosaminoglycans with the selectins—implications for the use of unfractionated and low molecular weight heparins as therapeutic agents. J Clin Invest 1998; 101:877–889.
46. Ma YQ, Geng JG. Heparan sulfate-like proteoglycans mediate adhesion of human malignant melanoma A375 cells to P-selectin under flow. J Immunol 2000; 165:558–565.
47. Xie X, Rivier AS, Zakrzewicz A, et al. Inhibition of selectin-mediated cell adhesion and prevention of acute inflammation by nonanticoagulant sulfated saccharides—studies with carboxyl-reduced and sulfated heparin and with trestatin A sulfate. J Biol Chem 2000; 275:34818–34825.
48. Folkman J, Shing Y. Control of angiogenesis by heparin and other sulfated polysaccharides. Adv Exp Med Biol 1992; 313:355–364.
49. Hu L, Lee M, Campbell W, Perez-Soler R, Karpatkin S. Role of endogenous thrombin in tumor implantation, seeding, and spontaneous metastasis. Blood 2004; 104:2746–2751.
50. Im JH, Fu W, Wang H, et al. Coagulation facilitates tumor cell spreading in the pulmonary vasculature during early metastatic colony formation. Cancer Res 2004; 64:8613–8619.
51. Vlodavsky I, Ishai-Michaeli R, Mohsen M, et al. Modulation of neovascularization and metastasis by species of heparin. Adv Exp Med Biol 1992; 313:317–327.
52. McEver RP. Selectin-carbohydrate interactions during inflammation and metastasis. Glycoconjugate J 1997; 14:585–591.
53. Kansas GS. Selectins and their ligands: current concepts and controversies. Blood 1996; 88:3259–3287.
54. Jung U, Ley K. Mice lacking two or all three selectins demonstrate overlapping and distinct functions for each selectin. J Immunol 1999; 162:6755–6762.
55. Ley K, Bullard DC, Arbonés ML, et al. Sequential contribution of L- and P-selectin to leukocyte rolling in vivo. J Exp Med 1995; 181:669–675.
56. Ley K. The role of selectins in inflammation and disease. Trends Mol Med 2003; 9:263–268.
57. Hafezi-Moghadam A, Thomas KL, Prorock AJ, Huo YQ, Ley K. L-selectin shedding regulates leukocyte recruitment. J Exp Med 2001; 193:863–872.
58. Varki A. Selectin ligands. Proc Natl Acad Sci USA 1994; 91:7390–7397.
59. Varki A. Selectin ligands: will the real ones please stand up? J Clin Invest 1997; 99:158–162.
60. Lowe JB. Selectin ligands, leukocyte trafficking, and fucosyltransferase genes. Kidney Int 1997; 51:1418–1426.
61. McEver RP, Cummings RD. Role of PSGL-1 binding to selectins in leukocyte recruitment. J Clin Invest 1997; 100:485–492.
62. McEver RP. Selectins: lectins that initiate cell adhesion under flow. Curr Opin Cell Biol 2002; 14:581–586.
63. Xia LJ, Sperandio M, Yago S, et al. P-selectin glycoprotein ligand-1-deficient mice have impaired leukocyte tethering to E-selectin under flow. J Clin Invest 2002; 109:939–950.
64. Kim YS, Gum J, Brockhausen I. Mucin glycoproteins in neoplasia. Glycoconjugate J 1996; 13:693–707.

65. Kim YJ, Varki A. Perspectives on the significance of altered glycosylation of glycoproteins in cancer. Glycoconjugate J 1997; 14:569–576.
66. Kim YJ, Borsig L, Han HL, Varki NM, Varki A. Distinct selectin ligands on colon carcinoma mucins can mediate pathological interactions among platelets, leukocytes, and endothelium. Am J Pathol 1999; 155:461–472.
67. Nakamori S, Kameyama M, Imaoka S, et al. Increased expression of sialyl Lewisx antigen correlates with poor survival in patients with colorectal carcinoma: clinicopathological and immunohistochemical study. Cancer Res 1993; 53:3632–3637.
68. Nakamori S, Kameyama M, Imaoka S, et al. Involvement of carbohydrate antigen sialyl Lewisx in colorectal cancer metastasis. Dis Colon Rectum 1997; 40:420–431.
69. Ogawa J, Tsurumi T, Yamada S, Koide S, Shohtsu A. Blood vessel invasion and expression of sialyl Lewisx and proliferating cell nuclear antigen in stage I non-small cell lung cancer: relation to postoperative recurrence. Cancer 1994; 73:1177–1183.
70. Ogawa J, Inoue H, Koide S. 2,3-sialyltransferase type 3N and -1,3-fucosyltransferase type VII are related to sialyl Lewisx synthesis and patient survival from lung carcinoma. Cancer 1997; 79:1678–1685.
71. Ura H, Denno R, Hirata K, Yamaguchi K, Yasoshima T, Shishido T. Close correlation between increased sialyl-Lewisx expression and metastasis in human gastric carcinoma. World J Surg 1997; 21:773–776.
72. Tatsumi M, Watanabe A, Sawada H, Yamada Y, Shino Y, Nakano H. Immunohistochemical expression of the sialyl Lewisx antigen on gastric cancer cells correlates with the presence of liver metastasis. Clin Exp Metast 1998; 16:743–750.
73. Jorgensen T, Berner A, Kaalhus O, Tveter KJ, Danielsen HE, Bryne M. Up-regulation of the oligosaccharide sialyl Lewisx: a new prognostic parameter in metastatic prostate cancer. Cancer Res 1995; 55:1817–1819.
74. Idikio HA. Sialyl-Lewis-X, Gleason grade and stage in non-metastatic human prostate cancer. Glycoconjugate J 1997; 14:875–877.
75. Renkonen J, Paavonen T, Renkonen R. Endothelial and epithelial expression of sialyl Lewisx and sialyl Lewisa in lesions of breast carcinoma. Int J Cancer 1997; 74:296–300.
76. Yamaguchi A, Ding KF, Maehara M, Goi T, Nakagawara G. Expression of *nm23-H1* gene and sialyl Lewis X antigen in breast cancer. Oncology 1998; 55:357–362.
77. Groves RW, Allen MH, Ross EL, Ahsan G, Barker JNWN, MacDonald DM. Expression of selectin ligands by cutaneous squamous cell carcinoma. Am J Pathol 1993; 143:1220–1225.
78. Ravindranath MH, Amiri AA, Bauer PM, Kelley MC, Essner R, Morton DL. Endothelial-selectin ligands sialyl Lewisx and sialyl Lewisa are differentiation antigens immunogenic in human melanoma. Cancer 1997; 79:1686–1697.
79. Tozawa K, Okamoto T, Kawai N, Hashimoto Y, Hayashi Y, Kohri K. Positive correlation between sialyl Lewisx expression and pathologic findings in renal cell carcinoma. Kidney Int 2005; 67:1391–1396.
80. Benharroch D, Dima E, Levy A, et al. Differential expression of sialyl and non-sialyl-CD15 antigens on Hodgkin-Reed-Sternberg cells: significance in Hodgkin's disease. Leuk Lymphoma 2000; 39:185–194.
81. Takahashi S, Oda T, Hasebe T, et al. Overexpression of sialyl Lewisx antigen is associated with formation of extratumoral venous invasion and predicts postoperative development of massive hepatic metastasis in cases with pancreatic ductal adenocarcinoma. Pathobiology 2001; 69:127–135.
82. Kannagi R. Carbohydrate-mediated cell adhesion involved in hematogenous metastasis of cancer. Glycoconjugate J 1997; 14:577–584.
83. Cameron MD, Schmidt EE, Kerkvliet N, et al. Temporal progression of metastasis in lung: cell survival, dormancy, and location dependence of metastatic inefficiency. Cancer Res 2000; 60:2541–2546.
84. Tanaka NG, Tohgo A, Ogawa H. Platelet-aggregating activities of metastasizing tumor cells. V. In situ roles of platelets in hematogenous metastases. Invasion Metast 1986; 6:209–224.
85. Honn KV, Tang DG, Crissman JD. Platelets and cancer metastasis: a causal relationship? Cancer Metast Rev 1992; 11:325–351.

86. Karpatkin S, Pearlstein E, Ambrogio C, Coller BS. Role of adhesive proteins in platelet tumor interaction in vitro and metastasis formation in vivo. J Clin Invest 1988; 81:1012–1019.
87. Nieswandt B, Hafner M, Echtenacher B, Männel DN. Lysis of tumor cells by natural killer cells in mice is impeded by platelets. Cancer Res 1999; 59:1295–1300.
88. Gasic GJ. Role of plasma, platelets, and endothelial cells in tumor metastasis. Cancer Metast Rev 1984; 3:99–114.
89. Fuster MM, Brown JR, Wang L, Esko JD. A disaccharide precursor of sialyl Lewisx inhibits metastatic potential of tumor cells. Cancer Res 2003; 63:2775–2781.
90. Borsig L. Selectins facilitate carcinoma metastasis and heparin can prevent them. News Physiol Sci 2004; 19:16–21.
91. Rickles FR. Mechanisms of cancer-induced thrombosis in cancer. Pathophysiol Haemost Thromb 2006; 35:103–110.
92. Wahrenbrock M, Borsig L, Le D, Varki N, Varki A. Selectin-mucin interactions as a probable molecular explanation for the association of Trousseau syndrome with mucinous adenocarcinomas. J Clin Invest 2003; 112:853–862.
93. Coussens LM, Werb Z. Inflammation and cancer. Nature 2002; 420:860–867.
94. Ley K. Integration of inflammatory signals by rolling neutrophils. Immunol Rev 2002; 186:8–18.
95. Worthylake RA, Burridge K. Leukocyte transendothelial migration: orchestrating the underlying molecular machinery. Curr Opin Cell Biol 2001; 13:569–577.
96. Wu QD, Wang JH, Condron C, Bouchier-Hayes D, Redmond HP. Human neutrophils facilitate tumor cell transendothelial migration. Am J Physiol Cell Physiol 2001; 280:C814–C822.
97. Bevilacqua MP, Nelson RM. Endothelial-leukocyte adhesion molecules in inflammation and metastasis. Thromb Haemost 1993; 70:152–154.
98. Wei M, Tai G, Gao Y, et al. Modified heparin inhibit P-selectin-mediated cell adhesion of human colon carcinoma cells to immobilized platelets under dynamic flow conditions. J Biol Chem 2004; 279:29202–29210.
99. Wang L, Brown JR, Varki A, Esko JD. Heparin's anti-inflammatory effects require glucosamine 6-O-sulfation and are mediated by blockade of L- and P-selectins. J Clin Invest 2002; 110:127–136.
100. Fidler IJ. The biology of cancer metastasis or, 'you cannot fix it if you do not know how it works.' Bio Essays 1991; 13:551–554.
101. Al-Mehdi AB, Tozawa K, Fisher AB, Shientag L, Lee A, Muschel RJ. Intravascular origin of metastasis from the proliferation of endothelium-attached tumor cells: a new model for metastasis. Nat Med 2000; 6:100–102.
102. Varki NM, Varki A. Heparin inhibition of selectin-mediated interactions during the hematogenous phase of carcinoma metastasis: rationale for clinical studies in humans. Semin Thromb Hemost 2002; 28:53–66.
103. Brown DC, Purushotham AD, Birnie GD, George WD. Detection of intraoperative tumor cell dissemination in patients with breast cancer by use of reverse transcription and polymerase chain reaction. Surgery 1995; 117:95–101.

8

The Burden of Cancer-Associated Venous Thromboembolism and Its Impact on Cancer Survival

Richard H. White
Department of Internal Medicine, Division of General Medicine, University of California, Davis, Sacramento, California, U.S.A.

Ted Wun
Department of Internal Medicine, Division of Hematology and Oncology, University of California, Davis, Sacramento, California, U.S.A.

- Most patients in whom acute venous thromboembolism (VTE) reflects the presence of a cancer have clinical, laboratory, or radiographic evidence of a cancer at the time they present with VTE. Epidemiologic evidence suggests that "occult" cancer is quite rare among patients with "idiopathic" VTE, and VTE patients who do harbor a cancer that is causally related to the VTE are almost always diagnosed with metastatic cancer in less than four months. Pancreatic cancer, gliomas, acute myelocytic leukemia, and stomach cancer are associated with the highest person-time incidence rate, with renal cell, lung, and ovarian cancer having lower but still very high incidence rates.
- The incidence rate of VTE decreases progressively after the cancer diagnosis date.
- The incidence of VTE appears to correlate more with how quickly the cancer spreads, not the extent of the spread.
- For most cancers, the incidence of VTE correlates with the percentage of cases that die within one year and the proportion of cases that present with metastatic cancer.
- Among patients with colon, breast, and lung cancer, major surgery is associated with a lower incidence of VTE, compared to patients who did not undergo surgery.
- For gliomas, however, the incidence of VTE is highest immediately following invasive neurosurgery.
- Survival of cancer patients who develop VTE is significantly reduced after adjusting for age, race, sex, cancer type, initial cancer stage, and medical comorbidity.
- The effect of VTE on reducing survival is greater among patients initially diagnosed with local- or regional-stage cancer compared to metastatic cancer.

INTRODUCTION

Based on astute clinical observation alone, a strong link between the presence of cancer and the development of symptomatic venous thromboembolism (VTE) was established nearly a century and a half ago (1). Since that time, numerous autopsy series, epidemiologic studies, and results of clinical trials have provided overwhelming evidence for this association (2–6). Despite this abundant evidence, many gaps remain in our knowledge linking malignancies and VTE. To date, all of the epidemiologic observations have had limitations or biases that have prevented the accurate assessment of the true incidence of symptomatic VTE, such as reporting the incidence of VTE in selected cases that have undergone autopsy (7), incomplete cancer case ascertainment (8,9), low power (10–12), and use of surrogate endpoints such as ultrasound evidence of VTE rather than clinically symptomatic VTE (13). Furthermore, the incidence, time course, and associated risk factors that contribute to VTE in particular tumor types have only recently been studied.

VTE complicates the management of patients with cancer, and there is intriguing evidence suggesting that VTE has a negative impact on the survival of cancer patients (14). It is not known whether this negative impact is related to a higher prevalence of medical comorbidities, is a reflection of the inherent aggressiveness of the cancer, or is simply due to pulmonary embolism. It is also possible that the prothrombotic and/or proinflammatory milieu that accompanies an acute thromboembolic event might actually promote tumor growth and metastases (5). Particularly provocative, but not yet proven, are the results of retrospective and prospective studies that have shown that administration of low-molecular-weight heparin may result in improved survival among certain subgroups of patients with cancer (15).

In order to fill some of the gaps in our current knowledge, our group undertook a study that used two merged administrative datasets, the California Cancer Registry (CCR) (16) and the California Discharge Dataset (17), to determine the incidence, time course, and risk factors for VTE in patients with the most common tumor types (18). Furthermore, we explored the effect of VTE on cancer-related mortality, focusing on patients with colon cancer (19), breast cancer (20), gliomas (21), and ovarian cancer (22). In this chapter, we will review the results of these studies, as well as the work of others, and attempt to provide an understanding of the epidemiology of cancer-associated VTE and the impact of VTE on the survival of cancer patients. We will not review the pathophysiology of cancer-associated thrombosis, nor the mechanisms that might underlie the negative impact on survival, as these will be covered by other authors in this volume.

THE EPIDEMIOLOGY OF CANCER-ASSOCIATED VTE IN CALIFORNIA

To accurately define the incidence of symptomatic venous thrombosis and pulmonary embolism in patients with cancer, the following information must be available: (*i*) the total number of cases diagnosed with a specific type of cancer in a defined geographic region, (*ii*) the cancer histology, (*iii*) the initial cancer stage and any spread over time, (*iv*) all treatments used (surgery: date, type, and extent; radiation: date, amount, and field; chemotherapy: drug, amount, and duration of treatment), and (*v*) the incidence over time of all cases of symptomatic, objectively defined VTE. Moreover, information should be available regarding the location of the VTE (superficial vs. deep, upper extremity vs. lower extremity, catheter-associated vs. non–catheter related) and treatment of the event. Most of these criteria can be met if there is a population-based cancer registry that identifies all patients with cancer and that can be merged with a comprehensive hospital database, or even better, hospital charts.

The CCR gathers information about all patients in California who are diagnosed with specific types of cancer (16). By law, all hospitals and clinics are required to submit information to the registry about all patients diagnosed with cancer (except nonmelanoma skin cancer and in situ cervical cancer). Among registry cases, 95% have an antemortem tissue diagnosis, and the remaining 5% are diagnosed on the basis of radiographic findings, laboratory plus clinical findings, or autopsy information. It is estimated that 99% of all specified cancers are detected. A very small number of patients with cancer are not identified, such as those who avoid seeking medical care and then die outside the hospital, or who have an as yet undiagnosed cancer but die from another medical problem. The State of California's Patient Discharge Dataset (PDD) provides clinical information about all patients who are hospitalized in the state, except for those in Veterans Administration or military facilities (23). This information can be linked for each individual patient, showing serial hospitalizations from 1990 to the present. This dataset can be linked via the encrypted social security number with the CCR to provide a temporal record of all hospitalizations for individual cases with a specified type of cancer. The PDD includes information about all clinical diagnoses (up to 25) and all surgical or invasive procedures (up to 24), which allows identification of outcomes of interest, including VTE. The State of California Master Death Registry is also linked to these two databases, allowing identification of all deaths. Although there is information in the CCR about the initial type of therapy (radiation, surgery, or chemotherapy), specific information regarding treatment dates, drugs used, and details of radiation treatment is not collected. Various published articles have more details about the exact methods used in these analyses (18). The following summarizes the epidemiologic findings that relate to the development of VTE in patients with cancer.

THE BURDEN OF CANCER-ASSOCIATED VTE

Most review articles that focus on the topic of VTE in cancer patients acknowledge that the exact incidence of VTE is not well defined (5,24). One method of estimating the impact of cancer on the incidence of VTE is to determine the prevalence of cancer among patients with a first-time (incident) VTE event. Using the population-based PDD dataset, we determined how many people in California were diagnosed with a first-time VTE event in 1996 and then determined what percentage of these cases had cancer at the time of or within six months of the event. We also determined the percentage of cases that had another provoking risk factor (surgery less than three months, trauma less than three months, pregnancy, during a medical hospitalization, or within two months of a medical hospitalization, etc.) (25). Of the 21,003 new cases of VTE diagnosed in California in 1996, 4368 (20.8%) had a diagnosis of cancer either at the time of the VTE or within the previous six months, and 5418 had an idiopathic VTE. The overall age-standardized incidence of incident VTE events in one year was approximately 100 cases/100,000 adults over the age of 18, and the one-year incidence of VTE associated with cancer was 21 cases/100,000, or 0.02% of the adult population. This value did not include those VTE cases that were subsequently diagnosed with cancer a few days to months after the VTE. However, as described below, the number of cases that had an occult cancer causally associated with the VTE was likely to be very small, perhaps 100 cases a year. This finding that 21% of incident symptomatic VTE cases were associated with cancer is very close to the figure of 18% reported by Heit et al. in their analysis of the incidence of VTE in Olmsted County, MN (26).

VTE AS A HARBINGER OF THE PRESENCE OF CANCER

Based on the phenomenon reported by Trousseau, there has been a longstanding interest in knowing how often the development of VTE heralds the presence of an "occult" malignancy (27–31). Large epidemiology investigations by Sorensen and others have suggested that the incidence of cancer among patients diagnosed with acute VTE is increased by approximately 30%, and that most of the excess cases are diagnosed with cancer within six months (29,32). If one classifies "occult" cancer cases as all of the patients who are diagnosed with cancer during the index hospitalization for VTE, the relative risk of cancer being present in a patient with acute VTE is much higher [relative risk (RR) = 4.4], over 400% higher compared to the general population (33). Indeed, Cornuz et al. showed that a routine medical evaluation at the time of hospitalization for VTE resulted in a diagnosis of cancer in 12% of their incident VTE cases, but that the incidence of cancer developing in the subsequent three years was low and no higher than in a control group (27). Thus, it appears that the incidence of an active cancer among patients who are hospitalized for acute VTE is quite high, but it is not clear how frequently patients with acute VTE, who appear otherwise healthy, harbor a clinically quiet "occult" cancer that is causally associated with the VTE. The results of a small and underpowered prospective study showed that extensive cancer screening of patients with acute VTE resulted in detection of some early-stage cancers, but resulted in no reduction in mortality compared to the control patients who did not undergo extensive screening (34).

In an effort to better quantify the risk of developing a cancer among patients with idiopathic VTE, we reversed the question and asked: how many patients with newly diagnosed cancer developed idiopathic VTE in the one-year period immediately preceding the cancer diagnosis? The six-year period between 1993 and 1999 was analyzed, and among 528,693 adults who were diagnosed with one of the 19 most common types of cancer (66% of all cancers diagnosed in California), there were 1113 (0.21%) cases who had been diagnosed with acute VTE during the previous year. Of these, 596 (0.11%) met criteria for idiopathic VTE, with no preceding (less than three months) provoking risk such as major surgery, trauma, pregnancy, or a medical hospitalization of over four days. Based on the known age-, sex-, and race-specific incidence of unprovoked VTE in the general population (25), the expected incidence of idiopathic VTE in this cohort of cancer patients was 447 cases. Thus, there were only 149 cases with first-time VTE that were not background or "expected" cases, which is just 25 cases each year in California. The standardized incidence ratio (SIR = observed VTE cases/expected VTE cases) for idiopathic VTE was SIR = 1.3 [confidence interval (CI): 1.2–1.5, $p < 0.001$], or 30% higher than expected. This is a value remarkably close to the SIR values for subsequent cancer reported by Murchison et al. (32) and Sorensen et al. (29). In this analysis, among the cases that were initially diagnosed with local-, regional-, or unknown-stage cancer, the SIR for an incident VTE in the year prior to the cancer diagnosis was 1.07 (CI = 0.97–1.18, $p = 0.09$), which was not significantly higher than expected. However, among the cases with metastatic disease initially, the SIR was much higher, equal to 2.3 (CI = 2.0–2.6), or over two times higher than expected. Figure 1 shows the time that VTE was diagnosed in the year before the cancer diagnosis, stratified by the initial cancer stage. Among the cases that were eventually diagnosed with local- or regional-stage cancer, the incidence of idiopathic VTE was steady throughout the year. However, among the patients who were subsequently diagnosed with metastatic cancer, there was a sharp increase in the incidence about four months before the cancer diagnosis date. (These cases can be seen above the line in Fig. 1 that extrapolates incidence of cases diagnosed during the first 265 days of the preceding year.) Assuming that this relationship between VTE and cancer also holds true for all the other cancer types and cases

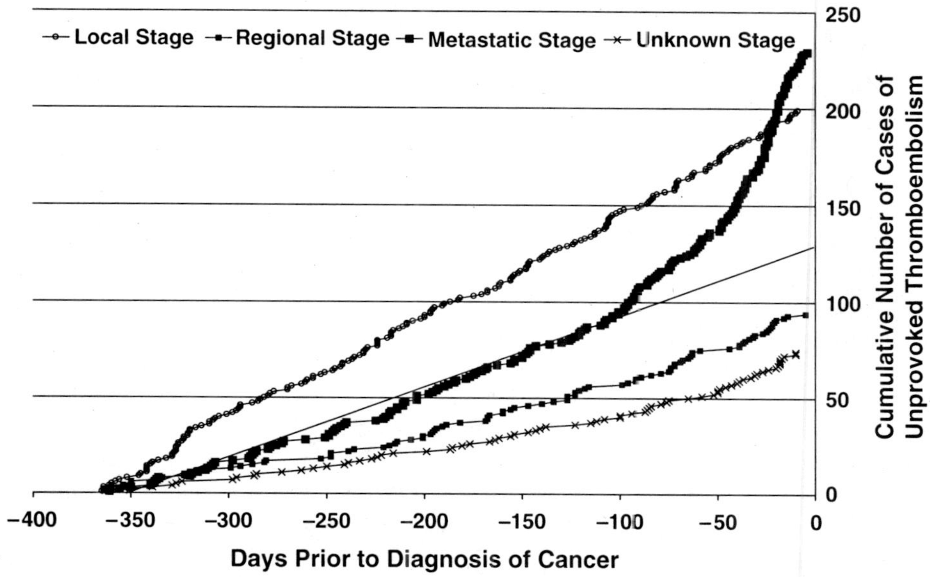

Figure 1 Plot of the time course of incident cases of unprovoked venous thromboembolism in the year prior to diagnosis of cancer, stratified by the stage of cancer at the time of diagnosis (local-, regional-, metastatic-, or unknown-stage cancer).

that were not included in our analysis, one can calculate that only about 36 (0.7%) of the 5000 patients diagnosed with first-time idiopathic VTE in California each year truly have an "occult" underlying malignancy that is causally related to the acute VTE. Conversely, 75% of all the cases that developed VTE in the year before cancer was diagnosed had background or "expected" cases of VTE, and most of these patients were subsequently diagnosed with local- or regional-stage cancer. It is worth stressing that in this large cancer cohort, there were 2246 patients who were diagnosed concurrently with VTE and cancer, or about 375 cases a year, which is approximately 15 times higher than the number of cases that appeared to have an unexpected "occult" cancer. These findings suggest that less than 1% of the approximately 5000 patients who develop a first-time idiopathic VTE each year in California have a truly "occult" cancer that is biologically responsible for the VTE. In summary, the data suggest that if a patient develops an "idiopathic" VTE and then subsequently develops a malignancy within one year, it is much more likely that the VTE event was a "normal" or expected VTE event rather than a VTE causally linked to the cancer. However, the exact number of cases that fit the criteria for having an "occult" cancer will clearly depend on how aggressively the treating physician evaluated the patient for an underlying malignancy. In our analysis, 2246 (0.4%) of the cancer cases were concurrently diagnosed with VTE, and of these, 412 (18%) were admitted with a principal diagnosis of acute VTE ("condition occasioning admission to the hospital").

TYPES OF CANCERS ASSOCIATED WITH ACUTE VTE THAT REMAIN CLINICALLY "OCCULT"

Only 7 of the 19 cancer types analyzed were associated with a higher-than-expected incidence of VTE in the year before cancer diagnosis. These cancers were: acute myelogenous leukemia (SIR = 4.2, CI: 2.4–6.8), ovarian cancer (SIR = 2.8, CI: 1.9–4.1), non-Hodgkins lymphoma (SIR = 2.7, CI: 1.9–3.7), pancreatic cancer (SIR = 2.6, CI: 1.8–3.6), renal cell cancer (SIR = 2.5, CI: 1.5–3.9), stomach cancer (SIR = 1.8, CI: 1.1–2.8), and lung cancer (SIR = 1.8, CI: 1.5–2.1). All of these cancers had SIR values for acute VTE that were significantly greater than 1.0. Notably missing were cancers of the prostate, breast, colon, bladder, brain, liver, and uterus. The implications of these findings are clinically important. If one makes a diagnosis of an idiopathic VTE, and if the patient has no signs or symptoms that suggest the presence of a cancer, then evaluation for breast, prostate, and colon cancer is probably not warranted unless it is part of adherence to cancer-screening guidelines. However, if there are some clues that make the clinician suspect the possibility of a cancer being present, a careful review of the blood smear and perhaps an abdominal–pelvic CT scan might be useful.

EFFECT OF CANCER TYPE ON THE INCIDENCE OF VTE AFTER THE CANCER DIAGNOSIS

Table 1 shows the one-year cumulative incidence of VTE for patients with 19 common types of cancers, using data analyzed from 1993 to 1995 (18). Cancers with the highest one-year incidence rate were, in decreasing order, pancreatic, brain, acute myelogenous leukemia, stomach, esophageal, renal, lung, ovary, liver, and lymphoma. There was a lower

Table 1 Incidence of VTE within One Year after Diagnosis of Cancer

Cancer	*N*	Year 1 incidence of VTE (%)	Year 1 rate VTE (/100 pt-yrs)	Year 1 deaths (%)[a]	Cases initially metastatic (%)[b]	Year 1 rate of VTE (/100 pt-yrs) initially metastatic (%)
Pancreas	6,524	5.3	14.0	85.3	43.5	28.32
Brain	3,775	6.9	11.1	56.3	0.7	6.12
AML	2,292	3.7	7.4	67.3	89.1	7.40
Stomach	5,766	4.5	7.4	57.6	28.9	16.67
Esophagus	2,491	3.6	5.8	60.5	19.1	10.40
Renal cell	4,891	3.5	4.3	23.6	18.2	12.10
Lung	44,497	2.4	4.3	64.2	47.0	7.39
Ovary	5,707	3.3	4.2	28.1	63.5	5.50
Liver	2,312	1.7	4.1	76.8	32.4	7.23
Lymphoma	9,003	2.8	3.7	34.8	45.3	3.95
CLL	2,023	2.7	3.1	16.6	90.3	2.83
ALL	1,058	2.6	3.1	23.6	89.5	3.29
Colon	32,611	2.3	2.7	23.8	19.0	5.72
CML	951	1.5	1.8	24.4	90.5	1.63
Bladder	7,138	1.5	1.7	18.7	4.7	11.15
Uterus	8,721	1.6	1.7	9.0	7.5	9.29
Prostate	51,362	0.9	1.0	6.2	6.8	1.34
Breast	44,707	0.9	0.9	5.7	4.6	3.84
Melanoma	9,497	0.5	0.5	6.5	4.7	5.33

[a] $r = 0.64$ vs. CI of VTE, $p = 0.002$; $r = 0.81$ vs. person-time rate of VTE, $p < 0.001$.
[b] $r = 0.60$ vs. CI of VTE, $p = 0.02$ (excluding brain and leukemias); $r = 0.55$ vs. person-time rate of VTE, $p = 0.04$ (excluding brain and leukemias).
Abbreviations: AML, acute myelogenous leukemia; ALL, acute lymphocytic leukemia; CML, chronic myelogenous leukemia; CLL, chronic lymphocytic leukemia; CI, confidence interval; VTE, venous thromboembolism.

incidence associated with colon, uterus, bladder, prostate, and breast cancer. It is noteworthy how variable the incidence rate of VTE was from one type of cancer to another, with an over 10-fold difference in the cumulative incidence when melanoma was compared to pancreatic cancer, and with over a 20-fold difference in the incidence rate of VTE (expressed as cases per 100 pt-yrs). The incidence figures cannot be readily compared to the findings from previous studies such as the report from Levitan et al. (8), who analyzed the incidence of VTE only among Medicare patients who were hospitalized with a cancer diagnosis. The results of the recent study of Blom et al. (2), which used a case–control design and a cohort that only included cases who were seen in an anticoagulation clinic, also cannot be directly compared. Using the National Hospital Discharge Survey Database, Stein et al. (39) recently reported the incidence of VTE during a hospital stay among patients who had a diagnosis of cancer. Although these data are also not directly comparable because the VTE incidence that was reported was the number of VTE diagnoses per 100 cancer cases hospitalized, the cancers they found to have the highest incidence of VTE were pancreatic, brain, and leukemias or myeloproliferative disorders, which is what we found. Cancers that had a large proportion of cases detected as local-stage disease, in general, had a very low overall incidence of VTE, with uterus, prostate, breast, and bladder being good examples.

MALIGNANT POTENTIAL OF CANCERS CORRELATES WITH THE HIGHEST INCIDENCE OF VTE

As shown in Table 1, for most of the cancer types capable of becoming metastatic (excluding brain and leukemias), the one-year VTE incidence rate was much higher among the patients who were initially diagnosed with metastatic cancer than for the cohort as a whole. Interestingly, the incidence of VTE for the different cancer types was directly proportional to both the one-year death rate and the percentage of cases that were initially diagnosed with metastatic cancer. The correlation between the percentage of cases that died within one year and the one-year incidence rate of VTE was very high ($r = 0.81$; $R^2 = 0.64$). Excluding brain cancer and leukemias, which do not fit the normal Surveillance Epidemiology and End Results (SEER) staging scheme, there was also a significant, albeit weaker, correlation between the percentage of cases initially diagnosed with metastatic stage cancer and the incidence of VTE ($r = 0.6$; $R^2 = 0.35$). Taken together, these findings simply indicate that the development of VTE is strongly associated with rapidly growing, biologically aggressive cancers that frequently are metastatic at the time of diagnosis, and that are associated with a shorter survival time.

THE INCIDENCE OF CANCER-ASSOCIATED VTE DECREASES OVER TIME

The incidence of VTE is highest in the first few months following the diagnosis of cancer, and it then decreases significantly over time. Figure 2 shows the incidence of VTE in the first year after diagnosis of colon cancer stratified by the initial cancer stage (19). The shapes of these plots are similar for the other types of cancer. For almost all of the cancer types, both the cumulative incidence of VTE and the VTE incidence rate fell dramatically over time, with a substantially lower incidence of VTE 7 to 12 months after cancer diagnosis compared to the incidence during the first six months. For example, among colon cancer patients, the incidence rate (per 100 pt-yrs) of VTE fell from 5.0% during the first six months after cancer diagnosis to 1.4% during follow-up months 7 to 12, and it fell even further 0.6% between follow-up months 13 and 24. There is indirect evidence that

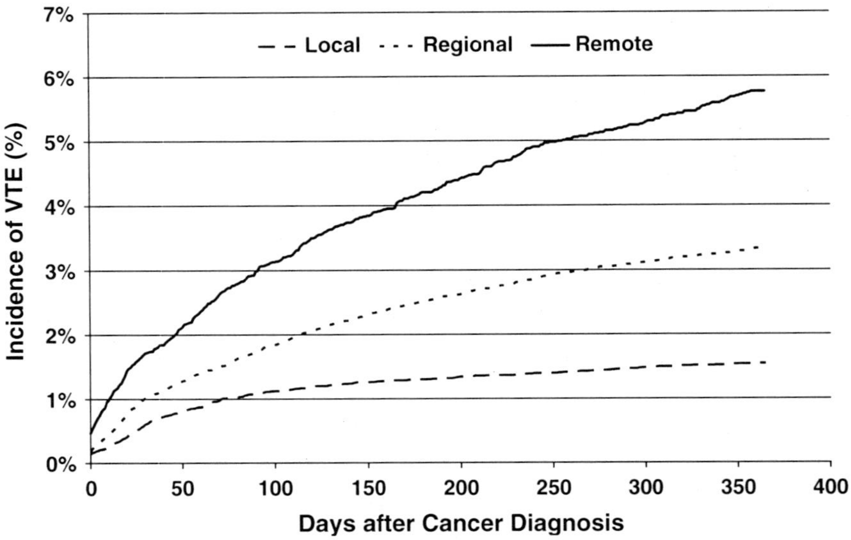

Figure 2 Kaplan Meier plot of the incidence of venous thromboembolism in patients with colon cancer, stratified by initial cancer stage.

suggests that the incidence of VTE is more closely related to the rate of cancer growth than the extent of cancer spread. For example, among patients with regional-stage colon cancer at the time of diagnosis, the incidence of VTE was 3.1% in the first 12 months after cancer diagnosis, during which time 14.7% of these cases died. On the other hand, during the second year of follow-up, when an additional 13.6% of the cases died, only 0.5% of these cases developed VTE. Thus, although the initial incidence rate of VTE correlated strongly with the initial (year 1) death rate among patients with solid organ malignancies, the longer that patients lived, the lower the incidence of VTE. One unifying hypothesis is that the incidence of VTE is closely linked to tumor biology, particularly the rate of growth of the cancer, and not simply the extent of metastatic dissemination. Patients who have fast-growing cancers at the outset are much more likely to develop VTE than patients with slower-growing (but still lethal) cancers.

EFFECT OF VTE ON THE SURVIVAL OF CANCER PATIENTS

Sorensen et al. were the first to report a negative effect of VTE on the survival of patients with cancer (14). However, their analysis did not specifically adjust for the effect of cancer stage or the presence of chronic comorbid medical conditions. In our studies, as shown in Table 2, the development of VTE was associated with reduced survival even after adjusting for age, race, sex, initial cancer stage, and presence of chronic comorbid medical conditions (18). Although somewhat counterintuitive, the reduced survival associated with VTE was greatest among cases diagnosed with local-stage cancer and was smallest among the cases that presented with metastatic cancer (18–20). Moreover, this detrimental effect of VTE on survival increased as the follow-up time after cancer diagnosis increased. Figure 3A shows the survival of patients diagnosed with local-stage breast cancer who either developed VTE or did not develop VTE during the first year after the cancer diagnosis. This survival plot is somewhat difficult to interpret because it is not clear when the patients developed the VTE. However, as shown in Figure 1, most of the cases with VTE were diagnosed in the

Table 2 Effect of the Diagnosis of VTE on Survival of Patients with Different Cancer Types, Stratified by Stage, Adjusted for Age, Race, and Sex [Hazard Ratio for Death within One year among Cases with Thromboembolism Diagnosed in Year 1 vs. Number of VTE (95% CI)]

Cancer type	Initial stage		
	Local	**Regional**	**Remote**
Prostate	5.6*** (3.8–8.5)	4.7*** (1.9–11.5)	2.8** (1.5–5.0)
Breast	6.6*** (3.7–11.8)	2.4** (1.3–4.5)	1.8* (1.1–2.9)
Lung	3.1*** (2.1–4.5)	2.9*** (2.3–3.5)	2.5*** (2.3–2.7)
Colon/rectum	3.2*** (1.8–5.5)	2.2*** (1.7–3.0)	2.0*** (1.7–2.4)
Melanoma	14.4*** (4.6–45.2)	—[a]	2.8** (1.5–5.3)
Non-Hodgkin's lymphoma	3.2*** (1.9–5.3)	2.0** (1.3–3.2)	2.3*** (1.7–3.1)
Uterus	7.0*** (3.4–14.2)	9.1*** (4.8–17.2)	1.7* (1.0–3.0)
Bladder	3.2*** (1.7–6.2)	3.3*** (1.7–6.4)	3.3*** (1.8–6.2)
Pancreas	2.3* (1.2–4.6)	3.8*** (2.8–5.1)	2.3*** (1.9–2.7)
Stomach	2.4* (1.1–5.1)	1.5* (1.0–2.1)	1.8*** (1.4–2.3)
Ovary	11.3** (2.5–51.7)	4.8* (1.1–20.4)	2.3*** (1.7–3.0)
Kidney	3.2* (1.2–8.8)	1.4 (0.6–3.2)	1.3 (0.9–2.0)

Note: VTE was modeled as a time-dependent covariate.
*$p < 0.05$; ** $p < 0.01$; *** $p < 0.001$.
[a]Not enough VTE cases to estimate.
Abbreviations: VTE, venous thromboembolism; CI, confidence interval.

first six months after the cancer diagnosis, yet there appears to be little effect of VTE on survival during this time period. Figure 3b helps to clarify this issue by showing the survival of patients with local-stage breast cancer who developed VTE, plotted from the date of the VTE event, not the cancer diagnosis date. For comparison, a cohort of patients was gathered that was matched for: (*i*) being alive the same number of days after cancer diagnosis as the patients with VTE, (*ii*) age, (*iii*) race, and (*iv*) their number of chronic medical conditions. This figure shows that the effect of VTE on reduced survival is most apparent in the first two-to-three months after VTE diagnosis.

Figure 4(A–C) shows the survival of breast cancer cases diagnosed with VTE 0 to 6 months, 7 to 12 months, and 13 to 24 months, respectively, after diagnosis of local-stage breast cancer. Although only a small number of patients developed VTE six months to two years after being diagnosed with breast cancer, a significant proportion of them died shortly after the VTE event. Review of hospital codes and death certificates indicated that many, but not all, of these cases died of breast cancer. Thus, it appears that at least one reason why VTE is more strongly associated with reduced survival among patients with early-stage cancer is that VTE frequently reflects the presence or emergence of a biologically aggressive cancer. The finding that most of the deaths associated with VTE occurred in the first 60 to 90 days after diagnosis of VTE suggests that the development of the VTE reflects significant and serious underlying comorbidity. This may be the presence of widely metastatic cancer, but it may also reflect the presence of other serious medical conditions; and it may simply reflect morbidity associated with the thromboembolic event. Among the cases that survived over 90 days after the VTE, which made up over 80% of all the VTE cases, there appeared to be little impact of VTE on subsequent survival. These latter cases of VTE may simply be background cases of VTE occurring in patients who were cured of breast cancer. This finding may also reflect the effect of chemotherapy regimens. Much more research is needed to tease out the clinical implications of a VTE developing in a patient initially

A

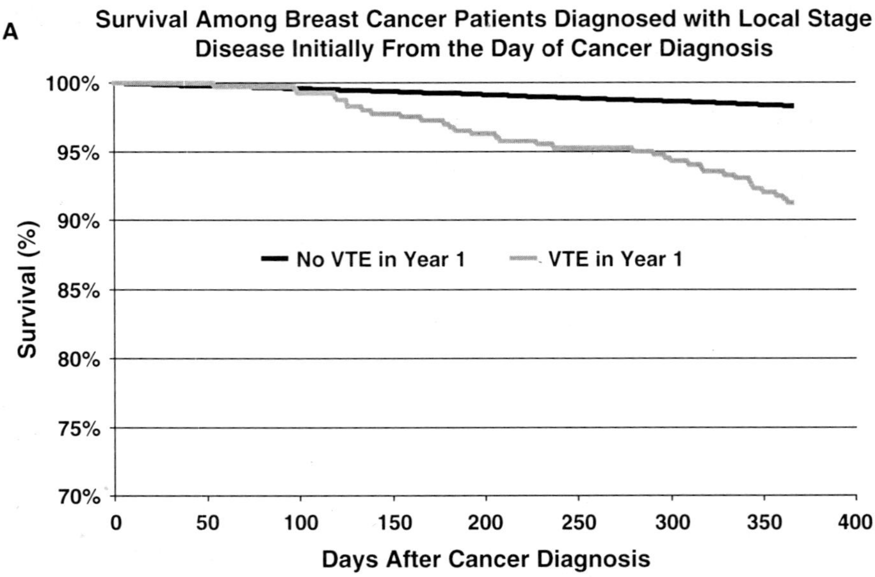

B

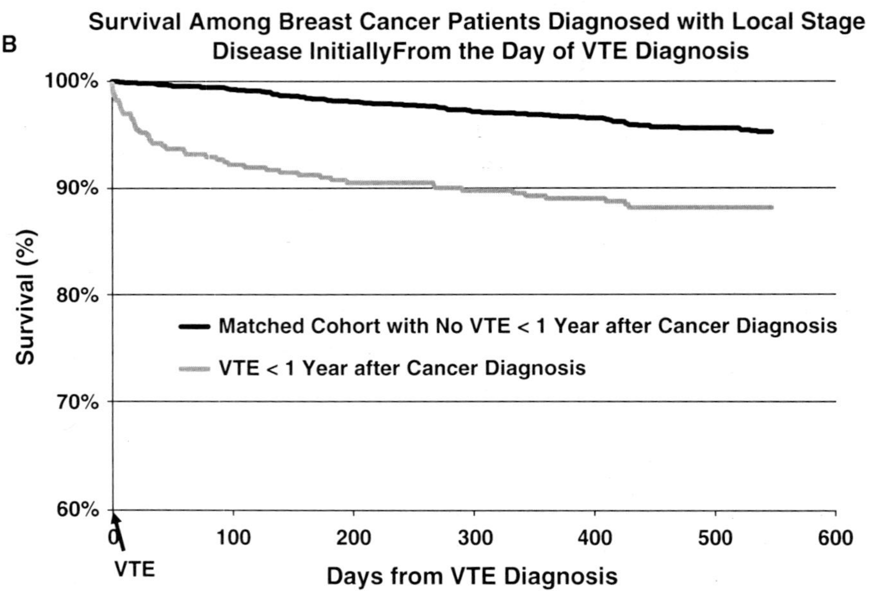

Figure 3 (**A**) Survival from the cancer diagnosis date among breast cancer patients with local-stage cancer who did or did not develop VTE within one year. (**B**) Comparison of survival from the date of diagnosis of VTE among breast cancer patients who developed VTE within one year of the diagnosis of local-stage breast cancer versus a matched sample of cases that were not diagnosed with VTE. *Abbreviation*: VTE, venous thromboembolism.

diagnosed with local- or regional-stage cancer. One thing is certain, however, it does not appear that cancer patients who develop VTE many months after their cancer diagnosis are a homogeneous group. Some die very quickly due to either metastatic cancer that has emerged or some chronic medical comorbidity, whereas others appear to do well.

Recent research on the relationship between cancer and thrombosis provides possible explanations for the epidemiological evidence that VTE is associated with a more aggressive cancer. The hypercoagulable state in patients with cancer is multifactorial, and

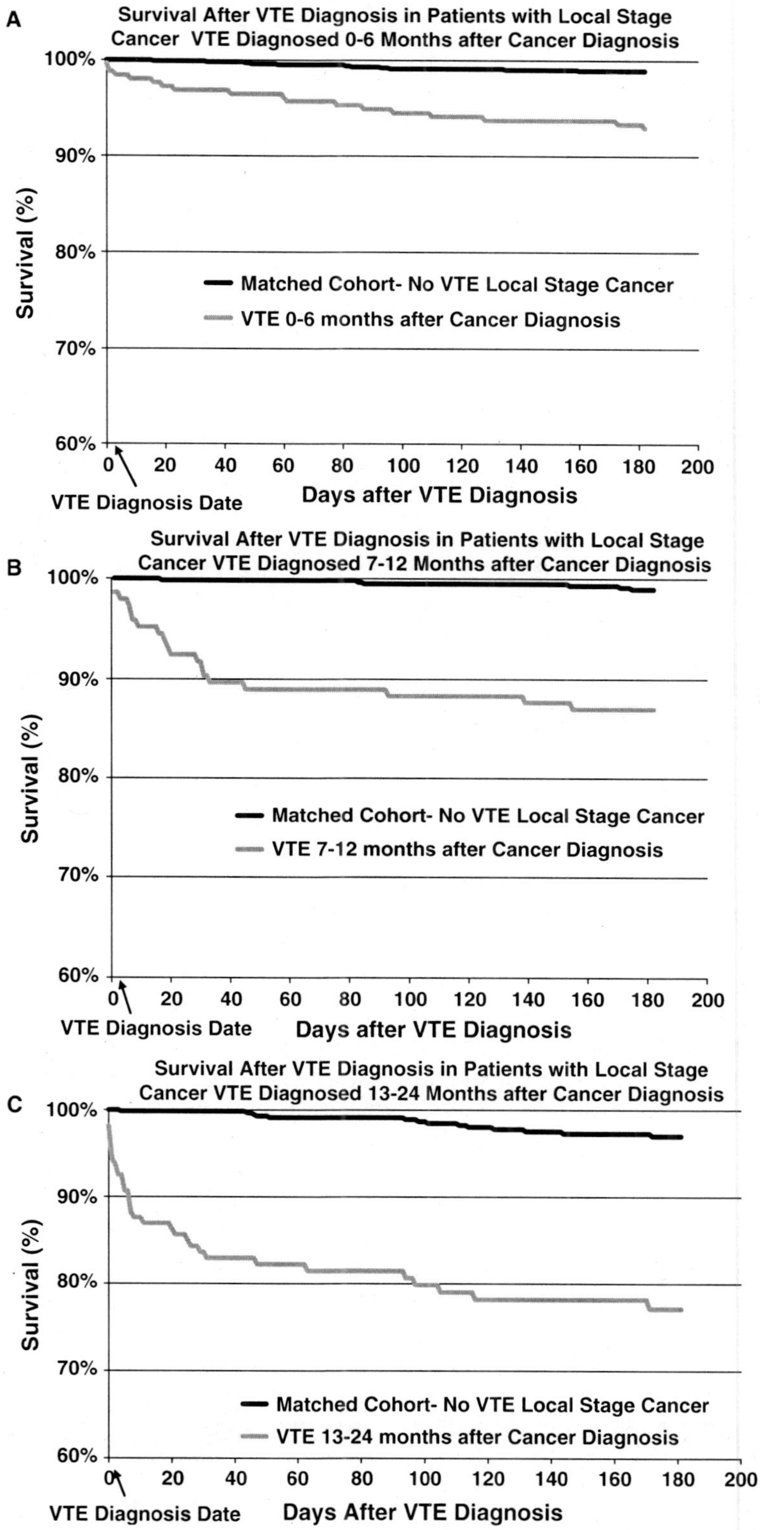

Figure 4 (**A–C**) Comparison of survival from the date of diagnosis of VTE among breast cancer patients who developed VTE at various time intervals after the diagnosis of local-stage breast cancer versus a matched sample of cases that were not diagnosed with VTE. *Abbreviation*: VTE, venous thromboembolism.

includes immobility, compression of vessels by a tumor mass and consequent low-flow states, host inflammatory response, and the effect of various therapies including surgery, radiation, systemic therapeutic agents, and hematopoietic growth factors. Elucidation of all these factors is beyond the scope of this review and the topic of other chapters in this volume. However, the inherent potential of tumor cells to activate the coagulation cascade may be intimately related to biological aggressiveness.

EFFECT OF MAJOR SURGERY ON THE INCIDENCE OF VTE

A number of studies have definitively shown that patients with cancer who undergo a specific type of operation have a higher incidence of postoperative VTE compared to patients without cancer who undergo the same operation (35). These data are generally interpreted as showing that surgery increases the risk of VTE in the postoperative period in cancer patients (24). However, our data suggest that surgery may actually *lower* the incidence of VTE, at least in patients who have breast or colon cancer. It is likely that when surgery is performed quite early after cancer is diagnosed, the high incidence of postoperative VTE may reflect the biology of the cancer, not the postoperative state. In addition, for patients in whom surgery cures the cancer, it is certainly plausible that surgery would be associated with a lower short-term incidence of VTE. Nevertheless, a final, definite answer about the effect of surgery on the incidence of VTE will require large randomized clinical trials designed to evaluate the effect of surgery on survival in patients with specific types of cancer.

The results of our analyses suggest that neurosurgery is a major risk factor for VTE among patients who develop a malignant glioma (21). Compared to patients who did not undergo surgery, patients who underwent major neuorsurgery or brain biopsy because of the presence of a glioma were 70% more likely to develop VTE within three months. However, major surgery does not appear to be a major risk factor for VTE in patients with organ system malignancies such as colon or ovarian cancer (19). In a multivariate analysis of patients with different types of cancer, after adjustment for age, race/ethnicity, gender, stage, histology, and the number of chronic comorbid conditions present, the effect of major surgery on the risk of subsequent VTE varied dramatically among different types of cancer. Patients undergoing breast surgery were 40% less likely to develop VTE, and patients with colorectal cancer were 60% less likely to develop VTE compared to patients who did not undergo major surgery. When VTE events were classified based on the presence or absence of a provoking risk factor such as major surgery, the proportions of all VTE cases that developed within three months of major surgery were 60% among the glioma cohort (21), 9% in the breast cohort (20), and 33% in the colorectal cancer cohort (19). Thus, the evidence appears to be quite compelling that invasive neurosurgery is indeed a major provoking risk factor for VTE among patients with a glioma, whereas the effect of surgery in patients with solid cancers remains unclear.

THE EFFECT OF CHRONIC MEDICAL CONDITIONS ON THE INCIDENCE OF VTE

The presence of chronic medical comorbid conditions has a dramatic effect on the incidence of cancer-associated thrombosis and survival (36). Use of administrative data allowed the identification of the presence or absence of chronic medical conditions using a set of specified ICD-9-CM codes (37). Both the Charlson Index and the Elixhauser Index are widely used software programs that identify important medical conditions (38), such as chronic renal disease, chronic liver disease, hypertension, chronic heart failure, psychiatric disease, etc. The Elixhauser index identifies 29 different conditions, but this can be modified to eliminate identification of disorders that are inappropriate, such as presence or absence of cancer (lymphoma, solid cancer without metastasis, cancer with metastasis) or conditions that may overlap with acute medical illness (anemia, electrolyte disorder, coagulopathy). In a detailed analysis of risk factors associated with the development of VTE within one year of the diagnosis of colorectal cancer, the strongest risk factor was the metastatic stage at the time of diagnosis [hazard ratio (HR) = 3.2, CI: 2.8–3.8], and the second strongest risk factor was the presence of three or more chronic medical conditions (HR = 2.0, CI: 1.7–2.3). In a similar analysis of risk factors in patients with breast cancer, ovarian cancer, and brain glioma, there was a steady increase in the risk of developing VTE as the number of chronic comorbid conditions increased, as shown in Table 3. The presence of three or more chronic medical conditions was the strongest risk factor for the development of VTE among the patients with glioma and ovarian cancer, whereas metastatic cancer was the strongest risk factor among patients with breast cancer and colon cancer. When a large percentage of cases were classified as having local or regional disease at the time of diagnosis, the presence of metastatic disease was the strongest risk factor for VTE. When the majority of the cases had metastatic disease, the presence of multiple comorbidities became the dominant predictor.

These findings suggest that the risk of developing VTE depends on the relative strength of the prothrombotic properties of the cancer and the host's defenses, which are weakened by the presence of an increasing number of chronic medical conditions. Further

Table 3 Predictors of Development of VTE after Diagnosis of Cancer

Variable	Breast hazard ratio (95% CI)	Glioma hazard ratio (95% CI)	Ovarian hazard ratio (95% CI)
Gender			
Female vs. male	–	0.8 (0.7–0.9)[a]	–
Age (vs. <45 yr)			
45–64 yr	1.4 (1.2–1.8)	2.4 (1.9–3.0)[a]	1.9 (1.3–2.6)[a]
65–74 yr	1.9 (1.5–2.4)[a]	2.6 (2.0–3.4)[a]	1.8 (1.3–2.6)[a]
>75 yr	2.0 (1.6–2.6)[a]	1.8 (1.4–2.5)[a]	1.5 (1.0–2.2)
Race (vs. Caucasian)			
Black	1.3 (1.0–1.5)	0.8 (0.6–1.2)	1.3 (1.0–1.8)
Hispanic	0.9 (0.8–1.1)	0.8 (0.6–1.0)	0.9 (0.7–1.1)
Asian American	0.3 (0.2–0.4)[a]	0.4 (0.2–0.6)[a]	0.8 (0.5–1.1)
Number of chronic comorbidities (vs. 0)			
1	1.9 (1.6–2.2)[a]	2.3 (1.9–2.8)[a]	2.1 (1.7–2.6)[a]
2	2.3 (1.9–2.7)[a]	2.8 (2.2–3.5)[a]	2.6 (2.0–3.3)[a]
3	2.9 (2.4–3.5)[a]	3.5 (2.8–4.3)[a]	3.9 (3.1–4.8)[a]
Stage (vs. localized)			
Regional	2.1 (1.8–2.3)[a]	N/A	1.7 (1.1–2.6)
Metastatic	6.3 (5.3–7.5)[a]	N/A	3.0 (2.1–4.2)[a]
Major cancer surgery			
Yes vs. no	0.6 (0.5–0.7)[a]	1.7 (1.3–2.3)[a]	0.7 (0.6–0.8)[a]

Abbreviations: VTE, venous thromboembolism; CI, confidence interval.
[a]$p < 0.0001$.

research is needed to determine which of the chronic medical conditions are the strongest risk factors for cancer-associated thrombosis.

REFERENCES

1. Trousseau A. Phlegmasia alba dolens. Clinique Medicale de l'Hotel-Dieu de Paris 1865; 3(94).
2. Blom JW, Vanderschoot JP, Oostindier MJ, Osanto S, van der Meer FJ, Rosendaal FR. Incidence of venous thrombosis in a large cohort of 66,329 cancer patients: results of a record linkage study. J Thromb Haemost 2006 Mar; 4(3):529–535.
3. Hansson PO, Welin L, Tibblin G, Eriksson H. Deep vein thrombosis and pulmonary embolism in the general population. 'The Study of Men Born in 1913'. Arch Intern Med 1997; 157(15):1665–1670.
4. Heit JA. Cancer and venous thromboembolism: scope of the problem. Cancer Control 2005; 12(suppl. 1):5–10.
5. Prandoni P, Falanga A, Piccioli A. Cancer and venous thromboembolism. Lancet Oncol 2005; 6(6):401–410.
6. Rickles FR, Levine MN. Epidemiology of thrombosis in cancer. Acta Haematol 2001; 106(1–2):6–12.
7. Ogren M, Bergqvist D, Wahlander K, Eriksson H, Sternby NH. Trousseau's syndrome—what is the evidence? A population-based autopsy study. Thromb Haemost 2006; 95(3):541–545.
8. Levitan N, Dowlati A, Remick SC, et al. Rates of initial and recurrent thromboembolic disease among patients with malignancy versus those without malignancy. Risk analysis using Medicare claims data. Medicine (Baltimore) 1999; 78(5):285–291.
9. Thodiyil PA, Kakkar AK. Variation in relative risk of venous thromboembolism in different cancers. Thromb Haemost 2002; 87(6):1076–1077.
10. Ambrus JL, Ambrus CM, Pickern J, Soldes S, Bross I. Hematologic changes and thromboembolic complications in neoplastic disease and their relationship to metastasis. J Med 1975; 6(5–6):433–458.
11. Fisher B, Costantino J, Redmond C, et al. A randomized clinical trial evaluating tamoxifen in the treatment of patients with node-negative breast cancer who have estrogen-receptor-positive tumors. N Engl J Med 1989; 320(8):479–484.
12. Sack GH Jr, Levin J, Bell WR. Trousseau's syndrome and other manifestations of chronic disseminated coagulopathy in patients with neoplasms: clinical, pathophysiologic, and therapeutic features. Medicine (Baltimore) 1977; 56(1):1–37.
13. Behrendt CE, Ruiz RB. Venous thromboembolism among patients with advanced lung cancer randomized to prinomastat or placebo, plus chemotherapy. Thromb Haemost 2003; 90(4):734–737.
14. Sorensen HT, Mellemkjaer L, Olsen JH, Baron JA. Prognosis of cancers associated with venous thromboembolism. N Engl J Med 2000; 343(25):1846–1850.
15. Kakkar AK. Low-molecular-weight heparin and survival in patients with malignant disease. Cancer Control 2005; 12(suppl. 1):22–30.
16. Kwong SL, Perkins CL, Morris CR, Allen M, Wright WE. Cancer in California: 1988–1999. Sacramento: Department of Health Services, Cancer Surveillance Section, December 2001.
17. White RH, Gettner S, Newman JM, Trauner KB, Romano PS. Predictors of rehospitalization for symptomatic venous thromboembolism after total hip arthroplasty. N Engl J Med 2000; 343(24):1758–1764.
18. Chew HK, Wun T, Harvey DJ, Zhou H, White RH. Incidence of venous thromboembolism and its effect on survival among patients with common cancers. Arch Intern Med 2006; 166(4):458–464.
19. Alcalay A, Wun T, Khatri V, et al. Venous thromboembolism in patients with colorectal cancer: incidence and effect on survival. J Clin Oncol 2006; 24(7):1112–1118.
20. Chew HK, Wun T, Harvey D, Zhou H, White RH. Incidence of venous thromboembolism and the impact on survival in breast cancer patients. J Clin Oncol 2007; 25(1): 70–76.

21. Semrad TJ, O'Donnell R, Wun T, Chew H, Harvey D, Zhou H, White RH. Epidemiology of venous thromboembolism in 9489 patients with malignant glioma. J Neurosurg 2007; 106(4):601–608.
22. Rodriguez AO, Wun T, Chew H, Zhou H, Harvey D, White RH. Venous thromboembolism in ovarian cancer. Gynecologic oncology 2007; 105(3):784–790.
23. Romano PS, Zach A, Luft HS, Rainwater J, Remy LL, Campa D. The California Hospital Outcomes Project: using administrative data to compare hospital performance. The Joint Commission Journal on Quality Improvement 1995; 21(12):668–682.
24. Prandoni P, Piccioli A, Girolami A. Cancer and venous thromboembolism: an overview. Haematologica 1999; 84(5):437–445.
25. White RH, Zhou H, Murin S, Harvey D. Effect of ethnicity and gender on the incidence of venous thromboembolism in a diverse population in California in 1996. Thromb Haemost 2005; 93(2):298–305.
26. Heit JA, O'Fallon WM, Petterson TM, et al. Relative impact of risk factors for deep vein thrombosis and pulmonary embolism: a population-based study. Arch Intern Med 2002; 162(11):1245–1248.
27. Cornuz J, Pearson SD, Creager MA, Cook EF, Goldman L. Importance of findings on the initial evaluation for cancer in patients with symptomatic idiopathic deep venous thrombosis. Ann Intern Med 1996; 125(10):785–793.
28. Monreal M, Prandoni P. Venous thromboembolism as first manifestation of cancer. Semin Thromb Hemost 1999; 25(2):131–136.
29. Sorensen HT, Mellemkjaer L, Steffensen FH, Olsen JH, Nielsen GL. The risk of a diagnosis of cancer after primary deep venous thrombosis or pulmonary embolism. N Engl J Med 1998; 338(17):1169–1173.
30. Ahmed Z, Mohyuddin Z. Deep vein thrombosis as a predictor of cancer. Angiology 1996; 47(3):261–265.
31. Bastounis EA, Karayiannakis AJ, Makri GG, Alexiou D, Papalambros EL. The incidence of occult cancer in patients with deep venous thrombosis: a prospective study. J Internal Med 1996; 239(2):153–156.
32. Murchison JT, Wylie L, Stockton DL. Excess risk of cancer in patients with primary venous thromboembolism: a national, population-based cohort study. Br J Cancer 2004; 91(1):92–95.
33. Baron JA, Gridley G, Weiderpass E, Nyren O, Linet M. Venous thromboembolism and cancer. Lancet 1998; 351(9109):1077–1080.
34. Piccioli A, Lensing AW, Prins MH, et al. Extensive screening for occult malignant disease in idiopathic venous thromboembolism: a prospective randomized clinical trial. J Thromb Haemost 2004; 2(6):884–889.
35. White RH, Zhou H, Romano PS. Incidence of symptomatic venous thromboembolism after different elective or urgent surgical procedures. Thromb Haemost 2003; 90(3):446–455.
36. Piccirillo JF, Tierney RM, Costas I, Grove L, Spitznagel EL Jr. Prognostic importance of comorbidity in a hospital-based cancer registry. JAMA 2004; 291(20):2441–2447.
37. Project HCaU. Comorbidity Software, Version 3.1. 2005 Fiscal Year 2006 [cited April 3, 2006]; available from: http://www.hcup-us.ahrq.gov/toolssoftware/comorbidity/comorbidity.jsp.
38. Elixhauser A, Steiner C, Harris DR, Coffey RM. Comorbidity measures for use with administrative data. Med Care 1998; 36(1):8–27.
39. Stein PD, Beemath A, Meyers FA, Skaf E, Sanchez J, Olson RE. Incidence of venous thrombolism in patients hospitalized with cancer. Am J Med 2006; 119(1):60–68.

9

Thromboembolism in Hematologic Malignancies

Anna Falanga and Marina Marchetti
Hematology Division, Ospedali Riuniti di Bergamo, Bergamo, Italy

- The rate of VTE in acute leukemias and lymphomas is comparable to that of other "high-risk" cancer types.
- Chemotherapy and antiangiogenic drugs increase the thrombotic risk in patients with lymphomas, acute leukemias, and multiple myeloma.
- Patients with hematologic malignancies present with a hypercoagulable state, or chronic DIC, in the absence of active thrombosis and/or bleeding.
- Malignant-cell procoagulant properties, cytotoxic therapies, and concomitant infections are the major determinants for the pathogenesis of clotting activation in hematologic malignancies.
- In acute leukemia, clinical manifestations range from localized venous or arterial thrombosis to diffuse life-threatening bleeding. ATRA has greatly improved the management of APL but has not significantly changed the rate of early hemorrhagic deaths.
- Studies of thromboprophylaxis to prevent VTE are needed, particularly in lymphomas and in multiple myeloma during treatment.
- Anticoagulant therapy of VTE is difficult in oncology/hematology patients who are at very high hemorrhagic risk. No guidelines for treatment of VTE in these types of cancers are available.

INTRODUCTION

Patients with cancer are at high risk for thrombosis as well as hemorrhagic complications (1). According to previous observations, venous thromboembolism (VTE) is more frequent in patients with solid tumors, whereas hemorrhage and also uncompensated disseminated intravascular coagulation (DIC) are more frequent with hematologic malignancies, particularly acute leukemias (2,3). However, recent studies indicate that the rate of VTE in acute leukemias and lymphomas is comparable to that of other "high-risk" types of cancers (4). In addition, in a large population study, acute myeloblastic leukemia and non-Hodgkin lymphoma were among the types of malignancies most frequently preceded by an idiopathic VTE episode in the year immediately before their diagnosis (5).

Current data allow estimation of thrombotic rates in hematologic malignancies, particularly lymphomas, acute leukemias, and multiple myeloma (MM). As in other cancers, the thrombotic risk in these conditions is increased by antitumor drugs and surgical procedures as well as by general risk factors, including immobility, advanced age, previous thromboses, venous stasis, and sepsis. In patients with non-Hodgkin and Hodgkin lymphomas, a significantly high risk for venous and arterial thrombosis during chemotherapy has been reported and confirmed by recent studies (6,7). Additionally, the clotting/bleeding syndrome of patients with acute leukemias is exacerbated during induction chemotherapy when large numbers of tumor cells are destroyed rapidly (8). In MM, new therapies with thalidomide and lenalidomide significantly increase the risk of VTE, especially when administered in combination with chemotherapy and steroids (9,10).

In patients with cancer, the use of central venous catheters (CVCs) contributes to the thrombotic risk. Two studies have addressed this issue in hematological patients, demonstrating a rate of symptomatic CVC-associated VTE of 3.1% and 4.4%, respectively (11,12).

The development of cancer is accompanied by derangement of the hemostatic system. Nearly all patients with malignancy show evidence of subclinical activation of clotting, or chronic DIC, in the absence of active bleeding and/or thrombosis (13,14). In patients with lymphomas, leukemias, and MM, laboratory hemostatic abnormalities underlying a subclinical hypercoagulable condition are common (1).

The patients with acute leukemia are unique in that they may present with different degrees of laboratory abnormalities of DIC and different clinical manifestations, ranging from localized venous or arterial thrombosis to diffuse life-threatening bleeding. The incidence of these complications varies according to the type of leukemia and the phase of treatment. Thrombotic events have been considered less common than hemorrhage in acute leukemia, but recently, a significant rate has been shown in all types of adult acute leukemias (15), including acute promyelocytic leukemia (APL), in which hemorrhage is usually prominent (16). In APL patients, thrombosis and bleeding manifestations may occur concomitantly as a part of the same thrombohemorrhagic syndrome typical of this disease. Before the introduction of all-trans retinoic acid (ATRA) for the management of APL, fatal hemorrhages were a major cause of induction remission failure (17). ATRA has produced a high rate of complete remission and a rapid resolution of the coagulopathy (18).

Major determinants on the pathogenesis of clotting activation in hematologic malignancies are (*i*) factors associated with malignant cells, i.e., the expression of procoagulant, fibrinolytic and proteolytic properties, and the secretion of inflammatory cytokines; (*ii*) cytotoxic therapies; and (*iii*) concomitant infectious complications.

Thrombotic complications can affect morbidity and mortality in cancer patients. No ad hoc studies or guidelines are available for prophylaxis or treatment of VTE in patients with hematologic malignancies. The use of low-molecular-weight heparins (LMWHs) has improved VTE treatment in patients with solid tumors, but no experience has been accumulated in patients with acute leukemia, who have a high risk of hemorrhage due to severe thrombocytopenia. This is an important problem for most of the patients with hematologic malignancies, who often undergo high-dose chemotherapy followed by hematopoietic stem-cell transplantation with prolonged and severe pancytopenias.

In this chapter, we will briefly summarize the current knowledge on the epidemiology, mechanisms, prophylaxis, and treatment of thrombosis, particularly VTE, in hematological malignancies.

EPIDEMIOLOGY

Lymphoma

Lymphoma is one of the malignancies associated with a high incidence of thrombosis, being at the fourth risk level after ovarian, brain, and pancreatic cancers, in the first large-scale trial on the rate of VTE among cancer patients (4). Published studies specifically evaluating the risk of VTE in lymphoma suggest an increased incidence of thrombosis with non-Hodgkin's lymphomas (NHLs) (6,19–21), Hodgkin's disease (HD) (6), large B cell lymphoma (22), and central nervous system (CNS) lymphoma (23). The results of studies performed to assess the rate of thrombosis in lymphoma are shown in Table 1 showing the VTE risk between 1.5% and 59.5%. A thrombogenic effect of weekly chemotherapy was suggested by a retrospective survey of patients receiving systemic chemotherapy as treatment for NHL. VTE occurred in patients receiving weekly chemotherapy but not in those who received less-intensive schedules. In addition, VTE developed when patients were in complete remission and between the fourth and the eighth cycle of weekly chemotherapy (19). A very high incidence of thrombosis (i.e., 59.5%) has been observed in CNS lymphoma patients (23), which is not surprising as patients with brain tumors are at particularly high risk (24). In CNS lymphoma, thrombosis occurred during the early period of intensive chemotherapy and the event was fatal in the 7%.

A VTE incidence of 7.7%, comparable to that observed in solid tumors (25), was found in the retrospective analysis of Mohren et al. (21), who also found a rate significantly higher in the high-grade (10.6%) than in the low-grade NHL (5.8%) and HD (7.25%). In hospitalized patients receiving chemotherapy, the rate of thrombosis in NHL patients was 5.01% for venous and 1.33% for arterial thromboembolism (7). In this study, the thrombosis rate was lower in patients with HD (i.e., 3.87% VTE and 0.54% arterial thromboembolism) compared to those with NHL. In diffuse large B-cell lymphoma, a 12.8% incidence of VTE was reported (22). In this study, VTE occurred during the first cycles of chemotherapy, and patients with VTE had a worse prognosis than those without VTE.

Two prospective studies are available in the setting of VTE in lymphoma patients. One study showed a 6.6% incidence in patients with high-grade NHL, with 77% of

Table 1 Incidence of Thrombosis in Patients with Lymphoma

References	Type of study	Patients (n)	Therapy	VTE [n (%)]
Clarke et al., 1990 (19)	Retrospective	75 NHL	CT	11 (14.6)
Goldschmidt et al., 2003 (23)	Retrospective	42, CNS lymphoma	CT	25 (59.5), fatal VTE 3 (7)
Mohren et al., 2005 (21)	Retrospective	1,038	CT	80 (7.7)
Khorana et al., [a]2006 (7)	Retrospective	12,977 NHL; 2,042 HD	CT	650 (5.01); 79 (3.87)
Komrokji et al., 2006 (22)	Retrospective	211	CT	27 (12.7)[c]
Ottinger et al., 1995 (20)	Prospective observational	593, NHL–HD	CT	39 (6.6)
Khorana et al., [b]2005 (6)	Prospective observational	267 NHL; 49 HD	CT	4 (1.5); 4 (8.6

[a]Ambulatory cancer patients (n = 3,003).
[b]Hospitalized neutropenic patients (n = 66,106) with different types of cancer.
[c]4.7% VTE occurred at diagnosis and 8% during CT.
Abbreviations: NHL, non-Hodgkin's lymphoma; CNS, central nervous system; HD, Hodgkin's disease; CT, chemotherapy; VTE, venous thromboembolism.

cases occurring before or within the first three months of chemotherapy (20). The VTE-related fatality was low in the clinical trial (1.7%) and at necropsy (8.5%); however, the occurrence of VTE was associated with an unsatisfactory response to chemotherapy and higher treatment-related mortality. In the other prospective study, the rate of VTE in ambulatory lymphoma patients initiating a new chemotherapy regimen was 8.16% in HD and 1.5% in NHL (6). Analysis of risk factors showed a role for elevated prechemotherapy platelet counts of above 350,000/mm^3 (OR 2.81; 95% CI 1.63–4.93; $p = 0.0002$).

In conclusion, VTE is a frequent complication in lymphoma, particularly when localized in the brain, and mainly occurs during chemotherapy.

Acute Leukemia

Patients with acute leukemias are at high risk of both hemorrhage and thrombosis. This risk varies according to (*i*) the type of leukemia and (*ii*) the phase of treatment, i.e., onset of the disease, induction, and consolidation.

Most patients with acute leukemias present with mild mucocutaneous bleeding, which readily responds to platelet transfusion. However, severe life-threatening bleeding can develop. Although the most common cause of bleeding in acute leukemia is thrombocytopenia, an underlying DIC can also contribute. Disordered hemostasis is prevalent in patients with APL, the M3 subtype of acute myeloid leukemia (AML), and other acute hyperleukocytic leukemias, particularly during induction chemotherapy. In recent years, DIC complicating the presentation of APL has received new interest, due to important advances, including (*i*) enhanced understanding of the biology of the disorder, (*ii*) greater sensitivity of diagnostic tests for subclinical DIC, and (*iii*) changes in management with the use of ATRA.

Clinical manifestations of DIC in acute leukemias range from bleeding to thrombosis of large vessels. Thrombosis is thought to be less common than bleeding; however, recent data indicate that it can be the presenting symptom. The principal data are summarized in Table 2. A large retrospective study has shown a VTE rate of 2.09% at the onset of the disease, with no significant differences between AML and acute lymphoblastic leukemia

Table 2 Thrombosis Rate in Adult Patients with Different Types of Acute Leukemias

References	Type of study	Leukemia phenotype	Patients (*n*)	Thrombosis at diagnosis (%)	Thrombosis in induction (%)
Zigler et al., 2005 (15)	Retrospective	AML (non-M3)	485	1.74	ND
		ALL	185	2.16	ND
		APL	49	6.12	ND
Mohren et al., 2006 (26)	Retrospective	AML	310	–	13[a]
		ALL	108	0.9	13[b]
De Stefano et al., 2005 (16)	Cohort observational	AML (non-M3)	279	3.2	1.7
		ALL	69	1.4	10.6
		APL	31	9.6	8.4

[a]57% = CVC-associated VTE.
[b]28.4% = CVC-associated VTE.
Abbreviations: AML, acute myeloid leukemia; ALL, acute lymphoblastic leukemia; APL, acute promyelocytic leukemia; ND, not determined; CVC, central venous catheters; VTE, venous thromboembolism.

(ALL) (15). In a cohort observational study, the thrombosis rate at diagnosis was 3.2% in AML (excluding APL), 1.4% in ALL, and 9.4% in APL. Thrombotic events at diagnosis included four arterial ischemic strokes. In the same study, the rate of thrombosis during induction was 1.7% in AML, 10.6% in ALL, and 8.4% in APL (16). All but one episode in induction involved the venous thrombosis. Another retrospective analysis of 455 patients did not confirm the data on thrombosis at presentation, but demonstrated a 12.1% VTE event rate during induction, about 30% to 50% of which were CVC-associated VTE, with no differences between AML and ALL (26).

In a cohort of 42 newly diagnosed consecutive APL patients, prospectively followed at our center from 2000 to 2006, 4.7% had thrombosis at presentation and 9.5% during induction therapy (Falanga, unpublished data, 2006). Thrombotic complications occurred in conjunction with bleeding as a part of the hemostatic derangement. Three early deaths occurred in this cohort of APL patients including three cerebral hemorrhages and one Budd–Chiari syndrome. Before the introduction of ATRA, fatal hemorrhages were a major cause of induction of remission failure (17). ATRA promotes the terminal differentiation of leukemic promyelocytes and has increased the rate of complete remission up to more than 90%. ATRA-induced remission of APL is accompanied by prompt improvement of the coagulopathy (18), although the rate of early fatal hemorrhages still ranges between 2.4% and 6.5%.

In acute ALL, a syndrome characterized by bleeding and thrombosis can also occur. It was first recognized by Priest et al. in 18 out of 1370 (1.2%) children with ALL treated with protocols including L-Asparaginase (L-Ase) (27). Of the 18, 14 had thrombohemorrhagic events in the CNS including dural sinus thrombosis and cerebral hemorrhagic infarction. Subsequently, others have confirmed these observations, reporting cerebral thrombohemorrhagic accidents and peripheral deep vein thrombosis (DVT) in 2.4% to 11.5% of children with ALL (28,29). A recent meta-analysis of 17 studies in pediatric patients showed a rate of thrombosis of 5.2%, with the majority occurring during induction therapy, including L-Ase (30). In adult ALL, hemorrhage was the main cause of early death in 170 ALL patients treated with an intensive regimen including L-Ase (31). A comparable rate of vascular complications (12%) was also reported in ALL patients not receiving L-Ase (32) and was significantly higher in patients with laboratory signs of DIC.

During consolidation, patients in remission must be considered in a different perspective. Currently, postremission therapy is administered at increased intensity, including protocols for transplantations in first remission. Therefore, the coagulation abnormalities or blast cell number play a minor role in this phase, with the exception of cases of thrombotic thrombocytopenic purpura secondary to bone marrow transplantation. During consolidation, the role of chemotherapy and concurrent infections becomes prominent in the pathogenesis of thrombosis.

Multiple Myeloma

MM represents about 10% of hematologic malignancies, and its prognosis remains generally poor. Recently, the search for new active drugs prompted the use of thalidomide in advanced and refractory MM, which resulted in an overall response rate of 32% to 37% in these patients (33,34). Thalidomide and its analog lenalidomide have produced major therapeutic responses in patients with MM, particularly when used in combination with steroids and chemotherapy but have remarkably increased the risk of VTE (34). In Table 3 are summarized the main prospective studies reporting the incidence of VTE in MM treated with thalidomide. In two of phase II studies of thalidomide as a single agent

Table 3 Thrombosis in Patients with Multiple Myeloma: Prospective Phase II and III Trials of Thalidomide Alone or in Combination

References	Study	Patients (n)	Therapy[b]	Thrombosis [n (%)]
Barlogie et al., 2001 (35)—CT refractory	Phase II	169	T	2 (1)
Rajkumar et al., 2003 (36)—New diagnosis	Phase II	31	T	1 (3)
Cavo et al., 2002 (10)—new diagnosis age < 65 yr	Phase II	19	DX + T	5 (26)
Urbauer et al., 2002 (37)—CT refractory	Phase II	14	CT + DX + T	3 (21)
Osman et al., 2001 (38)—First line,	Phase II	15	T + DX + CT	4 (27
new diagnosis)		45	T + DX	3 (7)
Zangari et al., 2001 (39)	Randomized	50	CT + DX	2 (4)
	Phase III	50	CT + DX + T	14 (28)[a]
Zangari et al., 2002 (40)	Randomized	31	Intensive CT	1 (3)
	Phase III	31	Intensive CT + T	11 (36)[a]
Rus et al., 2004 (41)	Randomized	64	MP	–
	Phase III	67	MP + T	11 (16.4)[a]
Rajkumar et al., 2006 (42)	Randomized	102	DX	3 (3)
	Phase III	102	DX + T	17 (17)[a]

[a]$p < 0.01$.
[b]DX+T = Anagnostopoulos, 2003; CT+DX+T = Dimopoulos 2004.
Abbreviations: T, thalidomide; DX, dexamethasone; CT, chemotherapy; M, melphalan; P, prednisone.

for refractory myeloma (35,36), the reported VTE rate was 1.2% and 3.2%. The incidence of VTE was significantly greater when thalidomide was given in combination with steroids and chemotherapy. Indeed, the VTE incidence was 26% in newly diagnosed patients receiving thalidomide in combination with dexamethasone (10) and 21% in patients with advanced/refractory patients receiving thalidomide in combination with chemotherapy (37). In a trial of thalidomide/doxorubicin/dexamethasone, a 27% incidence of VTE was reported in newly diagnosed patients, whereas the VTE rate was 7% when thalidomide and dexamethasone were given without chemotherapy (38). The data from phase III studies confirm the results of phase II trials. In newly diagnosed patients, a VTE incidence of 28% was found in patients receiving thalidomide + repeated cycles of combination chemotherapy versus 4% in patients receiving the same cycles without thalidomide (39). In another trial of thalidomide given in combination with intensive chemotherapy, the VTE incidence was 33% (40). Recently, two trials of thalidomide in combination with melphalan or dexamethasone gave a 16.4% and 17% incidence rate, respectively (41,42). The results of the interim analysis of two trials comparing lenalidomide in combination with dexamethasone versus dexamethasone alone in relapsed/refractory myeloma show an incidence of VTE of 11.3% in the lenalidomide arm versus 3.8% in the arm without lenalidomide (43). A high incidence of VTE (75%) was reported in a group of 12 newly diagnosed patients treated with lenalidomide and dexamethasone (44). The thrombogenic potential of thalidomide may not be associated only with treatment of MM, as there are reports of an increased thrombotic risk in patients receiving thalidomide for systemic lupus erythematosus and in prostate cancer patients given thalidomide in combination with docetaxel.

PATHOGENESIS OF THROMBOSIS IN HEMATOLOGICAL MALIGNANCIES

The Hypercoagulable State

Even in the absence of thrombosis, cancer patients commonly present with abnormalities of coagulation tests. This subclinical hypercoagulable condition is characterized by various degrees of blood clotting activation (8,13,14). The results of laboratory tests in cancer patients demonstrate that a process of fibrin formation and removal is actively ongoing during the development of malignancy. Fibrin and other clotting factors can play a role not only in thrombogenesis but also in tumor progression (45). This supports the hypothesis that inhibition of blood clotting in cancer patients may control the malignant disease.

Lymphoma

Activation of coagulation occurs in patients with lymphoma, as observed by several authors (14,46–48). An early study from our group evaluated the levels of hypercoagulation plasma markers in five patients with NHL before and during weekly chemotherapy. Two of the five patients had DVT during chemotherapy. Eight weeks of chemotherapy increased the levels of prothrombin fragment F1 + 2 (F1 + 2) and thrombin–antithrombin complex (TAT) by approximately 1.5- and 2.9-fold, respectively (14). In another study of cerebral lymphoma patients who had suffered from transient ischemic attack or stroke, an increased activated protein C resistance (APC-R) was observed in 44% and in 82% of the cases was not associated with factor V Leiden. The patients with increased APC-R showed the highest values of F1 + 2 and plasminogen activator inhibitor 1 (PAI-1) (47). In 30 patients with NHL, significant elevations of fibrinopeptide A, TAT, and D-dimer were observed (46). In addition, in 217 patients with different types of lymphoma, the plasma levels of fibrinogen/fibrin degradation products (FDPs), D-dimer, leukocyte tissue factor (TF) mRNA, and plasma TF antigen were not only abnormally elevated but also were significantly higher in stage IV than in stage I, II, or III patients (48).

In our laboratory, the plasma levels of hemostatic variables were prospectively evaluated in patients with hematologic malignancies receiving two different high-dose chemotherapy regimens for autologous hemopoietic stem cells (HSCs) transplantation, i.e., cyclophosphamide (Endoxan, EDX) or cytarabine (ARA-C), followed by granulocyte-colony stidulating factor, for hematopoietic progenitor cells mobilization. The EDX group consisted of 38 consecutive patients (20 with NHL and 18 with MM); and the ARA-C group included 19 consecutive patients (15 with NHL and four with AML). Plasma samples were collected at the following time intervals: (*i*) before therapy; (*ii*) after therapy (EDX or ARA-C), before starting G-CSF; (*iii*) at the end of G-CSF (~two weeks), before leukapheresis; (*iv*) before pretransplant chemotherapy conditioning regimen; (*v*) before autologous HPC transplantation; and, (*vi*) on weeks 1, 3, and 6 after transplantation. Hypercoagulation markers (i.e., F1 + 2, TAT, and D-Dimer) and markers of endothelial activation [i.e., thrombomodulin (TM) antigen and von Willebrand factor (vWF)] were measured. As shown in Figures 1 and 2, before high-dose chemotherapy for HPC mobilization (EDX or ARA-C), all the patients had significantly elevated plasma levels of either hypercoagulation (Fig. 1) or endothelial markers (Fig. 2). These parameters further increased after therapy with both EDX and ARA-C. The increments were transient, as all the values were reduced toward the basal level before transplant. No significant modifications occurred following the conditioning chemotherapy regimen and autologous transplantation, but all the parameters tended to increase again during the six weeks after transplantation, with the D-Dimer and vWF levels reaching statistical significance. In summary, at entry into the study, all patients showed a hypercoagulable state; high-dose chemotherapy regimens worsened this

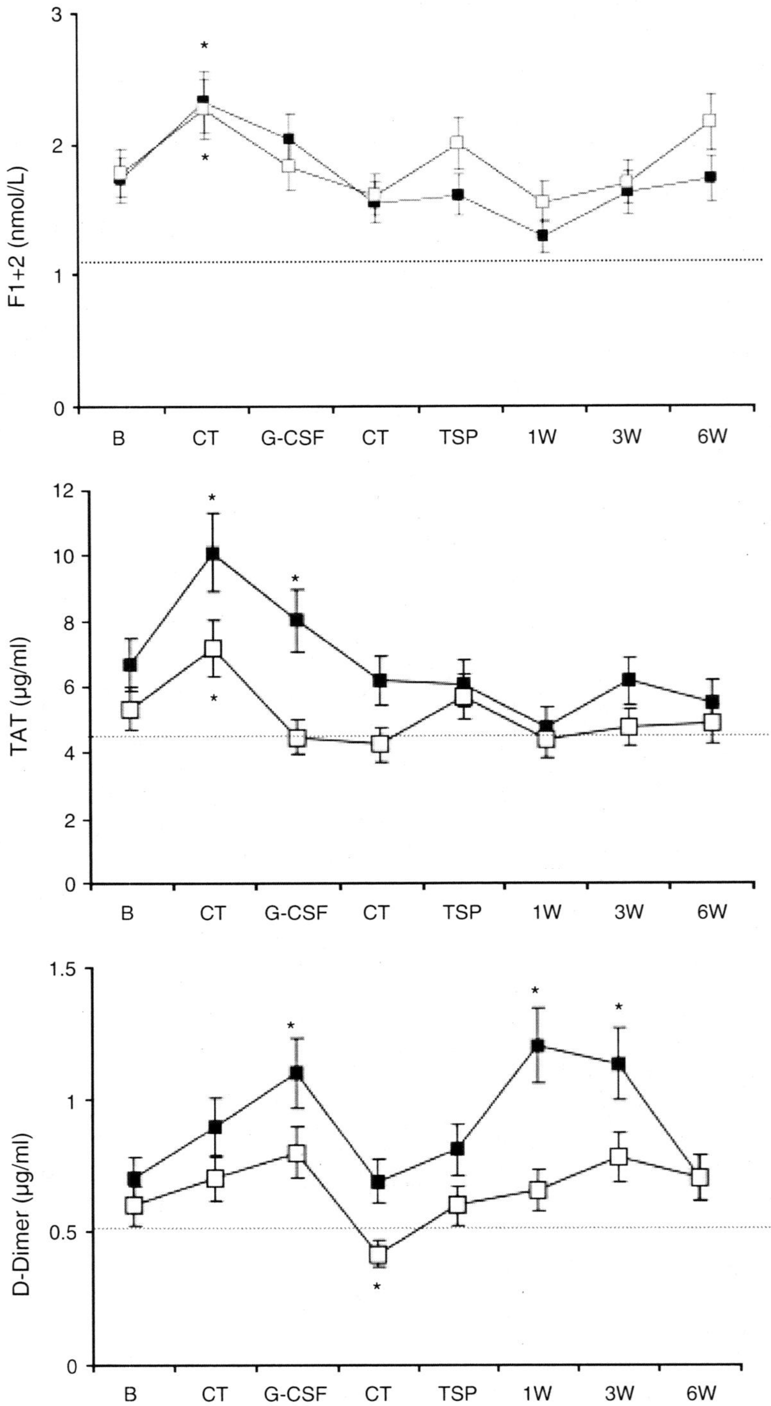

Figure 1 Plasma levels of hypercoagulation markers in patients with hematologic malignancy receiving two different high-dose chemotherapy regimens for autologous HPC transplantation, cyclophosphamide (EDX), or cytarabine (ARA-C). *Black square*, ARA-C group; *open square*, EDX group. Asterisk indicates $p < 0.05$ versus B. *Abbreviations*: B, baseline; CT, after high-dose chemotherapy (EDX or ARA-C), before starting G-CSF; G-CSF, at the end of G-CSF (~two weeks), before leukapheresis; CT, before pretransplant chemotherapy-conditioning regimen; TSP, before autologous HPC transplantation; 1W, 2W, and 3W, one, three, and six weeks after transplantation; HPC, hematopoietic progenitor cells. Data are expressed as mean ± SD.

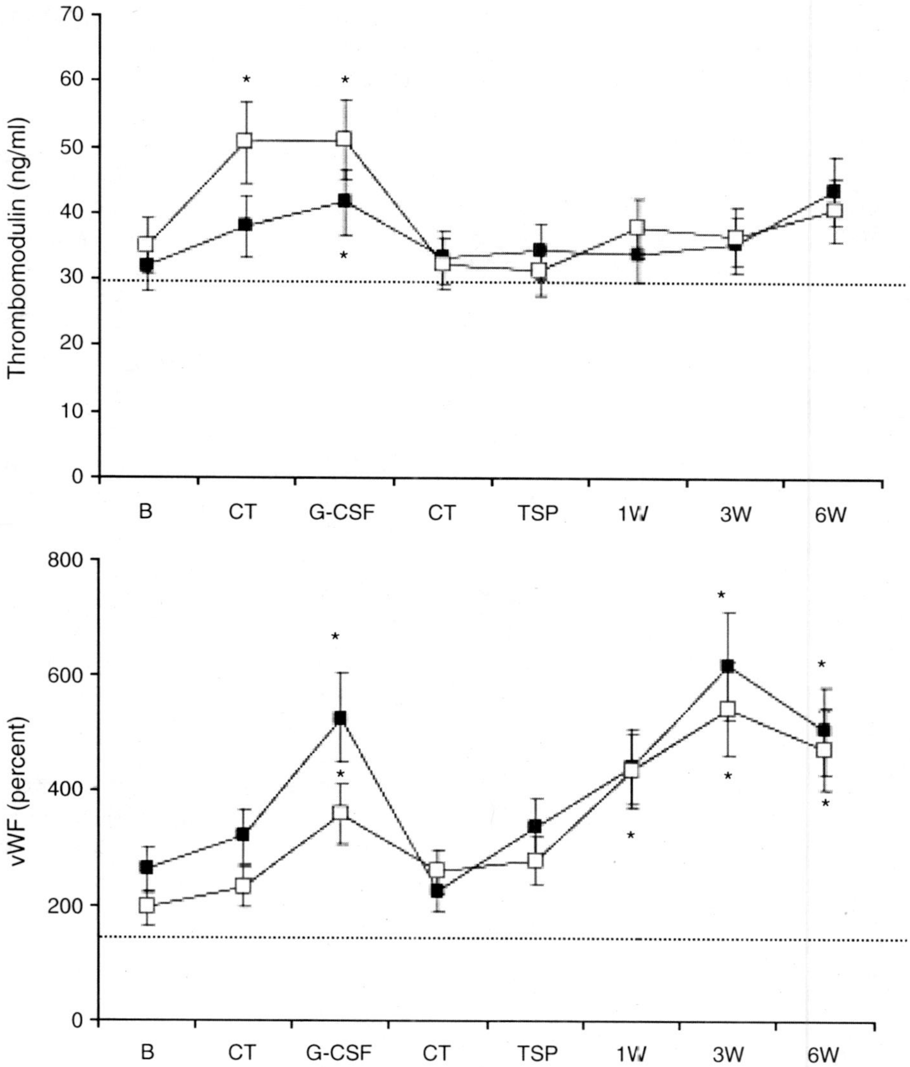

Figure 2 Plasma levels of endothelial cell activation markers in patients with hematologic malignancies receiving two different high-dose chemotherapy regimens for autologous HPC transplantation, cyclophosphamide (EDX), or cytarabine (ARA-C). *Black square*, ARA-C group; *open square*, EDX group. Asterisk indicates $p < 0.05$ versus B. *Abbreviations*: B, baseline; CT, after high-dose chemotherapy (EDX or ARA-C), before starting G-CSF; G-CSF, at the end of G-CSF (~two weeks), before leukapheresis; CT, before pretransplant chemotherapy-conditioning regimen; TSP, before autologous HPC transplantation; 1W, 2W, and 3W, one, three, and six weeks after transplantation; HPC. Data are expressed as mean ± SD.

condition regardless of the drugs used (EDX or ARA-C). In the posttransplant period, alterations of markers of endothelial damage were apparent, with no differences between the two types of regimens.

Multiple Myeloma

Several hemostatic alterations occur in patients with MM, i.e., high levels of factor VIII (FVIII) and vWF (49), acquired APC-R, the production of procoagulant autoantibodies, and high levels of PAI-1 (40,50–53). Given the significant increase of VTE in MM during thalidomide treatment combined with chemotherapy and/or dexamethasone, several studies have focused on the evaluation of thalidomide effect.

A cross-sectional study of 20 MM patients treated with thalidomide for refractory/relapsed disease (49) showed the presence of very high levels of FVIII-coagulant activity and vWF antigen in all patients on thalidomide compared to those without thalidomide. Other studies have focused on the search for acquired APC-R, a mechanism of hypercoagulability described in other cancer patients (54,55). In a prospective trial of 62 patients receiving intensive chemotherapy with or without thalidomide, 14 (23%) presented with APC-R in the absence of factor V Leiden. The occurrence of DVT was increased in patients with APC-R, irrespective of thalidomide administration. Interestingly, in carriers of APC-R, thalidomide increased the risk of VTE up to 50%. None of the patients with normal activated protein C (APC) response and not receiving thalidomide developed DVT. Therefore, acquired APC-R was present in almost one-quarter of newly diagnosed myeloma patients and significantly increased the risk of DVT. Similar results were found in a prospective study of 52 patients with newly diagnosed MM (52). Of interest, in this study, the APC-R became negative upon response to therapy. Thus APC-R appears to be a transitional condition that may be related to the myeloma status. This observation has been confirmed by analysis of a large population of 1178 patients (53). A group of 109 (9.25%) had abnormal APC-R and one-third were carriers of the factor V Leiden mutation. A higher incidence of VTE was observed in patients with acquired APC-R (31%) compared with controls (12%). APC-R was normalized after treatment in 30 out of 31 subjects with abnormal baseline values, indicating that acquired APC-R is the most common single transitory baseline coagulation abnormality associated with VTE in myeloma.

The development of hypofibrinolysis during induction therapy has also been observed in MM patients undergoing HSC transplantation (56). No evidence of hypofibrinolysis was present either at the time of diagnosis or after transplantation. The occurrence of hypofibrinolysis during chemotherapy is likely to contribute to the increased thrombotic risk in MM during this stage of treatment. No hypofibrinolysis associated with thalidomide treatment was observed (56).

The Coagulopathy of Acute Leukemia

Laboratory abnormalities of the clotting system underlying the clinical pictures of DIC are observed in both AML and ALL (57) and worsen upon initiation of chemotherapy. Routine coagulation test alterations include hypofibrinogenemia, increased FDPs, and prolonged prothrombin and thrombin times (1–3,8). These reflect the activation of coagulation, fibrinolysis, and nonspecific proteolysis. Studies of new hypercoagulation markers including F1 + 2, TAT, fibrinopeptide A and B, and D-dimer clearly show that thrombin generation constantly occurs in acute leukemia. Particularly, the increase of D-dimer demonstrates ongoing hyperfibrinolysis in response to clotting activation (18,58).

The advent of ATRA for remission induction of APL has opened new perspectives in the management of the coagulopathy. Clinicians soon noted the rapid resolution of the bleeding symptoms in patients treated with ATRA (59,60). Different laboratories, including ours, have shown a decrease of clotting and fibrinolytic variables during the first weeks of ATRA therapy (58,61,62).

In our study (58), hemostatic variables measured at the onset of APL showed elevated hypercoagulability markers (TAT, F1 + 2, D-dimer), low mean protein C, normal antithrombin (AT), normal fibrinolysis proteins, and increased elastase. After starting ATRA, all markers dropped within the first two weeks, protein C was increased, the overall fibrinolytic balance was unchanged, and elastase remained elevated. The beneficial effect on hypercoagulation/hyperfibrinolysis parameters paralleled improvement of clinical signs of the coagulopathy. The benefit persisted when ATRA was given in combination with chemotherapy.

Pathogenetic Mechanisms

Many factors contribute to the activation of coagulation and the thrombotic diathesis, including general factors, anticancer therapy, and tumor-specific factors.

The host response to the tumor including the acute-phase reaction, paraprotein production, inflammation, necrosis, and hemodynamic disorders contribute to thrombotic risk. The procoagulant effects induced by chemotherapy are also important (8,63). Additionally, the hemostatic system activation in malignancy can be attributed to tumor-specific clot-promoting mechanisms, which include the prothrombotic properties expressed by cancer cells.

In MM, at least four possible mechanisms leading to hypercoagulation have been suggested (64). They include the interference of paraproteins with fibrin structure, the production of procoagulant autoantibody, the effects of inflammatory cytokines, and acquired APC-R. In addition, injury to the endothelium, either by tumor cells or by chemotherapy, may predispose to thrombosis by causing upregulation of adhesion molecules, which mediate the adhesion of tumor cells to vascular cells, attract platelets and leukocytes, and localize the secretion of thrombogenic and angiogenic substances released by tumor cell and inflammatory tissues. However, in most cases, the pathogenesis of thrombotic complications in myeloma remains unexplained. Because thrombotic complications become prominent after the start of treatment, it is conceivable that chemotherapy plays a more important role in the thrombotic process than tumor cell abnormalities.

Considerably more information is available on mechanisms of clotting activation in leukemias (1–3,18). Prothrombotic factors expressed by leukemic cells include the expression of procoagulant, fibrinolytic, and proteolytic properties and the secretion of inflammatory cytokines (Fig. 3).

Many studies have characterized the procoagulant activity (PCA) expressed by leukemic cells, particularly TF, the major activator of blood coagulation, and "cancer procoagulant" (CP), more typical of malignant cells (58). All AML subtypes express PCA, with the greatest expression in the M3 type (65); but ALL blasts also express measurable PCA (66). The cellular differentiation of APL induced by ATRA is associated with loss of PCA expression by leukemic blasts. The inhibitory effect of ATRA on PCA occurs in vivo as well as in vitro. Both TF and CP of APL blasts are progressively reduced in patients given ATRA (58). The demonstration that the PCA loss parallels improvement of the hypercoagulable condition provides the first evidence in vivo for a role of tumor-cell PCA in the clotting complications of malignancy. Reduction of leukemic cell PCA by ATRA appears to be one mechanism involved in the resolution of the coagulopathy (3,18).

Leukemic cells also express fibrinolytic and proteolytic activities, which might be involved in the pathogenesis of the bleeding. However, these activities are lower in APL blasts than in mature granulocytes and are not sensitive to ATRA in vitro (67). Another study demonstrated the expression of an annexin II–associated fibrinolytic activity in APL blasts, which is increased compared to other myeloid subtypes or lymphoid blasts. This activity is reduced by ATRA (68).

Leukemic cells produce inflammatory cytokines, including tumor necrosis factor-α (TNF-α) and interleukin (IL)-1β. A role for the blast cytokines in the pathogenesis of the acute leukemia coagulopathy was suggested by findings that leukemic promyelocytes

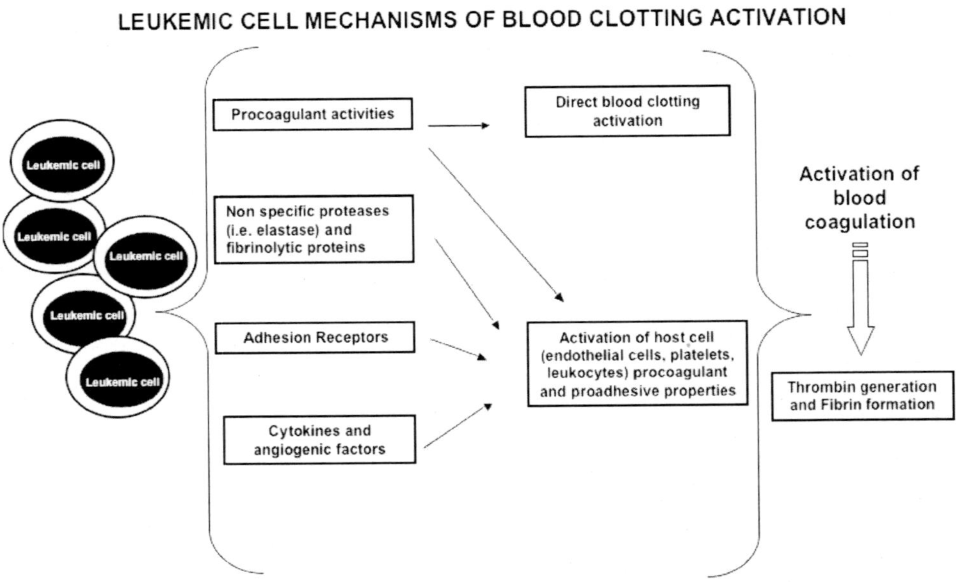

Figure 3 Leukemic cell mechanisms of blood clotting activation. Leukemic cells interact with the hemostatic system by (*i*) the expression of procoagulant activities (i.e., tissue factor, cancer procoagulant), which directly activate blood coagulation; (*ii*) the release of proinflammatory cytokines (i.e., interleukin 1-β, tumor necrosis factor α) and proangiogenic factors (i.e., vascular endothelial growth factor, fibroblast growth factor, interleukin 8), which induce the procoagulant and proadhesive properties of vascular blood cells; and (*iii*) the expression of cell membrane adhesion receptors (ICAM-1, Mac1, VLA4), which allow the direct interaction of leukemic cells with the vascular cells. *Abbreviations*: ICAM-1, intercellular cell adhesion molecule-1; Mac1; VLA4-very large antigen-4.

from patients with DIC secreted more IL-1β than APL blasts from patients without DIC (69). TNF-α, IL-1β, and endotoxin can induce the expression of the procoagulant TF by endothelial cells (ECs) (70). These cytokines also downregulate the expression of endothelial TM, the surface receptor for thrombin. The TM-thrombin complex activates the protein C system, which in turn functions as a potent anticoagulant. TF upregulation and TM downregulation lead to a prothrombotic condition of the vascular wall (71). In addition, TNF-α and IL-1β stimulate the endothelium to produce the tissue-type plasminogen activator inhibitor PAI-1 (72). Inhibition of fibrinolysis contributes to the prothrombotic potential of EC. ATRA upregulates the ability of leukemic cells to produce cytokines. In theory, this effect should favor the prothrombotic potential of the endothelium, but this does not happen because ATRA protects the endothelium against the prothrombotic assault of inflammatory cytokines (18).

Chemotherapy increases the risk of thrombosis (8,63). Among the postulated mechanisms for anticancer drug-related thrombosis are (*i*) release of procoagulants and cytokines from damaged malignant cells; (*ii*) direct drug toxicity on vascular endothelium; (*iii*) direct induction of monocyte or tumor-cell TF; and (*iv*) decrease in physiological anticoagulants. The release of procoagulants and cytokines by tumor cells that have been damaged by chemotherapy is considered responsible for the exacerbation of DIC observed upon starting chemotherapy, particularly in acute leukemias (3). The relation between the downregulation of TF and CP in APL blast cells in vivo and the resolution of the coagulopathy in the same subjects support the role of tumor cell PCA in the pathogenesis of DIC (58). The release of cytokines in response to chemotherapy may also be important in increasing thrombotic risk. The profound changes in the levels of markers of endothelium activation (i.e., vWF, TM, and PAI-1) in patients on chemotherapy demonstrate the direct endothelial damage. Another important prothrombotic mechanism involves the reduction in levels of physiological coagulation inhibitors (AT, protein C, and protein S), which occurs as a consequence of the hepatotoxicity of chemotherapy (73).

In this setting, it is important to mention hepatic veno-occlusive disease (VOD), a life-threatening thrombotic complication of HSC transplantation, which is characterized by the activation of blood coagulation, likely consequent to the endothelial damage (74,75). VOD occurs in about 50% of patients undergoing allogeneic transplantation but is also associated with autologous HSC transplants and represents an important cause of mortality (>30% of cases).

PROPHYLAXIS AND THERAPY OF THROMBOSIS IN HEMATOLOGIC MALIGNANCIES

Thrombotic complications can affect the morbidity and the mortality of cancer patients. No ad hoc studies or guidelines are available for prophylaxis or treatment of VTE in hematologic malignancies. The use of LMWHs has improved VTE management in patients with solid tumors, but no experience has been accumulated in patients with acute leukemia, who have a high risk of hemorrhage, due to thrombocytopenia secondary to chemotherapy. Therefore, the administration of anticoagulant treatments for VTE poses serious problems in this patient population and confers additional importance to the prevention of thrombotic complications.

Prophylaxis

Little information is available on thromboprophylaxis in acute leukemias and lymphoma, but some comes from studies on thromboprophylaxis of CVC-related thrombosis (11,12). In the randomized trial of 1 mg warfarin prophylaxis versus placebo, about 80% of patients had hematologic malignancies (12). This regimen was not effective in preventing CVC-related VTE but was safe. In the study conducted by the Italian CATHEM group, 14.2% of patients who entered were receiving thromboprophylaxis, mostly LMWH, but also unfractionated heparin (UFH), aspirin, or warfarin (11). In this subgroup, no increase in hemorrhagic complications was observed. More information is available on thromboprophylaxis in patients with MM, due to the high thrombotic risk associated with thalidomide and lenalidomide. Considering the advantages provided by these new drugs, the search for strategies of thomboprophylaxis in this setting is very active. Current data on thromboprophylaxis came from noncontrolled randomized clinical trials and are summarized in Table 4.

Prophylaxis with enoxaparin (40 mg/day), given to newly diagnosed MM patients enrolled in a trial of combination therapy of thalidomide with doxorubicin, reduced VTE during the first three months of treatment (76), whereas fixed low-dose warfarin (1 mg/day) did not. Similar results with LMWH have been reported in 209 newly diagnosed patients who received nadroparin prophylaxis during treatment with thalidomide + dexamethasone and doxorubicin. The VTE incidence was reduced to 10% without increasing bleeding (77). In another study, fixed low-dose warfarin (1.25 mg/day) prevented VTE in newly diagnosed patients treated with thalidomide and dexamethasone (78). Finally, the efficacy of aspirin prophylaxis has been suggested in patients given thalidomide + chemotherapy (79) (Table 4). Aspirin prophylaxis has been utilized with promising results also in patients treated with the thalidomide derivative lenalidomide (80,81). Recently, different thromboprophylaxis regimens have been retrospectively analyzed by Palumbo et al. (82). However, the most effective strategies to prevent VTE will come from ongoing prospective randomized studies.

Table 4 Thrombosis in Patients with Multiple Myeloma. Thromboprophylaxis: Prospective Phase II Studies

References	Study	Patients (*n*)	Therapy	Thrombosis [*n* (%)]
Zangari et al., 2004 (76)—newly diagnosed	Phase II	68	CT + DX + T + enoxaparin (40 mg/day)	10(14.7)
		35	CT + DX + T + warfarin (1 mg/day)	11(31.4)
Minnema et al., 2004 (77)—newly diagnosed	Phase II	209	CT + DX + T + Nadroparin	21(10)
Cavo et al., 2004 (78)—newly diagnosed, age < 65 yr	Phase II	19	DX + T	5 (26)
		52	DX + T + 1.2 mg warfarin	7 (13)
Baz et al., 2005 (79)— newly diagnosed and CT refractory	Phase II	19	CT + Dx + T	11 (58)
		84	CT + Dx + T + ASA	15 (17.8), $P < 0.001$

Abbreviations: CT, chemotherapy; DX, dexamethasone; T, thalidomide; ASA, aspirin.

Therapy of VTE

No studies have specifically addressed the issue of VTE treatment in patients with acute leukemia. In patients with solid tumors, a therapeutic strategy based on LMWH administered for six months after a VTE episode has been safe and superior to warfarin in preventing VTE recurrences and is currently recommended (83). This regimen was tested in a small group of patients with hematologic malignancies and VTE (84,85). The use of LMWH in these patients is an attractive choice due to their safety profile, no need for laboratory monitoring, and less sensitivity than warfarin to drug interference. Possibly, efforts should be made to standardize dose reductions or temporary suspensions of the drugs according to the degree of thrombocytopenia.

Treatment of the APL Coagulopathy

The role of heparin therapy in the treatment of the coagulopathy complicating acute leukemia, especially APL, remains uncertain. The old studies, which have used UFH, are small, retrospective, and not controlled. The benefit of UFH therapy has never been proved by prospective randomized trials. In a large retrospective analysis (17) of 268 patients, the results indicated no benefit from UFH with respect to early hemorrhagic deaths, CR rate, or overall survival. LMWHs have never been tested in this context.

Therapeutic regimens including antifibrinolytic agents such as epsilon-aminocaproic acid and tranexamic acid, or protease inhibitors such as aprotinin, have been suggested by studies of small series of patients (1–3,18). It is worth noting that thromboembolic events occur when antifibrinolytic agents are administered in conjunction with ATRA therapy (86).

Today, prophylactic platelet transfusions therapy represents an essential part of supportive care for patients with acute leukemia. This practice has resulted in a decrease in bleeding, prolonged survival, and allows for intensification of therapy (1). Current recommendations for patients with APL suggest that platelets should be transfused to maintain the platelet count above 20×10^9/L in those not actively bleeding and above 50×10^9/L with active bleeding (2,3). However, the advent of ATRA for remission induction has changed the natural history and has helped resolve the coagulopathy. Some of the mechanisms by which ATRA controls the hemostatic system have been elucidated (18). However, in spite of the improvement of the coagulopathy by ATRA, the rate of very early hemorrhagic deaths in APL has not been significantly changed. Additional efforts to develop therapies that rapidly correct the coagulopathy are required. New approaches of using anticoagulant and anti-inflammatory drugs should be considered.

ACKNOWLEDGMENTS

We wish to thank Prof. T. Barbui (Head of the Department of Hematology–Oncology of Ospedali Riuniti di Bergamo, Italy) for his continuing support to the research in the field of thrombosis in hematologic malignancies, Drs A. Vignoli, D. Balducci, and L. Russo for their contribution to studies performed in our laboratory and for revising the manuscript.

REFERENCES

1. Barbui T, Finazzi G, Falanga A. The management of bleeding and thrombosis in acute leukemia and chronic myeloproliferative disorders. In: Henderson ES, Lister TA, Greaves MF, eds. Leukemia. 7th ed. Saunders Company WB, 2001:363–382.
2. Tallman MS, Kwaan HC. Reassessing the hemostatic disorder associated with acute promyelocytic leukemia. Blood 1992; 79:543–553.
3. Barbui T, Finazzi G, Falanga A. The impact of all-trans-retinoic acid on the coagulopathy of acute promyelocytic leukemia. Blood 1998; 91:3093–3102.
4. Levitan N, Dowlati A, Remick SC, et al. Rates of initial and recurrent thromboembolic disease among patients with malignancy versus those without malignancy. Risk analysis using Medicare claims data. Medicine 1999; 78(5):285–291.
5. White RH, Chew HK, Zhou H, et al. Incidence of venous thromboembolism in the year before the diagnosis of cancer in 528693 adults. Arch Intern Med 2005; 165:1782–1787.
6. Khorana AA, Francis CW, Culakova E, et al. Risk factors for chemotherapy-associated venous thromboembolism in a prospective observational study. Cancer 2005; 104:2822–2829.
7. Khorana AA, Francis CW, Culakova E, et al. Thromboembolism in hospitalized neutropenic cancer patients. J Clin Onc 2006; 24:484–490.
8. Falanga A. Mechanisms of hypercoagulation in malignancy and during chemotherapy. Haemostasis 1998; 2(suppl 3):50–60.
9. Barbui T, Falanga A. Thalidomide and thrombosis in multiple myeloma. J Thromb Haemost 2003; 1:421–422.
10. Cavo M, Zamagni E, Cellini C, et al. Deep vein thrombosis in patients with multiple myeloma receiving first-line thalidomide-dexamethasone therapy. Blood 2002; 100:2272–2273.
11. Cortelezzi A, Moia M, Falanga A, et al. Incidence of thrombotic complications in patients with haematological malignancies with central venous catheters: a prospective multicentre study. Br J Hematol 2005; 129:811–817.
12. Couban S, Goodyear M, Burnell M, et al. Randomized placebo-controlled study of low-dose warfarin for the prevention of central venous catheter–associated thrombosis in patients with cancer. J Clin Oncol 2005; 23:4063–4069.
13. Rickles FR, Levine MN, Edwards RL. Hemostatic alterations in cancer patients. Cancer Metastasis Rev 1992; 11:237–248.
14. Falanga A, Ofosu FA, Delaini F, et al. The hypercoagulable state in cancer: evidence for impaired thrombin inhibition. Blood Coagul Fibrinolysis 1994; 5:S19–S23.
15. Zigler S, Sperr WR, Knobl P, et al. Symptomatic venous thromboembolism in acute leukemia. Incidence, risk factors, and impact on prognosis. Thromb Res 2005; 115:59–64.
16. De Stefano V, Sora F, Rossi E, et al. The risk of thrombosis in patients with acute leukemia: occurrence of thrombosis at diagnosis and during treatment. J Thromb Haemost 2005; 3:1985–1992.

17. Rodeghiero F, Avvisati G, Castaman G, et al. Early deaths and anti-hemorrhagic treatments in acute promyelocytic leukemia. A GIMEMA retrospective study in 268 consecutive patients. Blood 1990; 75:2112–2117.
18. Falanga A, Rickles FR. Pathogenesis and management of the bleeding diathesis in acute promyelocytic leukaemia. Best Pract Res Clin Haematol 2003; 16(3):463–482.
19. Clarke CS, Otridge BW, Carney DN. Thromboembolism. A complication of weekly chemotherapy in the treatment of non-Hodgkin's lymphoma. Cancer 1990; 66(9):2027–2030.
20. Ottinger H, Belka C, Kozole G, et al. Deep venous thrombosis and pulmonary artery embolism in high-grade non Hodgkin's lymphoma: incidence, causes and prognostic relevance. Eur J Haematol 1995; 54(3):186–194.
21. Mohren M, Markmann I, Jentsch-Ullrich K, et al. Increased risk of thromboembolism in patients with malignant lymphoma: a single-centre analysis. Br J Cancer 2005; 92(8):1349–1351.
22. Komrokji RS, Uppal NP, Khorana AA, et al. Venous thromboembolism in patients with diffuse large B-cell lymphoma. Leuk Lymphoma 2006; 47(6):1029–1033.
23. Goldschmidt N, Linetsky E, Shalom E, et al. High incidence of thromboembolism in patients with central nervous system lymphoma. Cancer 2003; 98(6):1239–1242.
24. Marras LC, Geerts WH, Perry JR. The risk of venous thromboembolism is increased throughout the course of malignant glioma. Cancer 2000; 89(3):640–646.
25. Ditcher SR. Cancer and thrombosis: mechanism and treatment. J Thromb Thrombolysis 2003; 16(1–2):21–31.
26. Mohren M, Markmann I, Jentsch-Ullrich K, et al. Increased risk of venous thromboembolism in patients with acute leukemia. Br J Cancer 2006; 94:200–202.
27. Priest JR, Ramsay NKC, Steinherz PG, et al. A syndrome of thrombosis and hemorrhage complicating L-asparaginase therapy for childhood acute lymphoblastic leukemia. J Pediatr 1982; 100:984–989.
28. Pui CH, Jackson CW, Chesney C, et al. Sequential changes in platelet function and coagulation in leukemic children treated with L-asparaginase, prednisone and vincristine. J Clin Oncol 1983; 1:380–385.
29. Nowak-Gottl U, Wermes C, Junker R, et al. Prospective evaluation of the thrombotic risk in children with acute lymphoblastic leukemia carrying the MTHFR TT 677 genotype, the prothrombin G20210A variant, and further thrombotic risk factors. Blood 1999; 93:1595–1599.
30. Caruso V, Iacoviello L, Di Castelnuovo A, et al. Thrombotic complications in childhood acute lymphoblastic leukemia: a meta-analysis of 17 prospective studies comprising 1752 pediatric patients. Blood 2006; 108(7):2216–2222.
31. Annino L, Vegna ML, Camera A, et al. GIMEMA group. Treatment of adult acute lymphoblastic leukemia (ALL): long-term follow-up of the GIMEMA ALL 0288 randomized study. Blood 2002; 99(3):863–871.
32. Sarris AH, Kempin S, Berman E, et al. High incidence of disseminated intravascular coagulation during remission induction of adult patients with acute lymphoblastic leukemia. Blood 1992; 79:1305–1310.
33. Singhal S, Mheta J, Desikan R, et al. Antitumor activity of thalidomide in refractory multiple myeloma. N Engl J Med 1999; 341:1565–1571.
34. Barlogie B, Tricot G, Anaissie E, et al. Thalidomide and hematopoietic-celltranplantation for multiple myeloma. N Engl J Med 2006; 354(10):1021–1030.
35. Barlogie B, Desikan R, Eddlemon P, et al. Extended survival in advanced and refractory multiple myeloma after single-agent thalidomide: identification of prognostic factors in a phase 2 study of 169 patients. Blood 2001; 98(2):492–494.
36. Rajkumar SV, Gertz MA, Lacy MQ, et al. Thalidomide as initial therapy for early-stage myeloma. Leukemia 2003; 17(4):775–779.
37. Urbauer E, Kaufmann H, Nosslinger T, et al. Thromboembolic events during treatment with thalidomide. Blood 2002; 99:4247–4248.
38. Osman K, Comenzo R, Rajkumar SV. Deep venous thrombosis and thalidomide therapy for multiple myeloma. N Engl J Med 2001; 344(25):1951–1952.

39. Zangari M, Anaissie E, Barlogie B. Increased risk of deep vein thrombosis in patients with multiple myeloma receiving thalidomide and chemotherapy. Blood 2001; 98:1614–1615.
40. Zangari M, Saghafifar F, Anaissie E, et al. Acivated protein C in the absence of factor V Leiden mutation is a common finding in multiple myeloma and is associated with an increased risk of thrombotic complications. Blood Coagul Fibrinolysis 2002; 13:187–192.
41. Rus C, Bazzan M, Palumbo A, et al. Thalidomide in front line treatment in multiple myeloma: serious risk of venous thromboembolism and evidence for thromboprophylaxis. J Thromb Haemost 2004; 2(11):2063–2065.
42. Rajkumar SV, Blood E, Vesole D, et al. Eastern Cooperative Oncology Group. Phase III clinical trial of thalidomide plus dexamethasone compared with dexamethasone alone in newly diagnosed multiple myeloma: a clinical trial coordinated by the Eastern Cooperative Oncology Group. J Clin Oncol 2006; 24(3):431–436.
43. Niesvizky R, Spencer A, Wang M, et al. Increased risk of thrombosis with lenalidomide in combination with dexamethasone and erythropoietin. Proc Am Soc Clin Oncol. J Clin Oncol 2006; 24(18S):7506.
44. Zonder JA, Durie BGM, McCoy J, et al. High incidence of thrombotic events observed in patients receiving lenalidomide (L) + dexamethasone (D) (LD) as first-line therapy for multiple myeloma (MM) without aspirin (ASA) prophylaxis [abstr]. ASH Annual Meeting. Blood 2005; 106:3455.
45. Falanga A, Marchetti M, Vignoli A, Balducci D. Clotting mechanisms and cancer: implications in thrombus formation and tumor progression. Clin Adv Hematol Oncol 2003; 1:673–678.
46. Zurborn KH, Duscha H, Gram J, et al. Investigations of coagulation system and fibrinolysis in patients with disseminated adenocarcinomas and non-Hodgkin's lymphomas. Oncology 1990; 47(5):376–380.
47. De Lucia D, De Francesco F, Marotta R, et al. Phenotypic APC resistance as a marker of hypercoagulability in primitive cerebral lymphoma. Exp Oncol 2005; 27(2):159–161.
48. Sase T, Wada H, Yamaguchi M, et al. Haemostatic abnormalities and thrombotic disorders in malignant lymphoma. Thromb Haemost 2005; 93:153–159.
49. Minnema MC, Fijnheer R, De Groot PG, et al. Extremely high levels of von Willebrand factor antigen and of procoagulant factor VIII found in multiple myeloma patients are associated with activity status but not with thalidomide treatment. J Thromb Haemost 2003; 1:445–449.
50. Deitcher SR, Choueiri T, Srkalovic G, et al. Acquired activated protein C resistance in myeloma patients with venous thromboembolic events. Br J Haematol 2003; 123(5):959.
51. Yagci M, Sucak GT, Haznedar R. Fibrinolytic activity in multiple myeloma. Am J Hematol 2003; 74:231–237.
52. Hugo JZ, Jeanet DM. Acquired activated protein C resistance and thrombosis in multiple myeloma patients. Thromb J 2006; 21:4–11.
53. Elice F, Fink L, Tricot G, et al. Acquired resistance to activated protein C (aAPCR) in multiple myeloma is a transitory abnormality associated with an increased risk of venous thromboembolism. Br J Haematol 2006; 134(4):399–405.
54. Haim N, Lanir N, Hoffman R, et al. Acquired activated protein C resistance is common in cancer patients and is associated with venous thromboembolism. Am J Med 2001; 110(2):91–96.
55. Nijziel MR, van Oerle, Christella M, et al. Acquired resistance to activated protein C in breast cancer patients. Br J Hematol 2003; 120(1):117–122.
56. van Marion AM, Auwerda JJ, Minnema MC, et al. Hypofibrinolysis during induction treatment of multiple myeloma may increase the risk of venous thrombosis. Thromb Haemost 2005; 94(6):1341–1343.
57. Leone G, Gugliotta L, Mazzucconi MG, et al. Evidence of a hypercoagulable state in patients with acute lymphoblastic leukemia treated with low dose of *E. coli* L-Asparaginase: a GIMEMA study. Thromb Haemost 1993; 69:12–15.
58. Falanga A, Iacoviello L, Evangelista V, et al. Loss of blast cell procoagulant activity and improvement of hemostatic variables in patients with acute promyelocitic leukemia given all-trans-retinoic acid. Blood 1995; 86:1072–1084.
59. Warrell RP, de The H, Wang ZY, Degos L. Acute promyelocytic leukemia. N Engl J Med 1993; 329:177–189.

60. Castaigne S, Chomienne, Daniel MT, et al. All-trans retinoic acid as a differentiation therapy for acute promyelocytic leukemia. Blood 1990; 76(9):1704–1709.
61. Tallman MS, Lefebvre P, Baine RM, et al. Effects of all-trans retinoic acid or chemotherapy on the molecular regulation of systemic blood coagulation and fibrinolysis in patients with acute promyelocitic leukemia. J Thromb Haemost 2004; 2:1341–1350.
62. Dombret H, Scrobahaci ML, Daniel MT, et al. In vivo thrombin and plasmin activities in patients with acute promyelocytic leukemia (APL): effect of all-trans retinoic acid (ATRA) therapy. Leukemia 1995; 9:19–24.
63. Lee AY, Levine MN. The thrombophilic state induced by therapeutic agents in the cancer patient. Semin Thromb Hemost 1999; 25(2):137–145.
64. Zangari M, Saghafifar F, Mehta P, et al. The blood coagulation mechanism in multiple myeloma. Semin Thromb Hemost 2003; 29(3):275–282.
65. Falanga A, Alessio MG, Donati MB, et al. A new procoagulant in acute leukemia. Blood 1988; 71:870–875.
66. Alessio MG, Falanga A, Consonni R, et al. Cancer Procoagulant in acute lymphoblastic leukemia. Eur J Haematol 1990; 45:78–81.
67. De Stefano V, Teofili L, Sica S, et al. Effect of all-trans-Retinoic Acid on procoagulant and fibrinolytic activities of cultured blast cells from patients with acute promyelocytic leukemia. Blood 1995; 86(9):3535–3541.
68. Menell JS, Cesarman GM, Jacovina AT, et al. Annexin II and bleeding in acute promyelocytic leukaemia. N Engl J Med 1999; 340(13):994–1004.
69. Cozzolino F, Torcia M, Miliani A, et al. Potential role of interleukin -1 as the trigger for diffuse intravascular coagulation in acute nonlymphoblastic leukemia. Am J Med 1988; 84(2):240–250.
70. Bevilacqua MP, Pober JS, Majeau GR, et al. Recombinant tumor necrosis factor induces procoagulant activity in cultured human vascular endothelium: characterization and comparison with the actions of interleukin-1. Proc Natl Acad Sci 1986; 83(12):4533–4537.
71. Moore KL, Esmon CT, Esmon NL. Tumor necrosis factor leads to the internalization and degradation of thrombomodulin from the surface of bovine aortic endothelial cells in culture. Blood 1989; 73(1):159–165.
72. Nachman RL, Hajar KA, Silverstein RL, et al. Interleukin 1 induces endothelial cell synthesis of plasminogen activator inhibitor. J Exp Med 1986; 163(3):1595–1600.
73. Harper PL, Jarvis J, Jennings I, et al. Changes in the natural anticoagulants following bone marrow transplantation. Bone Marrow Transpl 1990; 5(1):39–42.
74. Bearman SI. The syndrome of veno-occlusive disease after bone-marrow transplantation. Blood 1995; 85(11):3005–3020.
75. Falanga A, Vignoli A, Marchetti M, et al. Defibrotide reduces procoagulant activity and increases fibrinolytic properties of endothelial cells. Leukemia 2003; 17:1636–1642.
76. Zangari M, Barlogie B, Anaissie E, et al. Deep vein thrombosis in patients with multiple myeloma treated with thalidomide and chemotherapy: effects of prophylactic and therapeutic anticoagulation. Br J Haematol 2004; 126(5):715–721.
77. Minnema MC, Breitkreutz I, Auwerda JJ, et al. Prevention of venous thromboembolism with low molecular-weight hepatin in patients with multiple myeloma treated with thalidomide and chemotherapy. Leukemia 2004; 18(12):2044–2046.
78. Cavo M, Zamagni E, Tosi P, et al. First-line therapy with thalidomide and dexamethasone in preparation for autologous stem cell transplantation for multiple myeloma. Haematologica 2004; 89(7):826–831.
79. Baz R, Li L, Kottke-Marchant K, et al. The role of aspirin in the prevention of thrombotic complications of thalidomide and anthracycline-basedchemotherapy for multiple myeloma. Mayo Clin Proc 2005; 80(12):1568–1574.
80. Rajkumar SV, Hayman S, Lacy MQ, et al. Combination therapy with lenalidomide plus dexamethasone (rev/dex) for newly diagnosed myeloma [abstr]. ASH Annual Meeting. Blood 2005; 106:781.
81. Niesvizky R, Martinez-Banos DM, Gelbshtein UY, et al. Prophylactic low-dose aspirin is effective as antithrombotic therapy in patients receiving combination thalidomide or lenalidomide [abstr]. ASH Annual Meeting. Blood 2005; 106:3454.

82. Palumbo A, Rus C, Zeldis JB, et al. Italian Multiple Myeloma Network, Gimema. Enoxaparin or aspirin for the prevention of recurrent thromboembolism in newly diagnosed myeloma patients treated with melphalan and prednisone plus thalidomide or lenalidomide. J Thromb Haemost 2006; 4(8):1842–1845.
83. Lee AYY, Levine MN, Baker RI, et al. Low-molecular-weight heparin versus a coumarin for the prevention of recurrent venous thromboembolism in patients with cancer. N Engl J Med 2003; 349:146–153.
84. Herishanu Y, Misgav M, Kirgner I, et al. Enoxaparin can be used safely in patients with severe thrombocytopenia due to intensive chemotherapy regimens. Leukemia Lymphoma 2004; 45(7):1407–1411.
85. Imberti D, Vallisa D, Anselmi E, et al. Safety and efficacy of enoxaparin treatment in venous thromboembolic disease durino acute leukemia. Tumori 2004; 90(4):1–4.
86. Hashimoto S, Koike T, Tatewaki W, et al. Fatal thromboembolism in acute promyelocytic leukemia during all-trans-Retinoic Acid therapy combined with antifibrinolytic therapy for prophylaxis of hemorrhage. Leukemia 1994; 8(7):1113–1115.

10

Diagnosing Cancer in Patients with Venous Thromboembolism

A. Piccioli
Department of Medical and Surgical Sciences, University of Padua, Padua, Italy

Anna Falanga
Division of Hematology, Ospedali Riuniti di Bergamo, Bergamo, Italy

P. Prandoni
Department of Medical and Surgical Sciences, University of Padua, Padua, Italy

- The clinical association between cancer and VTE is clearly established.
- VTE, and especially idiopathic VTE, is associated with an increased risk of newly discovered cancers during follow-up, with an incidence of approximately 10%.
- The performance of extensive screening procedures for cancer identification at the time of VTE diagnosis appears advisable if it improves cancer-related mortality.
- Recent prospective trials have observed that most hidden cancers are detected at an earlier stage, with extensive screening procedures.
- Data from these studies do not conclusively demonstrate that earlier diagnosis prolongs life, but the collective observations make such a beneficial effect likely.

INTRODUCTION

Since Trousseau's time, the strong clinical association between cancer and venous thromboembolism (VTE) has been frequently observed and documented, and cancer patients clearly exhibit a higher risk of developing a thrombotic event when compared to noncancer patients. The risk is substantial, particularly in the presence of well-known risk factors such as prolonged immobilization, surgery, and chemo-radio-hormonal therapy. VTE, especially in its idiopathic presentation, may represent an epiphenomenon of yet undisclosed cancer, offering possible chances for early diagnosis and treatment.

The incidence of newly diagnosed cancer during follow-up of patients with VTE is high compared to the general population. In particular, the risk of cancer following a thrombotic event is higher among patients without any known risk factor for thrombosis (so-called idiopathic VTE) when compared with patients suffering from a secondary VTE. Newly discovered malignancies are not confined to certain subtypes, but involve virtually all body systems. Some of these malignancies can be identified by routine assessments at the time of the diagnosis of the thrombotic event. However, in patients with idiopathic VTE, who are apparently cancer free at baseline, there remains an approximate 10% incidence of clinically overt malignant disease during the follow-up period after the thrombotic event (1)[a].

CANCER DIAGNOSIS IN PATIENTS WITH VTE

The awareness that an episode of idiopathic VTE could signal the presence of a hidden cancer has generated interest in assessing the prevalence of either cancer diagnosed concomitantly with VTE or malignancy during the follow-up of VTE patients.

The risk of concomitant cancer, defined as cancer not known before the thrombotic event and discovered by routine exams at the time of idiopathic VTE diagnosis, varies among studies. This may be related either to the completeness of screening studies performed or to the demographic characteristics, especially in relation to age, of the population. It has been noted that the risk of concomitant cancer was increased 3- to 19-fold among patients with idiopathic VTE, whereas the prevalence of concomitant cancer in patients with secondary VTE was low and fully comparable to that observed in the general population after middle age (2).

Moreover, studies performed in the last two decades have demonstrated that patients with idiopathic VTE exhibit a higher risk of harboring a neoplasm when compared with patients with secondary VTE (Table 1) (3–9). The incidence of newly discovered malignancies during follow-up of patients with idiopathic VTE, in whom a routine initial screening for cancer identification is negative, is consistently around 10% (1).

The risk is even higher in patients presenting with bilateral idiopathic deep vein thrombosis (DVT) (10) and in patients with recurrent episodes of VTE (4). In a study by Bura et al., the incidence of newly discovered cancers during one-year follow-up after a thrombotic event was as high as 40% among patients with bilateral idiopathic DVT (10).

Clear evidence has been provided in four large population-based studies conducted in Denmark, Sweden, Scotland, and California (11–14). These reported data from cancer and thromboembolic disease national registries. All found a significantly increased risk of developing cancer in patients discharged with VTE, particularly in the first one-year period after the thrombotic event and remained substantial for quite a long time after. In all studies, the risk was higher in patients with idiopathic VTE, and cancers involved virtually all body systems. Notably, the study by White et al. found that acute myelogenous leukemia, non-Hodgkin lymphoma, renal cell cancer, ovarian cancer, pancreatic cancer, stomach cancer, and lung cancer were the most commonly involved cancer types.

Very recently, the association between VTE and subsequent incident cancer has been extended to patients who have already had a cancer diagnosis. Sorensen et al., using the Danish Cancer Registry and National Registry of patients, showed an excess risk of a second cancer among patients with malignancy in whom an episode of VTE occurred more than one year after the initial cancer, suggesting that the second VTE is an epiphenomenon of the second occult cancer. The overall relative risk for a second cancer in this setting was 1.4 [confidence interval (CI): 1.2–1.7], whereas the overall relative risk for patients experiencing an episode of VTE during the first year after cancer diagnosis was 1.0 (CI: 0.9–1.3). The risk was higher for cancers of the upper gastrointestinal tract, ovary, and prostate (15).

[a] Ref. 1 outlines the important two-way clinical association between cancer and venous thromboembolism.

Table 1 Incidence of Occult Cancer in the Follow-up of Patients with VTE

References	All VTE	Cancer	
		Secondary VTE	Idiopathic VTE
Aderka et al., 1986 (3)	11/83 (13.3%)	2/48 (4.2%)	9/35 (25.7%)
Prandoni et al., 1992 (4)	13/250 (5.2%)	2/105 (1.9%)	11/145 (7.6%)
Ahmed and Mohuddin 1996 (5)	3/196 (1.5%)	0/83 (0%)	3/113 (2.7%)
Monreal et al., 1997 (6)	8/659 (1.2%)	4/563 (0.7%)	4/96 (4.2%)
Hettiarachchi et al., 1998 (7)	13/326 (4.0%)	3/171 (1.8%)	10/155 (6.5%)
Rajan et al., 1998 (8)	21/264 (8.0%)	8/112 (7.1%)	13/152 (8.6%)
Schulman and Lindmarker 2000 (9)	111/854 (13.0%)	18/320 (5.6%)	93/534 (17.4%)

Abbreviation: VTE, venous thromboembolism.

PROGNOSIS OF PATIENTS DIAGNOSED WITH CANCER AT THE TIME OF OR FOLLOWING VTE

Despite the clear association between cancer and VTE, little is known about the prognosis of patients in whom cancer is discovered at the time of or following the thrombotic event. The need to screen for occult malignancy in this category of patients is, therefore, still under evaluation. Since extensive screening for cancer identification is associated with high costs and is itself associated with some morbidity and discomfort for the patient, it is acceptable only if it is shown to be cost-effective, with an impact on cancer-related mortality.

Some authors have raised concern about the utility of screening all patients with idiopathic VTE for occult malignancy. There is question whether early detection of cancer in patients with VTE may improve longterm survival. A retrospective study by Sorensen et al. (16) assessed the survival rate of patients with cancer diagnosed in the first year following the thrombotic event in comparison to that of cancer patients without thrombosis, and found an increased mortality in the former group. Moreover, patients in whom cancer was detected at the time of the thrombotic event experienced a poor prognosis as well. The results seem discouraging, as it appears that whenever cancer is preceded by a clinical manifestation of thrombosis, its prognosis is worse. Moreover, a retrospective study by White et al. found that most of the cancers diagnosed in the period from four months to one year after idiopathic VTE were at an advanced stage. These authors found a relative risk of having advanced cancer in this setting of 2.3 (CI: 2.0–2.6) (14). However, given the retrospective nature of these observations, it is likely that the cancers were already symptomatic at the time thrombosis occurred, and, therefore, easily detectable by routine tests. The crucial point may be that only patients in whom there is no evidence of malignancy at the time of VTE could benefit from early diagnosis by extensive screening (17).

RECENT STUDIES

Two prospective studies have recently been reported. Monreal et al. (18)[b] published the results of a prospective cohort follow-up study of consecutive patients with acute VTE. All patients underwent a routine clinical evaluation for malignancy, which included a thorough history, physical examination, laboratory testing including sedimentation rate, complete

[b] Ref. 18 is a prospective clinical evaluation assessing that a limited diagnostic work-up for occult cancer has the capacity of identifying approximately one half of hidden malignancies.

Table 2 Extensive Screening Strategy According to the SOMIT Study

Procedures
Ultrasound of abdomen and pelvis
CT scanning of abdomen and pelvis
Gastroscopy or double contrast barium swallowing
Flexible sigmoidoscopy or rectoscopy followed by barium enema or colonoscopy
Hemoccult, sputum cytology, tumor markers (CEA, αFP, CA 125)
Mammography and pap smear in women
Transabdominal ultrasound of the prostate and PSA in men

Abbreviations: SOMIT, Extensive Screening for Occult Malignancy in Idiopathic venous Thromboembolism; CT, computed tomography; PSA, Prostate-specific Antigen.

blood count, liver and renal function tests, serum protein electrophoresis, and chest X ray. If these were negative, patients underwent additional diagnostic evaluation consisting of abdominal and pelvic ultrasound, and laboratory markers for malignancy, including serum levels of carcinoembryonic antigen, prostate-specific antigen, and CA-125. The routine clinical evaluation was performed in 864 patients and revealed malignancy in 34 (3.9%). Among the remaining 830 patients, the additional diagnostic work-up revealed 13 further malignancies. During follow-up, cancer became symptomatic in 14 patients who were negative for cancer at screening (sensitivity of the additional diagnostic work-up was 48%). Malignancies that were identified by the additional diagnostic work-up were early stage in 61% of cases compared with 14% in cases occurring during follow-up. Most patients with occult cancer had idiopathic VTE and were older than 70 years. This study found that a limited diagnostic work-up for occult cancer has the capacity to identify approximately one half of the malignancies, which were mostly at an early stage.

We have recently conducted a multicenter randomized trial (the Extensive Screening for Occult Malignancy in Idiopathic venous Thromboembolism (SOMIT) study) (19)[c] among apparently cancer-free patients with symptomatic idiopathic VTE. These patients were randomized either to the strategy of extensive screening for occult cancer (Table 2) or to no further testing. Patients had a two-year follow-up evaluation. Of the 201 patients, 99 were allocated to the extensive screening group and 102 to no further testing. In 13 patients (13.1%), the extensive screening strategy identified occult cancer [mostly detected by computed tomography (CT) scanning]. In the extensive screening group, a single (1.0%) malignancy became apparent during follow-up, whereas in the control group, a total of 10 (9.8%) malignancies become symptomatic. Overall, malignancies identified in the extensive screening group were at an earlier stage, and the mean delay to diagnosis was reduced from 11.6 to 1.0 months. Cancer-related mortality occurred in 2 of the 99 patients in the extensive screening group versus 4 (3.9%) of the 102 control patients. A selective diagnostic work-up is capable of identifying most cancers, whose earlier detection is likely to be associated with improved treatment possibilities and thus prognosis.

The data of the SOMIT trial were also used to perform a decision analysis. Tests in the extensive screening battery were divided into several possible strategies, and the number of detected cancers as well as the number of patients investigated further for an eventually benign condition were calculated for each strategy. Also, the total costs for each strategy and for each detected cancer were determined. The strategy, which included CT

[c] Ref. 19 is a prospective evaluation showing that extensive screening procedures are able to identify most of hidden cancers, whose early detection is likely to be associated with improved treatment possibilities and thus prognosis.

scan of abdomen and pelvis with or without mammography and/or sputum cytology, was found most useful and cost-effective (20).

Although data from either study do not conclusively demonstrate that early diagnosis ultimately prolongs survival, the collective observations make such a beneficial effect likely. The early discovery of cancer, which might mean identification of the disease at a stage more easily treated, could improve outcomes.

Recently, Shutgens et al. reported that high D-dimer concentrations (>4000 μg/L) at presentation of VTE or after four days of treatment are indicators of an increased probability of overt or occult form of cancer, especially among patients under 60 years of age. These results argue for further investigations to confirm this observation and to evaluate the possible cost-effectiveness of screening for occult malignancy patients with initially high and/or persistently high D-dimer levels (21).

FUTURE PROSPECTS

A step forward in this challenging field would be to implement an extensive screening strategy, using the minimum possible number of diagnostic procedures, to identify the vast majority of hidden cancers. These tests could be selected from those that have given the best yields in previous studies. Investigations are already underway to test the effect of performing CT scans of the thorax, abdomen, and pelvis in addition to, for example, mammography in women on cancer identification at baseline and on its impact on cancer-related mortality.

Following the identification of the "ideal" set of screening tests, another question will arise: are all patients with idiopathic VTE at the same risk for occult cancer? It may be most reasonable to direct extensive screening procedures to subgroups of patients considered most at risk for occult cancer according to the findings of available studies. In fact, since extensive screening procedures are costly and are associated with some discomfort (waiting list, minor test-related side effects, and emotional distress), a refinement of the definition of subgroups of idiopathic VTE patients with a higher risk of having occult cancer could be of clinical value. For example, it may be reasonable to recommend extensive procedures to patients with recurrent idiopathic VTE or bilateral idiopathic VTE. Another group of clinical interest in this setting is of patients 60 or greater years in age, following an episode of idiopathic VTE, because the risk of cancer in the follow-up of patients with idiopathic VTE increases with age and is substantial over 60 years of age. Conversely, younger patients with idiopathic VTE could undergo extensive screening procedures for cancer identification if additional predictors are present, such as a high D-dimer level. All these very interesting topics have to be confirmed in appropriate prospective evaluations.

CONCLUSION

The clinical relationship between cancer and VTE has been conclusively demonstrated.

The observation that a thrombotic event, especially in its idiopathic presentation, could be a harbinger of a yet undisclosed cancer has generated a long-standing debate related to the usefulness of performing screening tests to detect the neoplasm. Recent prospective studies have demonstrated that extensive screening for cancer identification is able to identify most occult cancers at baseline. Because extensive screening is associated with some morbidity as well as high costs, it could be widely recommended only if it clearly has a favorable impact on cancer outcomes. The usefulness of early cancer identification through extensive screening is still under evaluation, since a benefit in survival has not yet been adequately addressed. Further well-designed prospective clinical trials are necessary to define the value of screening in its impact on cancer related mortality.

REFERENCES

1. Prandoni P, Falange A, Piccioli A. Cancer and venous thromboembolism. Lancet Onc 2005; 6:401–410.
2. Otten HM, Prints MH. Venous thromboembolism and occult malignancy. Thromb Res 2001; 102:V187–V194.
3. Aderka D, Brown A, Zelikovski A, Pinkhas J. Idiopathic deep vein thrombosis in an apparently healthy patient as a premonitory sign of occult cancer. Cancer 1986; 57:1846–1849.
4. Prandoni P, Lensing AWA, Buller HR, et al. Deep vein thrombosis and the incidence of subsequent symptomatic cancer. N Engl J Med 1992; 327:1128–1133.
5. Ahmed Z, Mohuddin Z. Deep vein thrombosis as a predictor of cancer. Angiology 1996; 47:261–265.
6. Monreal M, Fernandez-Liamazares J, Perandreu J, et al. Occult cancer in patients with venous thromboembolism: which patients, which cancers. Thromb Haemost 1997; 78:1316–1318.
7. Hettiarachi RJK, Lok J, Prins MH, et al. Undiagnosed malignancy in patients with deep vein thrombosis. Cancer 1998; 83:180–185.
8. Rajan R, Levine M, Gent M, et al. The occurrence of subsequent malignancy in patients presenting with deep vein thrombosis: results from an historical cohort study. Thromb Haemost 1998; 79:19–22.
9. Shulman S, Lindmarker P. Incidence of cancer after prophylaxis with warfarin against recurrent venous thromboembolism. N Engl J Med 2000; 342:1953–1958.
10. Bura A, Cailleux N, Bienvenu B, et al. Incidence and prognosis of cancer associated with bilateral venous thrombosis: a prospective study of 103 patients. J Thromb Haemost 2004; 2:441–444.
11. Sorensen HT, Mellemkjaer L, Olsen, et al. The risk of a diagnosis of cancer after primary deep-venous thrombosis or pulmonary embolism. N Engl J Med 1998; 338:1169–1173.
12. Baron JA, Gridley G, Nyren G, Linet M. Venous thromboembolism and cancer. Lancet 1998; 351:1077–1080.
13. Murchison JT, Wylie L, Stockton DL. Excess risk of cancer in patients with primary venous thromboembolism: a national, population-based cohort study. Br J Cancer 2004; 91:92–95.
14. White RH, Chew HK, Zhou H, et al. Incidence of venous thromboembolism in the year before the diagnosis of cancer in 528,693 adults. Arch Intern Med 2005; 165:1782–1787.
15. Sorensen HT, Pedersen L, Mellemkjaer L, et al. The risk of a second cancer after hospitalization for venous thromboembolism. Br J Cancer 2005; 93:838–841.
16. Sorensen HT, Mellemkjaer L, Olsen JH, Baron JA. Prognosis of cancer associated venous thromboembolism. N Engl J Med 2000; 343:1846–1850.
17. Piccioli A, Prandoni P. Screening for occult cancer in patients with idiopathic venous thromboembolism: yes. J Thromb Haemost 2003; 1:2271–2272.
18. Monreal M, Lensing AWA, Prins MH, et al. Screening for occult cancer in patients with acute deep vein thrombosis or pulmonary embolism. J Thromb Haemost 2004; 2:876–881.
19. Piccioli A, Lensing AWA, Prins MH, et al. Extensive screening for occult malignant disease in idiopathic venous thromboembolism. J Thromb haemost 2004; 2:884–889.
20. Di Nisio M, Otten HM, Piccioli A, et al. Decision analysis for cancer screening in idiopathic venous thromboembolism. J Thromb Haemost 2005; 3:2391–2396.
21. Shutgens RE, Beckers MM, Haas FJ, Biemsa DH. The predictive value of D-dimer measurements for cancer in patients with deep vein thrombosis. Haematologica 2005; 90:214–219.

11

Prothrombotic Mutations and Cancer-Associated Venous Thrombosis

J. W. Blom
Department of Public Health and Primary Care, Leiden University Medical Center, Leiden, The Netherlands

C. J. M. Doggen
Department of Clinical Epidemiology, Leiden University Medical Center, Leiden, The Netherlands

F. R. Rosendaal
Department of Clinical Epidemiology, Hemostasis and Thrombosis Research Center, Leiden University Medical Center, Leiden, The Netherlands

- Factor V Leiden and prothrombin 20210A cause a two- to threefold increased risk of venous thrombosis in cancer patients.
- The overall absolute risk for cancer patients with factor V Leiden or prothrombin 20210A is 1% to 4 % per year.
- Screening for prothrombotic mutations may well be beneficial for cancer patients with a high risk of venous thrombosis; the cancers with the highest risk will be associated with the lowest number to screen.
- Prothrombotic mutations cause an increased risk of venous thrombosis of the arm in combination with a central venous catheter.

INTRODUCTION

Venous thrombosis has an incidence in the general population of 1 to 3 per 1000 per year (1). Venous thrombosis mostly manifests in the lower extremities and when migrating to the lungs, as pulmonary embolism. Other, more rare locations are the upper extremities, mesenteric veins, retinal veins, and cerebral sinus. For cancer patients, the incidence is much higher than in the general population, and depends on the type and stage of cancer and cancer treatment. In general, the risk of venous thrombosis in cancer patients is approximately seven times increased compared to the general population, while for patients with recently diagnosed cancer, the risk is even higher (2). Cumulative incidences vary from 6% to 10% in the first year after diagnosis (3,4).

The blood coagulation system is controlled by a combination of procoagulant and anticoagulant factors. An imbalance in the procoagulant and anticoagulant factors can cause either hemorrhagic or thrombotic disease. Several hereditary risk factors for venous thrombosis have been identified in the last few decades. The first hereditary disturbances in the b alance between procoagulant and anticoagulant factors were discovered in the 1960s; i.e., a deficiency in antithrombin, followed by the finding of protein C and S deficiency in the 1980s. Many mutations in the genes encoding for these proteins have been identified (5,6) that cause an imbalance in the coagulation system due to a decrease in anticoagulant proteins. In 1994, the factor V Leiden mutation, causing partial resistance of factor V to the inactivating effects of activated protein C, was identified (7). Approximately 5% of the Caucasian general population carries this mutation. The risk of venous thrombosis is three- to eightfold increased for carriers compared to noncarriers. The prothrombin 20210A mutation, identified in 1996, is associated with elevated prothrombin levels and increases the risk of venous thrombosis twofold (8). Two percent of the general population, again restricted to Caucasians, carry this mutation. The factor V Leiden mutation as well as the prothrombin 20210A mutation cause an imbalance toward the procoagulant system. Since the discovery of these genetic factors associated with venous thrombosis, more genetic factors have been described of which an overview is given by Bezemer and Rosendaal [Bezemer ID, Rosendaal FR. Predictive genetic variants for venous thrombosis: what's new? Scmin Hematol 2007; 44:85–92]. Antithrombin deficiency, protein C and S deficiency, factor V Leiden, and prothrombin 20210A, and the associated risk of venous thrombosis have been studied in cancer patients. The prevalences of these genetic factors in cancer patients are equivalent to the prevalences in the general population. Apart from these risk factors for venous thrombosis, the risk of venous thrombosis associated with *MTHFR C677T* mutation and the factor XIII Val34Leu polymorphism has been studied in cancer patients. *MTHFR C677T* has a prevalence of homozygous carriership of approximately 10% (9) in the general population. *MTHFR C677T* is associated with increased levels of homocysteine. Hyperhomocysteinemia increases the risk of venous thrombosis. However, *MTHFR C677T* is at most a weak risk factor for venous thrombosis (10) [Bezemer ID, Doggen CJ, Vos HL, Rosendaal FR. No association between the common MTHFR 677C->T polymorphism and venous thrombosis: results from the MEGA study. Arch Intern Med 2007; 167:497–501] . Factor XIII Val34Leu has a prevalence of 25% to 30% in the general population and has been found to have a protective effect (11). Factor XIII is involved in stabilizing the fibrin clot during the process of coagulation, and this mutation is associated with increased activity of factor XIII, leading to thinner fibrin fibers and less-stable clots.

Venous thrombosis is often caused by the presence and interaction of several risk factors (12). Clinical studies have investigated the magnitude of the risk of venous thrombosis in patients with cancer and a prothrombotic mutation compared to patients with cancer without hereditary risk factors for venous thrombosis. Determination of the magnitude of this risk may identify high-risk groups that may benefit from prophylactic anticoagulant therapy. In this chapter, the literature on the risk of venous thrombosis in cancer patients with prothrombotic mutations is summarized and a clinical inference is formulated.

RISK OF VENOUS THROMBOSIS IN CANCER PATIENTS WITH PROTHROMBOTIC MUTATIONS

In 1984, a first case report described pulmonary embolism in a patient with acute myeloid leukemia and antithrombin deficiency (13). Since then, other case reports of venous thrombosis in patients with cancer and prothrombotic mutations have been published (14–16).

Thereafter, several cohort and case–control studies on patients with cancer and prothrombotic mutations have been published. This review summarizes the results of studies in which the magnitude of the (relative) risk to develop venous thrombosis for patients with cancer and prothrombotic mutations is compared to cancer patients without a mutation. Factor V Leiden was the most-often evaluated prothrombotic mutation (Table 1), followed by the prothrombin 20210A mutation (Table 2) and other mutations, such as factor XIII, Val34Leu, and *MTHFR C677T* (Table 3).

Deep venous thrombosis of the leg or arm and pulmonary embolism was the most common endpoint, although in a few studies, more unusual locations were included, such as thrombosis in the portal vein, mesenteric thrombosis, and cerebral sinus thrombosis. All studies reported symptomatic deep venous thrombosis, mostly objectively diagnosed.

Most studies gave odds ratios (ORs) for cancer patients with a prothrombotic mutation compared to cancer patients without a mutation. ORs were calculated as an approximation of relative risks. The 95% confidence intervals (CIs) were wide in almost all studies due to the small numbers of patients.

ORs for factor V Leiden in cancer patients compared to cancer patients without factor V Leiden varied mostly from 0.4 to 6.9 (Table 1), with a Mantel-Haenszel pooled OR of 2.2 (OR 2.2, 95% CI: 1.2–3.9). One cohort study including only patients with hematological cancers with a small number of venous thrombotic events, including post-mortem diagnosed events, reported an OR of 21.3 (95% CI: 1.0–429.5) (18), and a study with patients with venous thrombosis of the arm reported an OR of 20.0 (95% CI: 1.5–273.7) (24). Including these studies leads to a pooled OR of 2.7 (OR 2.7, 95% CI: 1.6–4.5).

Cancer patients carrying the prothrombin 20210A mutation had ORs varying from 0.7 to 2.4 compared to cancer patients without the mutation (Table 2). The Mantel-Haenszel pooled OR is 2.1 (OR 2.1, 95% CI: 1.0–4.4).

Although the *MTHFR C677T* mutation is at most associated with a minor overall increase in risk of venous thrombosis, a few studies investigated the association of this mutation with venous thrombosis in cancer patients. No increased risk has been found for cancer patients with the mutation, compared to cancer patients without the mutation (Table 3). The same applies for the factor XIII Val34Leu mutation, where no decrease in risk has been found.

Prothrombotic mutations also cause an increased risk of venous thrombosis of the arm in combination with a central venous catheter (CVC) (Table 4).

In Chapter 15, the risk of venous thrombosis for cancer patients with a CVC will be further discussed. The ORs for cancer patients with a CVC and a prothrombotic mutation compared to cancer patients with a CVC but without a mutation varied from 0.6 to 7.7 (Table 4). The Mantel-Haenszel pooled OR shows a four times increased risk (OR 5.2, 95% CI: 3.0–9.0).

CONCLUSION

Factor V Leiden and prothrombin 20210A cause an increase in the risk of venous thrombosis in cancer patients. Due to the low prevalence of patients with cancer and a prothrombotic mutation, few studies have reported on this issue, and CIs of the ORs are wide. However, when ORs are pooled, a two- to threefold increased risk of venous thrombosis is found for patients with either the factor V Leiden or the prothrombin 20210A mutation.

For clinical decision making regarding prophylactic anticoagulant treatment, it is important to estimate the absolute risk of venous thrombosis in cancer patients. Assuming a six- to sevenfold increased risk of venous thrombosis (2,35) for cancer patients compared

(*Text continued on page 164.*)

Table 1 Studies Reporting OR for Venous Thrombosis in Cancer Patients with Factor V Leiden Compared to Cancer Patients without Factor V Leiden

Study	Type of study	Type of cancer	No. of patients with FVL/with VT	No. of patients with FVL/without VT	Type of thrombosis	OR (95% confidence interval)
Otterson et al., 1996 (17)	Cohort	All types of cancer	2/14	17/328	DVT	3.05 (0.63–14.73)
Chiusolo et al., 2000[a] (18)	Cohort	Hematological cancer + chemotherapy /stem cell	1/4	1/65	DVT, PE	21.3 (1.0–429.5)[b]
Pihusch et al., 2002 (19)	Cohort	Gastrointestinal	5/28	7/147	DVT, PE	4.4 (1.3–14.9)
Ravin et al., 2002 (20)	Case–control	Gynecologic	2/40	5/34	DVT, PE	0.4 (0.1–2.5)
Ramacciotti et al., 2003 (21)	Cohort	All types of cancer	1/64	4/147	DVT, PE	0.6 (0.06–5.35)
Kennedy et al., 2004 (22)	Case–control	Nonhematological cancer	5/101	3/101	DVT, PE, unusual locations	1.7 (0.3–10.7)
Eroglu et al., 2005 (23)	Case–control	All types of cancer	9/30	4/68	DVT, PE	6.9 (1.8–23.9)[b]
Blom et al., 2005 (2)	Case–control	All types of cancer	16/178	1/29	DVT, PE	2.2 (0.3–17.8)
Blom et al., 2005[a] (24)	Case–control	All types of cancer	3/12	1/29	DVT arm ± PE	20.0 (1.5–273.7)
Mandala et al., 2006 (25)	Nested case–control	Gastrointestinal	2/60	1/30	DVT, PE, unusual locations	0.95 (0.08–10.91)

[a]Factor V Leiden and prothrombin G20210A studied together.
[b]OR not mentioned in publication but calculated by author (by using data from original publication).
Abbreviations: VT, venous thrombosis; DVT, deep venous thrombosis; PE, pulmonary embolism; FVL, factor V Leiden; OR, odds ratio.

Table 2 Studies Reporting OR for Venous Thrombosis in Cancer Patients with Prothrombin 20210A Compared to Cancer Patients without Prothrombin 20210A

Study	Type of study	Type of cancer	No. of patients with PT/with VT	No. of patients with PT/without VT	Type of thrombosis	OR (95% confidence interval)
Pihusch et al., 2002 (19)	Cohort	Gastrointestinal	3/31	7/154	DVT, PE[a]	2.4 (0.6–9.9)[a]
Ramacciotti et al., 2003 (21)	Cohort	All types of cancer	1/64	2/147	DVT, PE	1.2 (0.10–13.13)
Kennedy et al., 2004 (22)	Case–control	Nonhematological cancer	5/101	0/101	DVT, PE, unusual locations	∞
Mandala et al., 2006 (25)	Nested case–control	Gastrointestinal	2/30	5/60	DVT, PE, unusual locations	0.74 (0.14–4.08)

[a]OR not mentioned in publication but calculated by author (by using data from original publication).
Abbreviations: VT, venous thrombosis; DVT, deep venous thrombosis; PE, pulmonary embolism; PT, prothrombin 20210A; OR, odds ratio.

Table 3 Other Mutations: OR for Venous Thrombosis in Cancer Patients with Mutation Compared with Cancer Patients without Mutation

Study	Type of study	Mutation	Type of cancer	No. of patients with mutation/ with VT	No. of patients with mutation/ without VT	Type of thrombosis	OR (95% confidence interval)
Ramaciotti et al., 2003 (21)	Cohort	FXIII Val34Leu	All types of cancer	19/64	42/147	DVT, PE	1.0 (0.55–2.01)
Ramaciotti et al., 2003 (21)	Cohort	*MTHFR C677T*	All types of cancer	34/64	89/147	DVT, PE	0.8 (0.40–1.38)
Mandala et al., 2006 (25)	Nested case-control	*MTHFR C677T*	Gastro-intestinal	2/28	15/147	DVT, PE, unusual locations	1.5 (0.3–6.9)[a]

[a]OR not mentioned in publication but calculated by author (by using data from original publication).

Abbreviations: VT, venous thrombosis; DVT, deep venous thrombosis; PE, pulmonary embolism; OR, odds ratio.

Table 4 Patients wWith CVC: OR for Venous Thrombosis in Cancer Patients with CVC and Mutation Compared to Cancer Patients with CVC without Mutation

Study	Type study	Type of cancer of	Mutation	No. of patients with mutation/ with VT	No. of patients without mutation/ without VT	Type of thrombosis	OR (or relative risk) (95% confidence interval)
Sifontes et al., 1997 (26)	Case–control	All types of cancer, mainly hematological	FVL	1/32	0/35	DVT, PE, unusual locations	∞
Fijnheer et al., 2002 (27)	Cohort	Hematological cancer	FVL	7/33	6/244	DVT arm	RR 7.7 (3.3–17.9)
Knoefler et al., 2003 (28)	Cohort	All types of cancer	FVL	3/11	3/56	DVT	OR 6.6 (1.1–38.7)
Mandala et al., 2004 (29)	Nested case –control	Breast cancer	FVL	5/25	2/50	DVT arm	OR 6.1 (1.1–34.3)
Ratcliffe et al., 1999 (30)	Cohort	All types of cancer	FVL	1/01	2/76	DVT arm and leg	OR 4.1 (0.3–50.0)
Mitchell et al., 2003 (31)	Cohort	Hematological cancer	FVL	0/3	2/62	DVT, unusual locations	OR 0
Knöfler et al., 1999 (32)	Cohort	All types of cancer	FVL, PT, protein C deficiency	5/8	7/64	DVT arm	OR 13.6 (2.7–69.6)[a]
Wermes et al., 1999 (33)	Cohort	All types of cancer	FVL, PT, protein C and S or antithrombin deficiency, *MTHFR C677T*	4/10	24/127	DVT arm	$OR_{overall}$ 2.9 (0.7–11.4)[a]
				4/18	2/55		OR_{ALL} 7.6 (1.3–44.4)[a]
Tesselaar et al., 2004 (34)	Cohort	All types of cancer	FVL, PT	1/18	7/83	DVT arm	OR 0.6 (0.1–5.5)

[a]OR not mentioned in publication but calculated by author (by using data from original publication).
Abbreviations: VT, venous thrombosis; DVT, deep venous thrombosis; PE, pulmonary embolism; ALL, acute lymphatic leukemia; FVL, factor V Leiden; PT, prothrombin 20210A; CVC, central venous catheter; OR, odds ratio.

to noncancer patients, for cancer patients with factor V Leiden or prothrombin 20210A, this means that the risk is approximately 12 to 21 times increased compared to noncancer patients without these mutations. This is completely in line with a large population-based case–control study that reported the OR for venous thrombosis in cancer patients with the factor V Leiden mutation or the prothrombin 20210A mutation compared to individuals with neither cancer or a mutation [(OR 12.1, 95% CI: 1.6–88.1) and (OR 17.5, 95% CI: 1.2–252.0), respectively] (2). With a baseline risk of venous thrombosis of 1 to 3 per 1000 per year (1), the overall absolute risk for cancer patients with factor V Leiden or prothrombin 20210A will be 12 to 36 per 1000 per year.

TO SCREEN OR NOT TO SCREEN

The risk of venous thrombosis in cancer patients varies with the type and stage of cancer, and therapy (2). Likewise, cancer patients with prothrombotic mutations such as factor V Leiden or prothrombin 20210A mutation have an increased risk of venous thrombosis compared to cancer patients without these mutations. Screening for prothrombotic mutations in cancer patients, and subsequent prophylactic treatment, could be a beneficial strategy to prevent morbidity and mortality due to venous thrombosis. To evaluate this screening strategy, the number needed to treat (NNT) and subsequently number needed to screen (NNS) (36) can be calculated. The NNT is the number of patients whom we need to treat to prevent one case of thrombosis. The NNS is the number of patients we need to screen to prevent one case of venous thrombosis. We assume that treatment with anticoagulants reduces risk by 80% (37). For those with cancer and factor V Leiden, the incidence lies between 12 and 36 per 1000, which will be reduced to 2 to 7 per 1000; i.e., if we give thromboprophylaxis to 1000 patients with cancer and factor V Leiden, we will prevent 10 to 29 events. This implies that to prevent 1 case (NNT), we need to treat 34 to 100 patients with factor V Leiden and cancer. Since factor V Leiden has a prevalence of 5%, we will need to screen 20 times as many patients, i.e., the NNS is 680 to 2000. In populations with a higher prevalence of factor V Leiden, the NNS will be reduced. Furthermore, simultaneous screening of factor V Leiden and prothrombin 20210A decreases the NNS.

To estimate the incidence of venous thrombosis in cancer patients with a prothrombotic mutation, we used an OR for venous thrombosis in all cancer patients (2,35). These were patients with all types of cancer. For certain types of cancer or different stages of cancer, the OR for venous thrombosis will vary, and the cancers with the highest ORs will be associated with the lowest number to screen. Lung cancer and hematological cancer have been reported to have a high risk of venous thrombosis, with ORs of 22.2 and 28.0, respectively, compared to noncancer patients (2). This OR is three to four times higher than the overall OR for all types of cancer, and presumably this will lead to a three to four times decreased NNT and NNS.

The NNS would be higher than the above-mentioned NNS for other prothrombotic mutations, due to the lower prevalence of these mutations and the lower associated risk of venous thrombosis (5,6). However, if one combines the tests into one screening test, then the NNS would be lower. Due to the high prevalence of factor V Leiden and prothrombin 20210A and the high associated risks of venous thrombosis, these genetic risk factors will be most crucial in the calculation of the NNS.

In 1968, Wilson and Jungner formulated 10 criteria for screening for disease that should be met before a screening program can be offered to patients (38):

1. The condition sought should be an important health problem
2. There should be an accepted treatment for patients with recognized disease

3. Facilities for diagnosis and treatment should be available
4. There should be a recognizable latent or early symptomatic stage
5. There should be a suitable test or examination
6. The test should be acceptable to the population
7. The natural history of the condition, including development from latent to declared disease, should be adequately understood
8. There should be an agreed policy on whom to treat as patients
9. The cost of case-finding (including diagnosis and treatment of patients diagnosed) should be economically balanced in relation to possible expenditure on medical care as a whole
10. Case-finding should be a continuing process and not a "once and for all" project

Venous thrombosis in cancer patients causes serious morbidity and mortality. The risk of venous thrombosis is increased in cancer patients, and survival for cancer patients with venous thrombosis is decreased compared to cancer patients without venous thrombosis (39,40). Prevention of venous thrombosis in patients with a prothrombotic mutation can be achieved by prophylactic treatment with anticoagulant therapy, with a success rate of approximately 80%. However, this treatment can be harmful due to the risk of bleeding. Cancer patients have an increased risk of major bleeding when using oral anticoagulants compared to noncancer patients. A risk of major bleeding, such as fatal or nonfatal intracranial hemorrhage, and intra-articular or retro-peritoneal hemorrhage, in cancer patients using oral anticoagulant therapy, has been described, and it varies from 5% to 12% (41,42). Identifying patients with a prothrombotic mutation is feasible due to the availability of laboratory tests, based on polymerase chain reaction methods (43). Earlier research has shown that knowledge about the presence of a prothrombotic mutation has few negative psychological consequences (44).

Certain subgroups of cancer patients, such as lung cancer patients, patients with hematological cancer, and patients with an advanced stage of cancer have a highly increased risk of venous thrombosis and therefore a low NNT and NNS. Screening for prothrombotic mutations may well be beneficial in these patient groups. Clinical studies into the risk–benefit ratio of the treatment need to be done as well as a cost-effectiveness analysis for screening for prothrombotic mutations in cancer patients.

REFERENCES

1. Nordström M, Lindblad B, Bergqvist D, Kjellström T. A prospective study of the incidence of deep-vein thrombosis within a defined urban population. J Intern Med 1992; 232:155–160.
2. Blom JW, Doggen CJM, Osanto S, Rosendaal FR. Malignancies, prothrombotic mutations, and the risk of venous thrombosis. JAMA 2005; 293:715–722.
3. Ottinger H, Belka C, Kozole G, et al. Deep venous thrombosis and pulmonary artery embolism in high-grade non-Hodgkin's lymphoma: incidence, causes and prognostic relevance. Eur J Haematol 1995; 54:186–194.
4. Blom JW, Osanto S, Rosendaal FR. High risk of venous thrombosis in patients with pancreatic cancer: a cohort study of 202 patients. Eur J Cancer 2006; 42:410–414.
5. Lane DA, Mannucci PM, Bauer KA, et al. Inherited thrombophilia: part 1. Thromb Haemost 1996; 76:651–662.
6. Lane DA, Mannucci PM, Bauer KA, et al. Inherited thrombophilia: Part 2. Thromb Haemost 1996; 76:824–834.
7. Koster T, Rosendaal FR, de Ronde H, Briët E, Vandenbroucke JP, Bertina RM. Venous thrombosis due to poor anticoagulant response to activated protein C: Leiden Thrombophilia Study. Lancet 1993; 342:1503–1506.

8. Poort SR, Rosendaal FR, Reitsma PH, Bertina RM. A common genetic variation in the 3'-untranslated region of the prothrombin gene is associated with elevated plasma prothrombin levels and an increase in venous thrombosis. Blood 1996; 88:3698–3703.
9. Rozen R. Genetic modulation of homocysteinemia. Semin Thromb Hemost 2000; 26:255–261.
10. den Heijer M, Rosendaal FR, Blom HJ, Gerrits WB, Bos GM. Hyperhomocysteinemia and venous thrombosis: a meta-analysis. Thromb Haemost 1998; 80:874–877.
11. Wells PS, Anderson JL, Scarvelis DK, Doucette SP, Gagnon F. Factor XIII Val34Leu variant is protective against venous thromboembolism: a HuGE review and meta-analysis. Am J Epidemiol 2006; 164:101–109.
12. Rosendaal FR. Venous thrombosis: a multicausal disease. Lancet 1999; 353:1167–1173.
13. Sheehan T, O'Donnell JR. Acute myeloid leukaemia in a patient with congenital antithrombin III deficiency. J Clin Pathol 1984; 37:838–839.
14. Weitz IC, Israel VK, Liebman HA. Tamoxifen-associated venous thrombosis and activated protein C resistance due to factor V Leiden. Cancer 1997; 79:2024–2027.
15. Deitcher SR, Erban JK, Limentani SA. Acquired free protein S deficiency associated with multiple myeloma: a case report. Am J Hematol 1996; 51:319–323.
16. Conlan MG, Mosher DF. Concomitant chronic lymphocytic leukemia, acute myeloid leukemia, and thrombosis with protein C deficiency. Case report and review of the literature. Cancer 1989; 63:1398–1401.
17. Otterson GA, Monahan BP, Harold N, Steinberg SM, Frame JN, Kaye FJ. Clinical significance of the FV:Q506 mutation in unselected oncology patients. Am J Med 1996; 101:406–412.
18. Chiusolo P, Sica S, De Stefano V, Casorelli I, Laurenti L, Leone G. Incidence of factor V Leiden and prothrombin G20210A in patients submitted to stem cell transplantation. Haematologica 2000; 85:670–671.
19. Pihusch R, Danzl G, Scholz M, et al. Impact of thrombophilic gene mutations on thrombosis risk in patients with gastrointestinal carcinoma. Cancer 2002; 94:3120–3126.
20. Ravin AJ, Edwards RP, Krohn A, Kelley JR, Christopherson WA, Roberts JM. The factor V Leiden mutation and the risk of venous thromboembolism in gynecologic oncology patients. Obstet Gynecol 2002; 100:1285–1289.
21. Ramacciotti E, Wolosker N, Puech-Leao P, et al. Prevalence of factor V Leiden, FII G20210A, FXIII Val34Leu morphisms in cancer patients with and without venous thrombosis. Thromb Res 2003; 109:171–174.
22. Kennedy M, Andreescu AC, Greenblatt MS, et al. Factor V Leiden, prothrombin 20210A and the risk of venous thrombosis among cancer patients. Br J Haematol 2005; 128:386–388.
23. Eroglu A, Kurtman C, Ulu A, Cam R, Akar N. Factor V Leiden and PT G20210A mutations in cancer patients with and without venous thrombosis. J Thromb Haemost 2005; 3:1323–1324.
24. Blom JW, Doggen CJM, Osanto S, Rosendaal FR. Old and new risk factors for upper extremity deep venous thrombosis. J Thromb Haemost 2005; 3:2471–2478.
25. Mandala M, Falanga A, Cremonesi M, et al. The extension of disease is associated to an increased risk of venous thromboembolism in patients with gastrointestinal carcinoma. Thromb Haemost 2006; 95:752–754.
26. Sifontes MT, Nuss R, Hunger SP, Wilimas J, Jacobson LJ, Manco-Johnson MJ. The factor V Leiden mutation in children with cancer and thrombosis. Br J Haematol 1997; 96:484–489.
27. Fijnheer R, Paijmans B, Verdonck LF, Nieuwenhuis HK, Roest M, Dekker AW. Factor V Leiden in central venous catheter-associated thrombosis. Br J Haematol 2002; 118:267–270.
28. Knoefler R, Ludwig K, Kostka H, Kuhlisch E, Siegert G, Suttorp M. The impact of single nucleotide polymorphisms of the thrombin activatable fibrinolysis inhibitor (TAFI) gene on TAFI antigen levels in healthy children and pediatric oncology patients. Semin Thromb Hemost 2003; 29:575–583.
29. Mandala M, Curigliano G, Bucciarelli P, et al. Factor V Leiden and G20210A prothrombin mutation and the risk of subclavian vein thrombosis in patients with breast cancer and a central venous catheter. Ann Oncol 2004; 15:590–593.
30. Ratcliffe M, Broadfoot C, Davidson M, Kelly KF, Greaves M. Thrombosis, markers of thrombotic risk, indwelling central venous catheters and antithrombotic prophylaxis using low-dose warfarin in subjects with malignant disease. Clin Lab Haematol 1999; 21:353–357.

31. Mitchell LG, Andrew M, Hanna K, Abshire T, Halton J, Anderson R. et al. A prospective cohort study determining the prevalence of thrombotic events in children with acute lymphoblastic leukemia and a central venous line who are treated with L-asparaginase: results of the Prophylactic Antithrombin Replacement in Kids with Acute Lymphoblastic Leukemia Treated with Asparaginase (PARKAA) Study. Cancer 2003; 97:508–516.
32. Knöfler R, Siegert E, Lauterbach I, et al. Clinical importance of prothrombotic risk factors in pediatric patients with malignancy—impact of central venous lines. Eur J Pediatr 1999; 158(suppl 3):S147–S150.
33. Wermes C, von Depka PM, Lichtinghagen R, Barthels M, Welte K, Sykora KW. Clinical relevance of genetic risk factors for thrombosis in paediatric oncology patients with central venous catheters. Eur J Pediatr 1999; 158(suppl 3):S143–S146.
34. Tesselaar ME, Ouwerkerk J, Nooy MA, Rosendaal FR, Osanto S. Risk factors for catheter-related thrombosis in cancer patients. Eur J Cancer 2004; 40:2253–2259.
35. Heit JA, Silverstein MD, Mohr DN, Petterson TM, O'Fallon WM, Melton LJ III. Risk factors for deep vein thrombosis and pulmonary embolism: a population-based case-control study. Arch Intern Med 2000; 160:809–815.
36. Rembold CM. Number needed to screen: development of a statistic for disease screening. BMJ 1998; 317:307–312.
37. Lee AY. Management of thrombosis in cancer: primary prevention and secondary prophylaxis. Br J Haematol 2005; 128:291–302.
38. Wilson JMG, Jungner G. Principles and practice of screening for a disease. World Health Organisation, Public Health Papers no.34.1968.
39. Blom JW, Osanto S, Rosendaal FR. The risk of a venous thrombotic event in lung cancer patients: higher risk for adenocarcinoma than squamous cell carcinoma. J Thromb Haemost 2004; 2:1760–1765.
40. Sörensen HT, Melemkjær L, Ölsen JH, Baron JA. Prognosis of cancers associated with venous thromboembolism. N Engl J Med 2000; 343:1846–1850.
41. Prandoni P, Lensing AW, Piccioli A, et al. Recurrent venous thromboembolism and bleeding complications during anticoagulant treatment in patients with cancer and venous thrombosis. Blood 2002; 100:3484–3488.
42. Palareti G, Legnani C, Lee A, et al. A comparison of the safety and efficacy of oral anticoagulation for the treatment of venous thromboembolic disease in patients with or without malignancy. Thromb Haemost 2000; 84:805–810.
43. Gomez E, van der Poel SC, Jansen JH, van der Reijden BA, Lowenberg B. Rapid simultaneous screening of factor V Leiden and G20210A prothrombin variant by multiplex polymerase chain reaction on whole blood. Blood 1998; 91:2208–2209.
44. van Korlaar IM, Vossen CY, Rosendaal FR, et al. Attitudes toward genetic testing for thrombophilia in asymptomatic members of a large family with heritable protein C deficiency. J Thromb Haemost 2005; 3:2437–2444.

12

Who's At Risk for Thrombosis? Approaches to Risk Stratifying Cancer Patients

Maithili V. Rao, Charles W. Francis, and Alok A. Khorana
James P. Wilmot Cancer Center and the Department of Medicine, University of Rochester, Rochester, New York, U.S.A.

- The risk of venous thromboembolism (VTE) varies across cancer subpopulations and over the natural history of the illness, although it is consistently higher in cancer patients when compared to noncancer patients.
- Metastatic disease is independently associated with a 2- to 20-fold increased risk of VTE.
- The highest risk for VTE is at the time of cancer diagnosis or within the first three months after diagnosis; up to 80% of events can occur in this initial period.
- Cancers of the brain, pancreas, stomach, lung, ovary, kidney, and lymphoma have been consistently shown in various series to confer the highest risk of VTE.
- Hospitalization and major surgical intervention further increase the risk of VTE.
- Anticancer therapies, particularly chemotherapy and hormonal therapy, add to the risk of VTE; antiangiogenic agents and red cell and myeloid growth factors may also be associated with an increased risk.
- Cancer patients with febrile neutropenia, concurrent infections, comorbidities, and implanted venous access devices are also at increased risk for VTE.
- The presence of inherited thrombophilia may increase the risk of VTE in cancer patients.
- A prechemotherapy platelet count of $\geq$350,000/mm^3 is a novel risk factor for chemotherapy-associated VTE.
- Risk assessment models that incorporate major risk factors can identify cancer patients at particularly high risk of VTE and are currently in development.

INTRODUCTION

The association of venous thromboembolism (VTE) with cancer has been known for many years (1). Recent estimates suggest that the annual incidence of VTE in the cancer population is 0.5%, compared with 0.1% in the general population (2). The actual frequency is probably even greater, given recent studies showing a rapid increase in incidence starting in the late 1990s (3,4). Cancer patients comprise a heterogeneous group including patients on active therapy, patients undergoing surgery, hospitalized patients, cancer survivors, and patients with terminal illness. The risk of VTE in some of these subgroups is substantially higher than that estimated for the general cancer population. Table 1 lists the established and possible risk factors for cancer-associated VTE. All of these risk factors must be taken into account when assessing risk for individual patients. Further, it is imperative to note that risk factor assessment is a dynamic process and can change rapidly over time based on multiple cancer- and treatment-related factors. This is illustrated in Figure 1, which describes changes in relative risk for a representative cancer patient over the natural course of the disease.

Much of the data regarding risk factors for cancer-associated VTE is derived from population-based case–control studies and retrospective cohort record-linkage studies. Such studies allow for the analysis of large study populations, such as hospital discharge databases and cancer registries, and can help identify risk factors for cancer-associated VTE. However, because patients in these studies are not actively screened for VTE, subclinical VTE may be missed, leading to an underestimation of risk. Also, the data are analyzed

Table 1 Risk Factors for Cancer-Associated VTE

Established risk factors
Older age (3)
Advanced stage of cancer (3,5–10)
Time from diagnosis of cancer (6,7,11–13)
Risk elevated during initial period after diagnosis
Site of cancer (Table 2)
Hospitalization (3,4,14–16)
Recent surgery (16–21)
Cancer therapy (Tables 3 and 4)
Chemotherapy
Hormonal therapy
Antiangiogenesis agents (for arterial TE)
Erythropoietin
Comorbid conditions (3,15)
Infection
Obesity
Renal disease
Pulmonary disease
Other risk factors
Central venous catheters (22–25)
Prothrombotic mutations (7,15,26,27)
Factor V Leiden
Prothrombin gene mutation
Vena cava filters (28–30)
Possible risk factors
Female gender (3)
Race
Elevated in African Americans and lower in Asians (6)
Antiangiogenesis agents (for VTE) (Table 3)
Myeloid growth factors (Table 4)
Elevated prechemotherapy platelet count (31)

Abbreviations: TE, thromboembolism; VTE, venous thromboembolism.

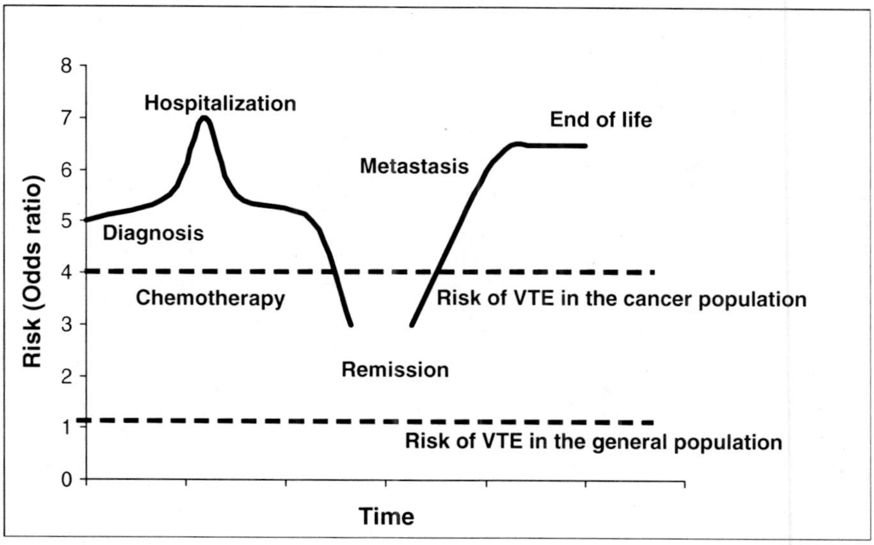

Figure 1 Changes in risk of VTE over the course of the illness in a representative cancer patient. *Abbreviation:* VTE, venous thromboembolism.

retrospectively and may rely on administrative coding without information regarding specific chemotherapy and supportive care agents that may influence the development of VTE. Prospective observational studies, although still not exempt from some of these limitations, enable comprehensive scrutiny of baseline or pretreatment information about patients and have led to identification of unique risk factors predisposing cancer patients to VTE.

In this chapter, we will review data from a variety of population-based studies, data from prospective registries, and toxicity data from clinical trials of anticancer agents to identify cancer patients most at risk for developing VTE. Overall, there are insufficient data on arterial thromboembolism (TE) in cancer patients. Hence our discussion will focus primarily on VTE, although the evidence on arterial TE is presented when available.

DEMOGRAPHICS

Age

In the general population, the incidence of VTE is higher in older patients (32). In a retrospective cohort study of hospitalized neutropenic cancer patients, those aged 65 years or older had a VTE rate of 6.18% per hospitalization compared to 5.1% in those younger than 65 years [odds ratio (OR) 1.23, 95% confidence interval (CI) 1.14–1.33] (3). The risk for arterial events among older patients was even greater (OR 3.0, 95% CI 2.64–3.40). However, in a separate study of all hospitalized cancer patients, there was no association of VTE with age (4).

Gender

Some evidence suggests that VTE in the general population is more common in women, particularly among older subjects (33). Among cancer patients, most studies do not identify gender as a significant predictor of VTE (4–6,31). Among older hospitalized neutropenic cancer patients, women were more likely to develop VTE (5.7% of men vs. 6.6% of women, OR 1.16, 95% CI 1.02–1.31), and the proportion was highest among black women over the age of 65 years (7.7% vs. 6.5% for other women aged ≥65 years; $P = 0.13$) (3). However, in multivariate analysis, this association was not significant.

Race

In the general population, the incidence of VTE is highest among blacks and lowest among Asian-Pacific Islanders (33). The latter may be a reflection of a lower prevalence of inherited genetic thrombophilic states, such as factor V Leiden in Asians as compared to Caucasians. In a retrospective record-linkage analysis of a cohort of 235,149 cancer patients in California, Asian-Pacific Islanders did indeed have a lower risk of VTE than Caucasians (6). This association was statistically significant in patients with prostate, breast, lung, colorectal, pancreatic, and stomach cancer and non-Hodgkin's lymphoma. In this study, the incidence of VTE was similar between Caucasians and African Americans except for a twofold higher risk in uterine cancer and a significantly lower risk of VTE in lung cancer and non-Hodgkin's lymphoma in black patients. In contrast, a large study of hospitalized cancer patients did not identify any racial disparities in the incidence of cancer-associated VTE (4).

STAGE OF CANCER

Multiple studies have shown an increased risk of VTE in cancer patients with advanced stage or metastatic disease. In a population-based case–control study of 3220 patients, including 389 cancer patients, those with distant metastases had a higher risk of VTE (adjusted OR 19.8, 95% CI 2.6–149.1) (7). Linking data from the Cancer Registry and an Anticoagulation Clinic in the Netherlands, the same investigators analyzed a cohort of 66,329 cancer patients (8). Again, patients with distant metastases had a twofold higher incidence of VTE in the first six months after a diagnosis of cancer than patients without metastases [adjusted risk ratio (RR_{adj}): 1.9, 95% CI 1.6–2.3].

Among hospitalized patients admitted to three medical centers, VTE occurred in 5.6% patients with early-stage cancers and in 10.3% patients with advanced disease ($P < 0.005$, OR 1.92, 95% CI 1.21–3.04) (5). Among a subgroup of hospitalized neutropenic cancer patients for whom information regarding presence or absence of metastatic disease was available, VTE was more common in patients with metastatic disease compared to those without metastases (OR 1.23, 95% CI 1.13–1.34) (3). However, in a prospective registry of ambulatory patients receiving chemotherapy, stage of disease was not a significant risk factor for VTE (31). Of note is the point that over 90% of patients in this registry had a performance status of 0 or 1, suggesting that the elevated risk of VTE in patients with metastatic disease may be attributable to poor functional status and immobilization and not simply to the burden of disease.

The association between metastatic disease and increased risk of VTE has also been reported in studies of specific cancers. In a retrospective cohort study of 537 non–small cell lung cancer (NSCLC) patients, those with distant metastases had a sixfold increased risk of VTE [hazard ratio (HR) 6.5, 95% CI 2.6–16.5] (9). Among patients in the California-based cohort study, metastatic disease at the time of cancer diagnosis was the strongest predictor for the development of VTE (6). Compared to patients with localized disease, the relative risk of developing symptomatic VTE was more than 20-fold higher for metastatic melanoma, ninefold higher for metastatic bladder cancer, five- to sixfold higher for metastatic breast or uterine cancer, and three- to fourfold higher for metastatic pancreas, lung, ovarian, and kidney cancer. A separate analysis of 68,142 colorectal cancer patients from the same database reported an increase in the two-year cumulative incidence of VTE from 1.8% in patients with localized disease to 4.7% in patients with metastatic disease ($P < 0.0001$) (10).

TIME AFTER DIAGNOSIS OF CANCER

The risk of VTE is not uniform over the natural history of cancer (Fig. 1) but appears to be highest during the first few months following a diagnosis of cancer. In the population-based study reported by Blom et al., the risk of VTE was highest in the first three months after initial diagnosis of cancer (OR 53.5, 95% CI 8.6–334.3) (7). The risk declined at the end of one year and again after three years, but continued to be increased compared with individuals without cancer (>3 months to ≤1 year: OR 14.3, 95% CI 5.8–35.2; >1 year to ≤3 years: OR 3.6, 95% CI 2.0–6.5). Only after 15 years did the risk subside to levels observed in the general population (OR 1.1, 95% CI 0.6–2.2). In this study, during the first year after diagnosis, 16.9% of patients received chemotherapy, 4.1% received radiotherapy, 23.8% underwent surgery, and an additional 36.6% had a combination of anticancer therapies. Many of these treatment modalities are themselves associated with an increased risk of VTE, and this may partly account for the increased risk observed in the initial period following diagnosis of malignancy. Similarly, in the California database study, VTE rates were higher in the first year of follow-up as compared to the second year (6). Unfortunately, information regarding the use and timing of chemotherapy that could further influence the risk of VTE in this population is not available.

Even in patients on chemotherapy, VTE rates are higher earlier in the course of therapy. In a retrospective review of patients with diffuse large B-cell lymphoma, 82% of VTE events occurred during the first three cycles of chemotherapy (11). Similarly, in patients with transitional cell carcinoma and lung cancer undergoing chemotherapy, the majority of VTE events (77% and 45% respectively) occurred during the first two cycles of therapy (12,13).

SITE OF CANCER

Certain sites of cancer, such as the brain, pancreas, ovary, kidney, stomach, and lung, have been consistently shown to be associated with the highest rates of VTE. However, data from more recent studies suggest that hematological malignancies, particularly myeloma and lymphoma, are also associated with high rates (3,7,11,34). Selected sites of malignancy and their associated risk of VTE are shown in Table 2.

In an analysis of the Medicare discharge database by Levitan et al., the highest incidence of VTE was observed in cancers of the ovary, brain, pancreas, lymphoma, stomach, kidney, leukemia, and colon (14). A similar distribution was observed in another large analysis of hospitalized patients in which the incidence of VTE was highest in patients with pancreatic cancer (4.3%), brain tumors (3.5%), myeloproliferative disorders (2.9%), stomach cancer (2.7%), and lymphoma (2.5%) (4). In the population-based study from the Netherlands, patients with hematological malignancies had the highest risk of VTE (OR 28, 95% CI 4.0–199.7), followed by lung (OR 22.2, 95% CI 3.6–136.1), and gastrointestinal (GI) cancers (OR 20.3, 95% CI 4.9–83.0) (7).

In a retrospective study by Sallah et al., multivariate analysis identified renal (RR 3.1, 95% CI 1.4–6.8), pancreatic (RR 8.8, 95% CI 3.5–22. 4), gastric (RR 3.3, 95% CI 1.3–8.5), and brain cancers (RR 9.0, 95% CI 3.1–26.4) as independent risk factors for

Table 2 Selected Sites of Cancer and Risk of VTE

Site of cancer	Study	OR (95% CI)	With event (%)	Type of study	Comments
Brain					
	Sallah, 2002 (5)	2.21 (0.74–6.59)	15*	Retrospective cohort	Hospitalized patients with solid tumors
	Khorana et al., 2006 (3)	2.23 (1.73–2.87)	9.5[c]		Hospitalized neutropenic cancer patients
	Blom et al., 2005 (7)	6.7 (1.0–45.4)	—	Retrospective case–control	OR in comparison to noncancer patients
Lung					
	Khorana et al., 2005 (31)	1.86 (0.99–3.49)	2.79[b]	Prospective cohort	Ambulatory cancer patients on chemotherapy
	Khorana et al., 2006 (3)	1.29 (1.14–1.46)	7[c]	Retrospective cohort	Hospitalized neutropenic cancer patients
	Blom et al., 2005 (7)	22.2 (3.6–136.1)	—	Retrospective case–control	OR in comparison to noncancer patients
Breast					
	Sallah et al., 2002 (5)	1.24 (0.67–2.31)	9.2	Retrospective cohort	Hospitalized patients with solid tumors
GI					
All GI	Blom et al., 2005 (7)	20.3 (4.9–83.0)	—	Retrospective case–control	OR in comparison to noncancer patients
Stomach/upper GI	Sallah et al., 2002 (5)	1.85 (0.70–4.87)	13[a]	Retrospective cohort	Hospitalized patients with solid tumors
	Khorana et al., 2005 (31)	3.88 (1.43–0.05)	5.62[b]	Prospective cohort	Ambulatory cancer patients on chemotherapy
	Khorana et al., 2006 (3)	1.60 (1.17–2.19)	7.4[c]	Retrospective cohort	Hospitalized neutropenic cancer patients
Pancreas	Sallah et al., 2002 (5)	2.18 (0.89–5.35)	15[a]	Retrospective cohort	Hospitalized patients with solid tumors
	Khorana et al., 2006 (3)	2.80 (2.09–3.76)	12.1[c]	Retrospective cohort	Hospitalized neutropenic cancer patients

Gynecological					
Ovary	Khorana et al., 2006 (3)	1.35 (1.12–1.63)	6.5[c]	Retrospective cohort	Hospitalized neutropenic cancer patients
	Blom et al., 2005 (7)	3.1 (0.6–15.3)	—	Retrospective case–control	OR in comparison to noncancer patients
Uterine/cervical	Khorana et al., 2006 (3)	1.98 (1.59–2.46)	8.96[c]	Retrospective cohort	Hospitalized neutropenic cancer patients
Cervix	Blom et al., 2005 (7)	2.9 (0.3–25.3)	—	Retrospective case–control	OR in comparison to noncancer patients
Genitourinary					
Kidney	Sallah et al., 2002 (5)	3.69 (1.54–8.85)	22[a]	Retrospective cohort	Hospitalized patients with solid tumors
	Blom et al., 2005 (7)	6.2 (0.8–46.5)	—	Retrospective case–control	OR in comparison to noncancer patients
Prostate	Khorana et al., 2006 (3)	1.39 (0.97–2.00)	7.29[c]	Retrospective cohort	Hospitalized neutropenic cancer patients
Hematological malignancies					
All	Blom et al., 2005 (7)	28.0 (4–199.7)	—	Retrospective case–control	OR in comparison to noncancer patients
Lymphoma	Khorana et al., 2005 (31)	1.50 (0.67–3.38)	1.5[a]	Prospective cohort	Ambulatory cancer patients on chemotherapy
	Komrokji et al., 2006 (11)	-	12.8	Retrospective single-institution cohort	DLBCL patients on first-line chemotherapy
	Mohren et al., 2005 (35)	-	7.7		All lymphoma patients

[a]Over median follow-up 26 mo.
[b]Median follow-up 2.4 mo.
[c]Over 8 yr of study.
Abbreviations: OR, odds ratio; CI, confidence interval; DLBCL, diffuse large B-cell lymphoma; VTE, venous thromboembolism; GI, gastrointestinal.

VTE, although this study did not include patients with prostate cancer and hematologic malignancies (5). In the retrospective cohort study of hospitalized neutropenic cancer patients by Khorana et al., the highest proportion of cancers in patients with VTE were pancreatic (12.1%), brain (9.5%), and endometrial or cervical (9%) (3). The highest proportions of cancers in patients with arterial TE were prostate (3.9%), lung (2.8%), bladder (2.8%), colon (2.6%), and leukemia (1.91%). Over one-third of VTE events and nearly half of arterial TE events occurred in patients with non-Hodgkin's lymphoma and leukemia, who constituted over 40% of the study population.

In a prospective observational study of ambulatory cancer patients on chemotherapy, the incidence of VTE again varied significantly by site of cancer ($P = 0.01$). Upper GI cancers (OR 3.88, 95% CI 1.43–10.05), lung cancer (OR 1.86, 95% CI 0.99–3.49), and lymphoma (OR 1.50, 95% CI 0.67–3.38) were independent predictors of VTE (31). However, certain malignancies known to be strongly associated with TE, such as brain tumors, were underrepresented in the study population.

HOSPITALIZATION

Hospitalized cancer patients are at substantially greater risk of developing VTE than noncancer patients (3,4,14). Most studies of cancer-associated VTE restrict themselves to either hospitalized or ambulatory cancer patients. However, the rate of VTE in hospitalized cancer patients is substantially greater than the rate in ambulatory cancer patients, suggesting that hospitalization and acute medical illnesses add to the risk of VTE in this population. Indeed, in a prospective cohort study of 507 cancer patients, inpatient treatment was identified as an independent predictor for VTE (OR 2.34, 95% CI 1.63–3.36, $P \leq 0.0001$) (15). Rates of VTE in hospitalized patients rose to approximately 4% per hospitalization in the late 1990s and were much higher in specific subgroups such as those on chemotherapy or with specific sites of disease (3,4). The American College of Chest Physicians Guidelines considers hospitalized cancer patients to have the "highest" risk of VTE (16).

SURGERY

The increased risk of VTE in the postoperative recovery period is well described in the general patient population. Patients with cancer have a further twofold increased risk of postoperative deep vein thrombosis (DVT) and pulmonary embolism (PE) compared to noncancer patients (17). In a prospective cohort of over 21,000 surgery patients, the presence of cancer was an independent predictor for postoperative VTE (OR 2.4, 95% CI 1.9–3.2) (18). In the American College of Chest Physicians Guidelines, cancer patients undergoing surgery are stratified into the "high" or "highest" risk category (16). The presence of other risk factors such as the type of cancer can further elevate the risk of postoperative VTE. Rates range from 0.16% in the postoperative setting in breast cancer (19) to 2.1% in patients undergoing general, urologic, or gynecologic surgery (20). Factors predictive for postoperative VTE in this latter cohort include age >60 years (OR 2.63, 95% CI 1.21–5.71), previous VTE (OR 5.98, 95% CI 2.13–16.80), advanced cancer (OR 2.68, 95% CI 1.37–5.24), anesthesia lasting more than two hours (OR 4.50, 95% CI 1.06–19.04), and bedrest longer than three days (OR 4.37, 95% CI 2.45–7.78). It should be noted that 40% of the VTE events occurred more than 21 days after surgery. In most studies, VTE events are recorded up to 30 postoperative days, but there is evidence to suggest that the increased risk of VTE in cancer patients can persist up to seven weeks after major surgery (21).

CANCER THERAPY

Chemotherapy

The association of VTE with chemotherapy has been documented in a variety of population-based studies, retrospective analyses, prospective observational studies, and toxicity data from clinical trials. Selected studies of chemotherapy and their associated risk of VTE are listed in Table 3.

In a population-based case–control study of 625 patients with a first VTE and matched controls without VTE, the presence of cancer was associated with a fourfold increased risk of VTE (OR 4.05, 95% CI 1.93–8.52), whereas treatment with cytotoxic or immunosuppressive chemotherapy was associated with a 6.5-fold increase (OR 6.5, 95% CI 2.1–0.2) (36). In a retrospective cohort study reported by Blom et al., patients on chemotherapy had a 2.2-fold increased risk for VTE (RR_{adj} 2.2, 95% CI 1.8–2.7) (8). Similar ORs for chemotherapy have been reported in analyses of retrospective cohorts as well as in a prospective observational study (5,15,47). In a large prospective, multicenter observational study of ambulatory patients starting a new chemotherapy regimen reported by Khorana et al., the overall incidence of VTE was 1.93% over a median follow-up period of 2.4 months (31). This translates into an incidence rate of 0.8%/mo, much greater than the estimated rate of 0.5%/yr (or 0.04%/mo) for the entire cancer population.

Similar conclusions can be derived from toxicity reporting in clinical trials conducted in specific cancer populations. In an analysis of seven consecutive Eastern Cooperative Oncology Group (ECOG) studies of adjuvant therapy in 2673 breast cancer patients, 5.4% of patients receiving adjuvant therapy developed VTE versus 1.6% of patients randomized to observation ($P = 0.0002$) (37). Menopausal status and concurrent tamoxifen use significantly influenced VTE risk in these patients. In a randomized trial of 205 women with stage II breast cancer that compared treatment with either 12 or 36 weeks of chemotherapy, the overall incidence of thrombosis was 6.8%, with all events occurring during the months of active chemotherapy (48). Chemotherapy can also further increase the risk of VTE in the postoperative setting. In a randomized European Organisation for Research and Treatment of Cancer (EORTC) study of over 2500 early stage breast cancer patients, the incidence of VTE within six weeks after surgery was significantly higher among patients assigned to perioperative chemotherapy as compared to those assigned to surgery alone (2.1% vs. 0.8%, $P = 0.004$) (49).

An analysis of data from lung cancer studies showed results similar to those reported for breast cancer. In a retrospective record-linkage study of a cohort of 537 patients newly diagnosed with NSCLC over a 10-year period in the Netherlands, the risk of VTE increased threefold with the initiation of chemotherapy (HR 3.2, 95% CI 2.1–4.3) and continued to increase further with increasing duration of chemotherapy when compared to the period when no chemotherapy was given (9). Numico et al. prospectively recorded vascular events in 108 unresectable NSCLC patients, treated consecutively with cisplatin and gemcitabine (13). Over a median follow-up of 8.7 months, 19 patients developed events (17.6%, 95% CI 10.3–24.8), including 10 arterial events and four related deaths (three arterial and one venous) for an overall mortality rate of 3.7%.

Results from lung cancer studies suggest that platinum compounds, the most frequently utilized drugs in the trials reviewed, may be a specific risk factor for chemotherapy-associated VTE. In the prospective registry study reported by Kroger et al., treatment with anthracyclines ($P = 0.04$), platinum-based drugs ($P = 0.01$), and nitrogen mustard analogs ($P = 0.04$) was significantly associated with the risk of VTE (15). However, in multivariate analysis, only platinum-based regimens were significantly associated with VTE ($P = 0.026$). The association of platinum drugs with VTE is supported by reports of high rates of VTE in

Table 3 Selected Anticancer Treatments and Risk of VTE

Cancer therapy	Reference	OR (95% CI)	With event (%)	Type of study	Comment
Chemotherapy					
	Heit et al., 2000 (36)	6.5 (2.1–20.2)	—	Population based case–control	Cancer patients on chemotherapy compared to general population
	Sallah et al., 2002 (5)	2.9 (1.8–4.6)	14[a]	Retrospective cohort	Hospitalized cancer patients on chemotherapy compared to those not on chemotherapy
	Blom et al., 2006 (8)	2.2 (1.8–2.7)	—	Retrospective cohort	Cancer patients on chemotherapy compared to those not chemotherapy
	Kroger et al., 2006 (15)	2.15, p= 0.0080	15[b]	Prospective cohort	Ambulatory and hospitalized cancer patients on chemotherapy compared to those not on chemotherapy
	Khorana et al., 2005 (31)	—	1.93%[c]	Prospective cohort	Ambulatory cancer patients on chemotherapy
Hormonal agents					
Tamoxifen	Saphner et al., 1991 (37)	5.5 (0.5–61.5)	—	Cohort study	Tamoxifen vs. observation
	Fisher et al., 1996 (38)	—	1.7 vs. 0.4	RCT	Tamoxifen vs. placebo
	Pritchard et al., 1996 (39)	—	13.6 vs. 2.6	RCT	Tamoxifen plus chemotherapy vs. tamoxifen
Aromatase inhibitors	Howell et al., 2005 (40)	0.61, $p = 0.0004$	4.5 vs. 2.8	RCT	Higher incidence of VTE in Tamoxifen treated patients compared to those on anastrozole

Antiangiogenesis agents					
Thalidomide	Rajkumar et al., 2006 (41)	—	17 vs. 3 $p < 0.001$	RCT	Thalidomide plus dexamethasone vs. dexamethasone
	Zangari et al., 2001 (42)	—	28 vs. 4 $p = 0.002$	RCT	Thalidomide plus chemotherapy vs. thalidomide
	Zangari et al., 2003 (34)	4.3, $p \leq 0.001$	—	Cohort	
Lenalidomide	Knight et al., 2006 (43)	3.51(1.77–6.97)	14 vs. 3.5 $p < 0.001$	RCT	Lenalidomide plus dexamethasone vs. dexamethasone
	Dimopoulos et al., 2005 (44)	—	8.5 vs. 4.5	RCT	
Bevacizumab	Kabbinavar et al., 2003 (45)	—	19 vs. 8.4	Phase II RCT	Bevacizumab plus chemotherapy vs. chemotherapy
	Hurwitz et al., 2004 (46)	—	19.4 vs.16.2	RCT	

[a]Over median follow-up 26 mo.
[b]Median follow-up 8 ± 5 mo.
[c]Median follow-up 2.4 mo.
Abbreviations: OR, Odds ratio; CI, confidence interval; VTE, venous thromboembolism; RCT, randomized controlled trial.

patients with other cancers receiving cisplatin or carboplatin. Retrospective reviews and one prospective analysis have recorded a VTE incidence of 12.9% in bladder cancer patients, 8.4% in male germ cell cancer patients, and 19% to 26% in patients with high-grade brain tumors, all receiving platinum-containing multiagent chemotherapy regimens (12,50–52).

HORMONAL THERAPY

Tamoxifen

Tamoxifen, a selective estrogen receptor modulator, is commonly used as adjuvant therapy for women with early stage hormone-receptor positive breast cancer. A systematic review of adjuvant hormonal therapy for breast cancer estimated that women treated with five years of tamoxifen have a 1.5-fold to 7.1-fold increased risk of VTE compared to women treated with placebo or observation (53). Selected studies of tamoxifen and the associated risk of VTE are listed in Table 3. In the NSABP B-14 trial, 1.7% of tamoxifen-treated patients had VTE compared to 0.4% in the placebo group (38). The risk of VTE associated with tamoxifen increased with age and was greatest in women over the age of 60 years (2.2%). Concurrent chemotherapy further increased the risk in tamoxifen-treated patients. In randomized trials of adjuvant therapy in early-stage breast cancer patients, those assigned to receive tamoxifen plus chemotherapy had significantly greater rates of VTE (range, 6.5–13.6%) compared to those receiving tamoxifen alone (range, 1.8–2.6%) (39,54). In a retrospective analysis of a cohort of over 2600 breast cancer patients from seven consecutive ECOG studies of adjuvant therapy, premenopausal women who received chemotherapy with tamoxifen had a higher frequency of VTE compared to patients who received chemotherapy alone (2.8% vs. 0.8%, $P = 0.03$) (37). Similarly, postmenopausal patients who received tamoxifen and chemotherapy had significantly higher rates than those who received tamoxifen alone (8% vs. 2.3%, $P = 0.03$).

Aromatase Inhibitors

Aromatase inhibitors (AIs) inhibit the peripheral conversion of testosterone and androstenedione to estradiol and estrone, respectively. Anastrozole, letrozole, and exemestane are commonly used AIs in breast cancer. The incidence of VTE appears to be lower in women receiving adjuvant AI therapy as compared to tamoxifen, although rates are still high in comparison to untreated, healthy women. The Arimidex, Tamoxifen alone or in Combination (ATAC) trial of over 9000 postmenopausal women assigned to receive five years of adjuvant tamoxifen or anastrozole reported significantly higher rates of VTE among tamoxifen users compared to anastrozole users after 68 months (4.5% vs. 2.8%, OR 0.61, $p = 0.0004$) (40). In other randomized trials, breast cancer patients assigned to sequential therapy of two to three years of tamoxifen followed by two to three years of AI had significantly lower rates of VTE as compared to those assigned to five years of tamoxifen (1.3% vs. 2.4%, $P = 0.007$; 0.19% vs. 0.75%) (55,56). When breast cancer patients who had completed five years of adjuvant tamoxifen were randomized to five additional years of letrozole or placebo, there were no significant differences in VTE rate between the two arms (57).

Hormonal Therapy in Prostate Cancer

Early studies of diethylstilbestrol (DES), a commonly used synthetic estrogen in the 1960s and 1970s for the treatment of prostate cancer, raised concerns of excess cardiovascular toxicity. Results from three major randomized clinical trials conducted by the Veterans Administration Cooperative Urological Research Group revealed an increased risk of cardiovascular death from DES, especially at a 5 mg daily dose (58). In randomized trials of metastatic prostate cancer patients, those receiving DES had significantly more thromboembolic events as compared to those receiving the Leuteinizing Hormone-Releasing Hormone (LHRH) agonist leuprolide ($P = 0.065$) (59) or the nonsteroidal, antiandrogen flutamide (33.3% vs. 17.6%, $P = 0.051$) (60). Steroidal antiandrogens such as megestrol acetate, cyproterone acetate, and medroxyprogesterone acetate also increase VTE risk but to a lesser extent than DES (61,62). High thrombosis rates of 31% and 11%, respectively, have been reported in DES-treated patients despite receiving concurrent prophylaxis with either fixed low-dose warfarin or low-dose aspirin (63,64). The risk of thrombosis is accentuated when DES is combined with chemotherapy as demonstrated in an ECOG study in which prostate cancer patients randomized to DES plus doxorubicin had a 10-fold increased rate of cardiovascular toxicity compared to those in the doxorubicin alone arm (6.75% vs. 0.7%) (65).

Antiangiogenesis Therapy

Recent reports indicate that drugs with antiangiogenic mechanisms of action can cause vascular toxicity, including arterial and venous events (Table 3). *Thalidomide* is an orally administered drug with immunomodulatory and antiangiogenic properties that is active in the treatment of multiple myeloma. When used as a single agent, the incidence of VTE is less than 2% (66). However, rates of VTE range from 17% to 26% in combination with dexamethasone (41,67), and 12% to 28% in combination with other chemotherapy agents including anthracyclines (42,68). In a multivariate analysis of 5354 myeloma patients, the combination of thalidomide with chemotherapy regimens containing doxorubicin was associated with the highest OR for VTE (4.3, $P < 0.001$) (34). Newly diagnosed disease (OR, 2.5; $P = 0.001$) and presence of chromosome 11 abnormality (OR, 1.8; $P = 0.048$) were also independent predictors for VTE. High rates of VTE have also been reported with thalidomide combinations used in other cancers. In a phase II study, 19% of patients with metastatic prostate cancer who received thalidomide with docetaxel developed VTE compared to none who received docetaxel alone (69). A remarkably high VTE rate of 25% was observed in a Cancer and Leukemia Group B (CALGB) phase II trial of thalidomide plus temozolomide in patients with brain metastases from melanoma (70).

Lenalidomide is a thalidomide analog recently approved in the United States for the second-line treatment of patients with multiple myeloma in combination with dexamethasone. In an initial phase II study, the combination of lenalidomide with dexamethasone and concurrent daily prophylactic aspirin reported only a 3% incidence of VTE (71). However, larger phase III studies of this combination without the use of prophylactic aspirin have shown higher rates of VTE. In one phase III study, relapsed refractory myeloma patients randomized to lenalidomide plus dexamethasone arm had an 8.5% incidence of thromboembolic events versus 4.5% in the dexamethasone-alone group (44).

Bevacizumab, a monoclonal antibody to vascular endothelial growth factor (VEGF), was the first antiangiogenic agent approved for cancer therapy. An early study reported a 19% rate of VTE events in patients treated with bevacizumab and chemotherapy compared to only 8.4% in patients treated with chemotherapy alone (45). A VTE rate of 24% was noted in another phase II trial of bevacizumab, irinotecan, and cisplatin in metastatic gastric cancer (6 of 24 patients, 95% CI 11–45) (72). Bevacizumab was also associated with a twofold increase in arterial TE (4.4% vs. 1.9% in control arm). However, later clinical trials have not reported significant differences in the incidence of VTE among patients receiving bevacizumab plus 5-fluorouracil–containing chemotherapy compared to those receiving chemotherapy alone (46,73). In 2005, the Food and Drug Administration issued safety warnings regarding the increased risk of arterial TE associated with bevacizumab (74). This may be a class effect of antiangiogenic therapy since other antiangiogenic agents still in development have also been associated with thrombosis. Patients receiving PTK787/ZK222584, a small molecule tyrosine kinase inhibitor of VEGF, in a recent phase III study had a 6% rate of PE compared to 1.4% in the placebo arm (75). In an early-phase study of the VEGF inhibitor SU5416, 17% of patients developed VTE (76). Much work remains to be done to understand the mechanisms involving venous and arterial toxicity of antiangiogenic therapy.

SUPPORTIVE THERAPY

Recombinant Erythropoietin

Epoetin and darbepoetin are two types of recombinant erythropoietins currently available. These agents are often used in cancer patients to increase hemoglobin levels and reduce the need for blood transfusions. Recent reports suggest an association between erythropoietins and thrombosis (Table 4).

A systematic review of 57 trials and 9353 cancer patients involved in randomized trials comparing the use of epoetin or darbepoetin plus red blood cell transfusions against red blood cell transfusions alone for prophylaxis or treatment of anemia in cancer patients with or without concurrent antineoplastic therapy was recently published (77). Among 6769 patients in 35 trials, 229 of the 3728 patients treated with darbepoetin or epoetin had TE events as compared to 118 events in 3041 untreated controls (4.5% vs. 1.4%, RR = 1.67, 95% CI = 1.35–2.06). This is in contrast to an earlier meta-analysis by the same group which did not show a significant association of erythropoietins with thrombosis (RR = 1.58, 95% CI = 0.94–2.66) (79). The strengthened association observed in the latest meta-analysis may be due to results from more recent trials of erythropoietins that enrolled nonanemic patients or targeted hemoglobin levels higher than the product label recommendations (13 g/dL). It should be noted that this latest meta-analysis also noted a trend towards decreased survival associated with erythropoietin treatment (HR 1.08, 95% CI 0.99–1.18), although it is unclear whether VTE events contributed to this trend. A second report describing an association with erythropoietin therapy involves a prospective registry of ambulatory cancer patients receiving chemotherapy. Patients with a baseline hemoglobin <10 g/dL or receiving red cell growth factors during their first cycle of chemotherapy were at increased risk of VTE (31). In multivariate analysis, a strong association between hemoglobin <10 g/dL and use of red cell growth factors ($p < 0.0001$) was found, and this combined variable was an independent predictor of VTE (OR 1.83, 95% CI 1.07–3.14). In a recent clinical trial comparing lenalidomide plus dexamethasone with dexamethasone alone in myeloma patients, concomitant use of erythropoietin in either group was significantly associated with VTE (16% vs. 2.6%, OR 3.21, 95% CI 1.72–6.01, $P < 0.001$) (43).

Myeloid Growth Factors

Myeloid growth factors are commonly used in cancer patients for prophylaxis or treatment of febrile neutropenia or to maintain dose intensity of specific chemotherapy regimens and may be associated with VTE (Table 4). In the early 1990s, the possibility of the increased risk of VTE in association with myeloid growth factor use was raised in anecdotal case reports and randomized clinical trials. A meta-analysis of 52 consecutive studies of 1846 cancer patients found that use of Granulocyte Macrophage Colony-Stimulating Factor (GM-CSF)

Table 4 Selected Supportive Therapy Agents and Risk of VTE

Supportive therapy	Reference	OR (95% CI)	With event (%)	Type of study	Comment
Erythropoietin	Bohlius et al., 2006 (77)	1.67 (1.35–2.06)	4.5 vs. 1.4	Meta-analysis	OR in comparison to untreated patients
	Khorana et al., 2005 (31)	1.83 (1.07–3.14)	8.75	Prospective cohort	Combined effect of hemoglobin <10 g/dL or erythropoietin use
Myeloid growth factors	Barbui et al., 1996 (78)	1.67 (0.92–3.04)	6.6 vs. 3.6	Meta-analysis	OR in comparison to untreated patients, GM-CSF therapy only
	Khorana et al., 2005 (31)	4.0 (1.8–8.7)	5.9 vs. 1.5	Prospective cohort	OR in comparison to untreated patients, in high-risk cancer sites only. No significant elevation of risk in other sites of cancer

Abbreviations: OR, Odds ratio; CI, confidence interval; VTE, venous thromboembolism; GM-CSF, Granulocyte Macrophage Colony-Stimulating Factor.

was associated with a significantly higher rate of thrombosis as compared to Granulocyte Colony-Stimulating Factor (G-CSF) (4.2% vs. 1.2%, $P < 0.01$) (78). Compared to untreated controls, cancer patients who received GM-CSF had a nonsignificant trend toward higher frequency of VTE (6.6% vs. 3.6%, OR 1.67, 95%, CI 0.92–3.04). Patients given GM-CSF in the setting of myeloablative chemotherapy also had an increased rate of thrombosis compared to those receiving conventional regimens (9.8% vs. 3.3%, $P < 0.01$).

In the prospective study of ambulatory cancer patients on chemotherapy by Khorana et al., VTE was noted in 28 (2.78%) of the 1007 patients who received white blood cell growth factors during their first cycle ($P = 0.02$) (31). In multivariate analyses, only patients with sites of cancer already associated with the highest risk of VTE, such as upper GI, lung, or lymphoma, had a significantly increased risk of VTE associated with myeloid growth factor use (VTE rate of 5.9% vs. 1.5% without growth factor use, $P = 0.0001$, OR 4.0, 95% CI 1.8–8.7). This study did not distinguish between use of G-CSF and GM-CSF.

BIOLOGICAL RISK FACTORS

D-Dimer

In a study of 32 metastatic breast cancer patients receiving chemotherapy, markers of hemostatic activation including D-dimer were elevated in cancer patients compared to normal controls, and declined in 16 patients receiving warfarin prophylaxis (80). Of note is the point that 2 of 16 patients not receiving prophylaxis with persistent hemostatic activation developed DVT. In a larger study of 223 patients with solid tumors diagnosed with a first episode of VTE, poor performance status and elevated D-dimer levels ($p = 0.001$) were also predictive of recurrent VTE (81). Similar results were reported in a trial analyzing the usefulness of D-dimer testing in cancer patients with suspected DVT (82). In a study of D-dimer testing in cancer patients with suspected DVT, only one episode of VTE occurred during a three-month follow-up period in patients in whom both D-dimer and ultrasonography results were normal (1.6%, 95% CI, 0.04–8.53%). These data suggest that D-dimer levels may be a predictor of VTE in cancer patients, although this needs to be established in a prospective study.

Tissue Factor

Tissue factor (TF) is a 47 kDa transmembrane protein that functions as the principal physiologic initiator of coagulation. TF expression is commonly observed in a variety of malignancies and is believed to contribute significantly to the prothrombotic state observed in cancer patients. In a recent retrospective analysis of resected pancreatic cancers, 54% of patients had high TF expression (defined as ≥grade 2, the median score), and 46% had low or no TF expression (83). Data regarding subsequent VTE were available for a subgroup of these patients ($n = 33$). Resected patients with high TF expression had a VTE rate of 20% compared to 5.5% in patients with low TF expression ($p = 0.04$), suggesting that the grade of TF expression by tumor cells is a predictor of subsequent clinical VTE. Although provocative, these results should be viewed as preliminary until confirmatory prospective studies have been performed.

COMORBID CONDITIONS

Certain comorbidities such as infection, obesity, immobilization, and smoking are known risk factors for VTE in the general population, but their significance in cancer-associated

VTE is not completely understood. In a retrospective review of hospitalized neutropenic cancer patients, obesity (OR 1.52, 95% CI 1.10–2.09), renal disease (OR 1.41, 95% CI 1.30–1.54), pulmonary disease (OR 1.57, 95% CI 1.45–1.70), and the presence of infection (OR 1.28, 95% CI 1.20–1.38) were identified as independent risk factors for VTE (3). Infection and its associated inflammatory milieu increase procoagulant activity and the propensity for thrombosis among the general patient population (84–86). Infection in cancer patients increases the risk for VTE as evidenced in the previous study and is also supported by another prospective cancer registry that reported fever ($P = 0.0093$) and elevated C-Reactive Protein >5 mg/L ($P < 0.001$) to be predictive for VTE (15). Arterial TE in itself is a risk factor for VTE in cancer patients. In a cohort of hospitalized neutropenic cancer patients, Khorana et al. found arterial TE to be an independent predictor for VTE (OR 1.36, 95% CI 1.09–1.71) (3). The effect of smoking on VTE occurrence in cancer patients is not known, as most risk assessment studies did not screen for smoking. Inferior vena cava obstruction by large abdominopelvic tumors causing stasis of blood in the lower extremities increases the risk of VTE in cancer patients. For instance, the VTE rate was 33% in a series of male germ cell tumor patients with such tumors (87).

OTHER RISKS

Central Venous Catheters

The occurrence of catheter-related thrombosis (CRT) is influenced by the type of catheter, patient factors, and treatment-related factors. The reported incidence of symptomatic CRT among cancer patients on chemotherapy followed prospectively ranges from 4.3% to 14% over 76,713 patient-days of follow-up (19 of 444 patients, 0.3 per 1000 catheter-days) with median time to thrombosis of 51 days (range 6–309 days, 33 of 243 patients) (22,23). Rates are lower in the most recent studies. Several catheter-related factors are associated with increased risk including more than one insertion attempt (OR 5.5, 95% CI 1.2–24.6, $P = 0.03$), previous central venous catheters (CVC) insertion (OR 3.8, 95% CI 1.4–10.4, $P = 0.01$), left-sided placement (OR 3.5, 95% CI 1.6–7.5), catheter tip position in the superior vena cava as compared with right atrium (OR 2.7, 95% CI 1.1–6.6), and arm ports as compared to chest ports (OR 8.1, 95% CI 3.5–19.1) (22,23). Of note is the point that ovarian cancer patients appear to have a 4.8- to 5.6-fold increased risk of CRT compared to other malignancies. Elevated plasma level of homocysteine, a marker of inflammation, has also been associated with increased incidence of CRT (OR 3.8, 95% CI 1.3–11.3). In a separate prospective study, cancer patients on chemotherapy with CVC-related infection had a higher risk of CRT compared to those without infection (RR 17.6, 95% CI 4.1–74.1) (24).

Several treatment-related factors associated with CRT were recently systematically reviewed (25). These include L-asparaginase for acute lymphoblastic leukemia induction, estrogen or progesterones in hematological malignancies, recombinant erythropoietin in combination with chemotherapy and radiation in women with cervical cancer, interleukin 2 in melanoma or renal cell carcinoma, GM-CSF during peripheral blood cell mobilization and collection, and thalidomide in combination with corticosteroids or additional agents for myeloma.

Prothrombotic Mutations

The prevalence of prothrombotic mutations in cancer populations is the same as in the general population. The association of prothrombotic mutations with cancer-associated VTE has been investigated in several small cohort and case–control studies. A population-based case–control study in the Netherlands estimated that patients with cancer and factor V Leiden have a twofold increased incidence of VTE compared to cancer patients without the mutation (OR 2.2, 95% CI 0.3–17.8) (7). Other studies have shown a similar increased risk (OR ranging from 0.4 to 6.9, pooled OR 2.2, 95% CI 1.2–3.9) (26–28). Similarly, cancer patients with prothrombin gene mutation also have an increased risk of VTE (OR range: 0.7–2.4, pooled OR 2.7, 95% CI 1.6–4.5) (26,28). Cancer patients with a prothrombotic mutation also have an increased risk of catheter-related upper extremity thrombosis compared to cancer patients without such mutations (29,30). A family history of VTE, which may be suggestive of underlying inherited thrombophilia, has been associated with an increased risk of VTE in cancer patients (15).

Inferior Vena Cava Filter

Filter-associated thrombosis and recurrent DVT and/or PE are some potential late complications of vena cava filter (VCF). The PREPIC study is the only prospective randomized controlled trial evaluating long-term outcomes of VCF (88). In this study, 200 patients (including 56 with cancer) were randomized to treatment with a VCF and anticoagulation versus anticoagulation alone. VCF provided short-term protection from PE, but at two-year follow-up, there were significantly more recurrent DVT and filter-site thrombosis in the VCF group (20.8% vs. 11.6%, OR 1.87, 95% CI 1.10–1.38). One retrospective study reported a 40% incidence (40 of 99) of recurrent DVT among cancer patients requiring VCF placement because of either failure of or contraindication for anticoagulation (89). Detection of new metastasis (OR 3.3, 95% CI 1.16–9.09, $P = 0.02$), prior history of VTE (OR 10.6, 95% CI 1.98–57.2, $P = 0.006$), and multiple neutropenic episodes ($P = 0.04$) were significant risk factors for recurrence. In another retrospective analysis of a cohort of over 500 consecutive cancer patients with DVT treated mostly with anticoagulation, the presence of VCF was again significantly associated with recurrent DVT (32%, $P < 0.001$) (90).

Platelet Count

In a prospective analysis of a cohort of cancer patients on chemotherapy, those with a baseline platelet count of 350,000/mm^3 or greater had a significantly higher incidence of VTE as compared to those with a platelet count of <200,000/mm^3 (3.98% vs. 1.25%, 1.66%/mo vs. 0.52%/mo, OR 2.81, $P = 0.0002$) (31). Patients who developed VTE also had higher mean platelet counts before each cycle of chemotherapy ($P = 0.001$) and higher minimum platelet counts ($P = 0.001$) when compared with patients without VTE. These results await further confirmation.

FUTURE DIRECTIONS: DEVELOPMENT OF RISK ASSESSMENT MODELS

It is evident from the extensive list of risk factors discussed above that cancer-associated thrombosis is a multifactorial disease, and that many risk factors can interact in the same patient. The failure of recent studies of thromboprophylaxis has shown that selection of patients based on site or stage alone is insufficient to identify a high-risk population (91). It is important, therefore, to study the interactions between risk factors in an effort to stratify patients into subgroups at high or low risk for VTE. Such a risk stratification approach could help identify ambulatory patients with risks of VTE high enough to justify the use of thromboprophylaxis. Formal risk assessment models for DVT in other high-risk populations have been developed and are used clinically (92–94). An initial effort at such a predictive risk assessment model designed specifically for cancer patients receiving outpatient chemotherapy has been presented in preliminary form (95). Incorporating variables such as site of cancer, prechemotherapy platelet counts, anemia, and use of growth factors, this model discriminated well between patients with low risk (score = 0, VTE incidence = 0.34%/mo), and those with higher risk (score = 3, 2.6%/mo or score = 4, 5.5%/mo). Further development and validation of this model is ongoing. Future directions in the field of cancer-associated thrombosis must include prospective testing of such risk stratification approaches in order to optimize the risk–benefit ratio of thromboprophylaxis.

REFERENCES

1. Khorana AA. Malignancy, thrombosis and trousseau: the case for an eponym. J Thromb Haemost 2003; 1(12):2463–2465.
2. Lee AY, Levine MN. Venous thromboembolism and cancer: risks and outcomes. Circulation 2003; 107(23 suppl 1):I17–I21.
3. Khorana AA, Francis CW, Culakova E, et al. Thromboembolism in hospitalized neutropenic cancer patients. J Clin Oncol 2006; 24(3):484–490.
4. Stein PD, Beemath A, Meyers FA, et al. Incidence of venous thromboembolism in patients hospitalized with cancer. Am J Med 2006; 119(1):60–68.
5. Sallah S, Wan JY, Nguyen NP. Venous thrombosis in patients with solid tumors: determination of frequency and characteristics. Thromb Haemost 2002; 87(4):575–579.
6. Chew HK, Wun T, Harvey D, et al. Incidence of venous thromboembolism and its effect on survival among patients with common cancers. Arch Intern Med 2006; 166(4):458–464.
7. Blom JW, Doggen CJ, Osanto S, et al. Malignancies, prothrombotic mutations, and the risk of venous thrombosis. JAMA 2005; 293(6):715–722.
8. Blom JW, Vanderschoot JP, Oostindier MJ, et al. Incidence of venous thrombosis in a large cohort of 66,329 cancer patients: results of a record linkage study. J Thromb Haemost 2006; 4(3):529–535.
9. Blom JW, Osanto S, Rosendaal FR. The risk of a venous thrombotic event in lung cancer patients: higher risk for adenocarcinoma than squamous cell carcinoma. J Thromb Haemost 2004; 2(10):1760–1765.
10. Alcalay A, Wun T, Khatri V, et al. Venous thromboembolism in patients with colorectal cancer: incidence and effect on survival. J Clin Oncol 2006; 24(7):1112–1118.
11. Komrokji RS, Uppal NP, Khorana AA, et al. Venous thromboembolism in patients with diffuse large B-cell lymphoma. Leuk Lymphoma 2006; 47(6):1029–1033.
12. Czaykowski PM, Moore MJ, Tannock IF. High Risk of Vascular Events in Patients with Urothelial Transitional Cell Carcinoma Treated with Cisplatin Based Chemotherapy. J Urol 1998; 160(6 Part 1):2021–2024.
13. Numico G, Garrone O, Dongiovanni V, et al. Prospective evaluation of major vascular events in patients with nonsmall cell lung carcinoma treated with cisplatin and gemcitabine. Cancer 2005; 103(5):994–999.
14. Levitan N, Dowlati A, Remick SC, et al. Rates of initial and recurrent thromboembolic disease among patients with malignancy versus those without malignancy. Risk analysis using medicare claims data. Medicine (Baltimore) 1999; 78(5):285–291.
15. Kroger K, Weiland D, Ose C, et al. Risk factors for venous thromboembolic events in cancer patients. Ann Oncol 2006; 17(2):297–303.
16. Geerts WH, Pineo GF, Heit JA, et al. Prevention of venous thromboembolism: the seventh ACCP conference on antithrombotic and thrombolytic therapy. Chest 2004; 126(suppl 3):338S–400S.
17. Bergqvist D. Venous thromboembolism and cancer: prevention of VTE. Thromb Res 2001; 102(6):V209–V213.
18. Kikura M, Takada T, Sato S. Preexisting morbidity as an independent risk factor for perioperative acute thromboembolism syndrome. Arch Surg 2005; 140(12):1210–1217; discussion 1218.

19. Andtbacka RH, Babiera G, Singletary SE, et al. Incidence and prevention of venous thromboembolism in patients undergoing breast cancer surgery and treated according to clinical pathways. Ann Surg 2006; 243(1):96–101.
20. Agnelli G, Bolis G, Capussotti L, et al. A clinical outcome-based prospective study on venous thromboembolism after cancer surgery: the @RISTOS project. Ann Surg 2006; 243(1):89–95.
21. Bergqvist D. Low-molecular-weight heparin for the prevention of postoperative venous thromboembolism after abdominal surgery: a review. Curr Opin Pulm Med 2005; 11(5):392–397.
22. Lee AYY, Levine MN, Butler G, et al. Incidence, risk factors, and outcomes of catheter-related thrombosis in adult patients with cancer. J Clin Oncol 2006; 24(9):1404–1408.
23. Tesselaar MET, Ouwerkerk J, Nooy MA, et al. Risk factors for catheter-related thrombosis in cancer patients. Eur J Cancer 2004; 40(15):2253–2259.
24. van Rooden CJ, Schippers EF, Barge RMY, et al. Infectious complications of central venous catheters increase the risk of catheter-related thrombosis in hematology patients: a prospective study. J Clin Oncol 2005; 23(12):2655–2660.
25. Linenberger ML. Catheter-related thrombosis: risks, diagnosis, and management. J Natl Compr Canc Netw 2006; 4(9):889–901.
26. Kennedy M, Andreescu AC, Greenblatt MS, et al. Factor V leiden, prothrombin 20210A and the risk of venous thrombosis among cancer patients. Br J Haematol 2005; 128(3):386–388.
27. Eroglu A, Kurtman C, Ulu A, et al. Factor V leiden and PT G20210A mutations in cancer patients with and without venous thrombosis. J Thromb Haemost 2005; 3(6):1323–1324.
28. Ramacciotti E, Wolosker N, Puech-Leao P, et al. Prevalence of factor V leiden, FII G20210A, FXIII Val34Leu and MTHFR C677T polymorphisms in cancer patients with and without venous thrombosis. Thromb Res 2003; 109(4):171–174.
29. Fijnheer R, Paijmans B, Verdonck LF, et al. Factor V leiden in central venous catheter-associated thrombosis. Br J Haematol 2002; 118(1):267–270.
30. Mandala M, Curigliano G, Bucciarelli P, et al. Factor V leiden and G20210A prothrombin mutation and the risk of subclavian vein thrombosis in patients with breast cancer and a central venous catheter. Ann Oncol 2004; 15(4):590–593.
31. Khorana AA, Francis CW, Culakova E, et al. Risk factors for chemotherapy-associated venous thromboembolism in a prospective observational study. Cancer 2005; 104(12):2822–2829.
32. Stein PD, Hull RD, Kayali F, et al. Venous thromboembolism according to age: the impact of an aging population. Arch Intern Med 2004; 164(20):2260–2265.
33. White RH. The epidemiology of venous thromboembolism. Circulation 2003; 107(90231):I-4–I-8.
34. Zangari M, Barlogie B, Thertulien R, et al. Thalidomide and deep vein thrombosis in multiple myeloma: risk factors and effect on survival. Clin Lymphoma 2003; 4(1):32–35.
35. Mohren M, Markmann I, Jentsch-Ullrich K, et al. Increased risk of thromboembolism in patients with malignant lymphoma: a single-centre analysis. Br J Cancer 2005; 92(8):1349–1351.
36. Heit JA, Silverstein MD, Mohr DN, et al. Risk factors for deep vein thrombosis and pulmonary embolism: a population-based case-control study. Arch Intern Med 2000; 160(6):809–815.
37. Saphner T, Tormey DC, Gray R. Venous and arterial thrombosis in patients who received adjuvant therapy for breast cancer. J Clin Oncol 1991; 9(2):286–294.
38. Fisher B, Dignam J, Bryant J, et al. Five versus more than five years of tamoxifen therapy for breast cancer patients with negative lymph nodes and estrogen receptor-positive tumors. J Natl Cancer Inst 1996; 88(21):1529–1542.
39. Pritchard KI, Paterson AH, Paul NA, et al. Increased thromboembolic complications with concurrent tamoxifen and chemotherapy in a randomized trial of adjuvant therapy for women with breast cancer. National cancer institute of canada clinical trials group breast cancer site group. J Clin Oncol 1996; 14(10):2731–2737.
40. Howell A, Cuzick J, Baum M, et al. Results of the ATAC (arimidex, tamoxifen, alone or in combination) trial after completion of 5 years' adjuvant treatment for breast cancer. Lancet 2005; 365(9453):60–62.
41. Rajkumar SV, Blood E, Vesole D, et al. Phase III clinical trial of thalidomide plus dexamethasone compared with dexamethasone alone in newly diagnosed multiple myeloma: a clinical trial coordinated by the eastern cooperative oncology group. J Clin Oncol 2006; 24(3):431–436.

42. Zangari M, Anaissie E, Barlogie B, et al. Increased risk of deep-vein thrombosis in patients with multiple myeloma receiving thalidomide and chemotherapy. Blood 2001; 98(5):1614–1615.
43. Knight R, DeLap RJ, Zeldis JB, et al. Lenalidomide and venous thrombosis in multiple myeloma. N Engl J Med 2006; 354(19):2079–2080.
44. Dimopoulos MA, Spencer A, Attal M, et al. Study of lenalidomide plus dexamethasone versus dexamethasone alone in relapsed or refractory multiple myeloma (MM): results of a phase 3 study (MM-010). ASH Annual Meeting Abstracts 2005; 106(11):6.
45. Kabbinavar F, Hurwitz HI, Fehrenbacher L, et al. Phase II, randomized trial comparing bevacizumab plus fluorouracil (FU)/leucovorin (LV) with FU/LV alone in patients with metastatic colorectal cancer. J Clin Oncol 2003; 21(1):60–65.
46. Hurwitz H, Fehrenbacher L, Novotny W, et al. Bevacizumab plus irinotecan, fluorouracil, and leucovorin for metastatic colorectal cancer. N Engl J Med 2004; 350(23):2335–2342.
47. Otten HM, Mathijssen J, ten Cate H, et al. Symptomatic venous thromboembolism in cancer patients treated with chemotherapy: an underestimated phenomenon. Arch Intern Med 2004; 164(2):190–194.
48. Levine MN, Gent M, Hirsh J, et al. The thrombogenic effect of anticancer drug therapy in women with stage II breast cancer. N Engl J Med 1988; 318(7):404–407.
49. Clahsen P, van de Velde C, Julien J, et al. Thromboembolic complications after perioperative chemotherapy in women with early breast cancer: a european organization for research and treatment of cancer breast cancer cooperative group study. J Clin Oncol 1994; 12(6):1266–1271.
50. Weijl NI, Rutten MF, Zwinderman AH, et al. Thromboembolic events during chemotherapy for germ cell cancer: a cohort study and review of the literature. J Clin Oncol 2000; 18(10):2169–2178.
51. Cheruku R, Tapazoglou E, Ensley J, et al. The incidence and significance of thromboembolic complications in patients with high-grade gliomas. Cancer 1991; 68(12):2621–2624.
52. Brandes AA, Scelzi E, Salmistraro G, et al. Incidence and risk of thromboembolism during treatment of high-grade gliomas: a prospective study. Eur J Cancer 1997; 33(10):1592–1596.
53. Deitcher SR, Gomes MP. The risk of venous thromboembolic disease associated with adjuvant hormone therapy for breast carcinoma: a systematic review. Cancer 2004; 101(3):439–449.
54. Fisher B, Dignam J, Wolmark N, et al. Tamoxifen and chemotherapy for lymph node-negative, estrogen receptor-positive breast cancer. J Natl Cancer Inst 1997; 89(22):1673–1682.
55. Coombes RC, Hall E, Gibson LJ, et al. A randomized trial of exemestane after two to three years of tamoxifen therapy in postmenopausal women with primary breast cancer. N Engl J Med 2004; 350(11):1081–1092.
56. Jakesz R, Jonat W, Gnant M, et al. Switching of postmenopausal women with endocrine-responsive early breast cancer to anastrozole after 2 years' adjuvant tamoxifen: combined results of ABCSG trial 8 and ARNO 95 trial. Lancet 2005; 366(9484):455–462.
57. Goss PE, Ingle JN, Martino S, et al. Randomized trial of letrozole following tamoxifen as extended adjuvant therapy in receptor-positive breast cancer: updated findings from NCIC CTG MA.17. J Natl Cancer Inst 2005; 97(17):1262–1271.
58. Byar DP, Corle DK. Hormone therapy for prostate cancer: results of the veterans administration cooperative urological research group studies. NCI Monogr 1988; (7):165–170.
59. The Leuprolide Study Group. Leuprolide versus diethylstilbestrol for metastatic prostate cancer, N Engl J Med 1984; 311(20):1281–1286.
60. Chang A, Yeap B, Davis T, et al. Double-blind, randomized study of primary hormonal treatment of stage D2 prostate carcinoma: flutamide versus diethylstilbestrol. J Clin Oncol 1996; 14(8):2250–2257.
61. Pavone-Macaluso M, de Voogt HJ, Viggiano G, et al. Comparison of diethylstilbestrol, cyproterone acetate and medroxyprogesterone acetate in the treatment of advanced prostatic cancer: final analysis of a randomized phase III trial of the european organization for research on treatment of cancer urological group. J Urol 1986; 136(3):624–631.
62. de Voogt HJ, Smith PH, Pavone-Macaluso M, et al. Cardiovascular side effects of diethylstilbestrol, cyproterone acetate, medroxyprogesterone acetate and estramustine phosphate used for the treatment of advanced prostatic cancer: results from european organization for research on treatment of cancer trials 30761 and 30762. J Urol 1986; 135(2):303–307.

63. Klotz L, Mcneill I, Fleshner N. A phase 1–2 trial of diethylstilbestrol plus low dose warfarin in advanced prostate carcinoma. J Urol 1999; 161(1):169–172.
64. Shahidi M, Norman AR, Gadd J, et al. Prospective review of diethylsilbesterol in advanced prostate cancer no longer responding to androgen suppression. Proc Am Soc Clin Oncol 2001; 20 (abstr 2455).
65. Leaf AN, Propert K, Corcoran C, et al. Phase III study of combined chemohormonal therapy in metastatic prostate cancer (ECOG 3882): an eastern cooperative oncology group study. Med Oncol 2003; 20(2):137–146.
66. Barlogie B, Desikan R, Eddlemon P, et al. Extended survival in advanced and refractory multiple myeloma after single-agent thalidomide: identification of prognostic factors in a phase 2 study of 169 patients. Blood 2001; 98(2):492–494.
67. Cavo M, Zamagni E, Cellini C, et al. Deep-vein thrombosis in patients with multiple myeloma receiving first-line thalidomide-dexamethasone therapy. Blood 2002; 100(6):2272–2273.
68. Facon T, Mary JY, Hulin C, et al. Major superiority of melphalan—prednisone (MP) +thalidomide (THAL) over MP and autologous stem cell transplantation in the treatment of newly diagnosed elderly patients with multiple myeloma. ASH Annual Meeting Abstracts 2005; 106(11):780.
69. Horne MK III, Figg WD, Arlen P, et al. Increased frequency of venous thromboembolism with the combination of docetaxel and thalidomide in patients with metastatic androgen-independent prostate cancer. Pharmacotherapy 2003; 23(3):315–318.
70. Krown SE, Niedzwiecki D, Hwu WJ, et al. Phase II study of temozolomide and thalidomide in patients with metastatic melanoma in the brain: high rate of thromboembolic events (CALGB 500102). Cancer 2006; 107(8):1883–1890.
71. Rajkumar SV, Hayman SR, Lacy MQ, et al. Combination therapy with lenalidomide plus dexamethasone (Rev/Dex) for newly diagnosed myeloma. Blood 2005; 106(13):4050–4053.
72. Shah MA, Ilson D, Kelson DP. Thromboembolic events in gastric cancer, high incidence in patients receiving irinotecan and bevacizumab-based therapy. J Clin Oncol 2005; 23(11):2574–2576.
73. Giantonio BJ, Catalano PJ, Meropol NJ, et al. High-dose Bevacizumab improves survival when combined with FOLFOX4 in previously treated advanced colorectal cancer: results from the eastern cooperative oncology group (ECOG) study E3200. J Clin Oncol 2005 ASCO Annual Meeting Proceedings Vol. 23. No 16S, Part I of II (June I suppl) 2005:2 (abstr).
74. Http://www.avastin.com/avastin/drugWarningPro.m, 2005.
75. Hecht JR, Trarbach T, Jaeger E, et al. A randomized double-blind placebo-controlled phase III study in patients with metastatic adenocarcinoma of the colon or rectum receiving first-line chemotherapy with oxaliplatin/5-fluorouracil/leucovorin and PTK787/ZK222584 or placebo (CONFIRM-1). J Clin Oncol, 2005 ASCO Annual Meeting Proceedings, Vol. 23, No. 16S, Part I of II (June I suppl), 2005:93.
76. Kuenen BC, Levi M, Meijers JC, et al. Analysis of coagulation cascade and endothelial cell activation during inhibition of vascular endothelial growth factor/vascular endothelial growth factor receptor pathway in cancer patients. Arterioscler Thromb Vasc Biol 2002; 22(9):1500–1505.
77. Bohlius J, Wilson J, Seidenfeld J, et al. Recombinant human erythropoietins and cancer patients: updated meta-analysis of 57 studies including 9353 patients. J Natl Cancer Inst 2006; 98(10):708–714.
78. Barbui T, Finazzi G, Grassi A, et al. Thrombosis in cancer patients treated with hematopoietic growth factors--a meta-analysis. On behalf of the subcommittee on haemostasis and malignancy of the scientific and standardization committee of the ISTH. Thromb Haemost 1996; 75(2):368–371.
79. Bohlius J, Langensiepen S, Schwarzer G, et al. Recombinant human erythropoietin and overall survival in cancer patients: results of a comprehensive meta-analysis. J Natl Cancer Inst 2005; 97(7):489–498.
80. Falanga A, Levine MN, Consonni R, et al. The effect of very-low-dose warfarin on markers of hypercoagulation in metastatic breast cancer: results from a randomized trial. Thromb Haemost 1998; 79(1):23–27.
81. Sallah S, Husain A, Sigounas V, et al. Plasma coagulation markers in patients with solid tumors and venous thromboembolic disease receiving oral anticoagulation therapy. Clin Cancer Res 2004; 10(21):7238–7243.

82. ten Wolde M, Kraaijenhagen RA, Prins MH, et al. The clinical usefulness of D-dimer testing in cancer patients with suspected deep venous thrombosis. Arch Intern Med 2002; 162(16):1880–1884.
83. Khorana AA, Francis CW, Ryan CK, et al. Tissue factor, angiogenesis and thrombosis in pancreatic cancer. J Clin Oncol 2006 ASCO Annual Meeting Proceedings 2006; Part I Vol 24, No 18S (June 20 suppl):4001 (abstr).
84. Bryant AE. Biology and pathogenesis of thrombosis and procoagulant activity in invasive infections caused by group A streptococci and clostridium perfringens. Clin Microbiol Rev 2003; 16(3):451–462.
85. Keller TT, Mairuhu AT, de Kruif MD, et al. Infections and endothelial cells. Cardiovasc Res 2003; 60(1):40–48.
86. Levi M, Keller TT, van Gorp E, et al. Infection and inflammation and the coagulation system. Cardiovasc Res 2003; 60(1):26–39.
87. Hassan B, Tung K, Weeks R, et al. The management of inferior vena cava obstruction complicating metastatic germ cell tumors. Cancer 1999; 85(4):912–918.
88. Decousus H, Leizorovicz A, Parent F, et al. A clinical trial of vena caval filters in the prevention of pulmonary embolism in patients with proximal deep-vein thrombosis. Prevention du risque d'embolie pulmonaire par interruption cave study group. N Engl J Med 1998; 338(7):409–415.
89. Lin J, Proctor MC, Varma M, et al. Factors associated with recurrent venous thromboembolism in patients with malignant disease. J Vasc Surg 2003; 37(5):976–983.
90. Elting LS, Escalante CP, Cooksley C, et al. Outcomes and cost of deep venous thrombosis among patients with cancer. Arch Intern Med 2004; 164(15):1653–1661.
91. Haas SK, Kakkar AK, Kemkes-Matthes B, et al. Prevention of venous thromboembolism with low-molecular-weight heparin in patients with metastatic breast or lung cancer - results of the TOPIC studies. J Thromb Haemost 2005; 3(suppl 1):abstract number OR059 (abstr).
92. Caprini JA, Arcelus JI, Hasty JH, et al. Clinical assessment of venous thromboembolic risk in surgical patients. Semin Thromb Hemost 1991; 17(suppl 3):304–312.
93. Ageno W. Applying risk assessment models in general surgery: overview of our clinical experience. Blood Coagul Fibrinolysis 1999; 10(suppl 2):S71–S78.
94. Heinemann LA, Dominh T, Assmann A, et al. VTE risk assessment—a prognostic model: BATER cohort study of young women. Thromb J 2005; 3(1):5.
95. Khorana AA, Francis CW, Culakova E, et al. Risk factors for chemotherapy-associated venous thromboembolism in a prospective observational study: a proposed predictive model. J Thromb Haemost 2005; 3(suppl 1): abstract number OR058 (abstr).

13
Thromboprophylaxis in Cancer Surgery

Gloria Petralia
Centre for Surgical Sciences, Institute of Cancer, Barts, and the London Queen Mary's School of Medicine and Dentistry, and Thrombosis Research Institute, London, U.K.

Aidan McManus
Thrombosis Research Institute, London, U.K.

Ajay Kakkar
Centre for Surgical Sciences, Institute of Cancer, Barts, and the London Queen Mary's School of Medicine and Dentistry, and Thrombosis Research Institute, London, U.K.

- Cancer patients undergoing surgery are at particular risk of venous thromboembolism (VTE) in the perioperative period.
- Low-dose unfractionated heparin (UFH) or low-molecular-weight heparins (LMWHs) are the most appropriate pharmacologic prophylactic agents.
- For patients with contraindications to pharmacologic prophylaxis, use of mechanical methods such as intermittent pneumatic compression stockings should be considered.
- Prophylaxis should be administered for at least the duration of the hospital stay, and up to four weeks in patients with persistent risk factors.

INTRODUCTION

The rationale for considering thromboprophylaxis routinely in patients undergoing major surgery is based on our understanding that

1. Venous thromboembolism (VTE) is a frequent complication in high-risk surgical populations.
2. VTE can lead unpredictably to a fatal outcome.
3. Thromboprophylaxis is not only effective but safe in preventing the mortality and morbidity associated with VTE.

Operation for cancer has long been recognized to be associated with a higher risk for the development of postoperative deep vein thrombosis (DVT) than for noncancer-related procedures (Table 1). In studies comparing patients with and without cancer, the risk of a fatal thromboembolic outcome in the cancer surgical population is threefold higher,

Table 1 Incidence of Postoperative VTE: Cancer Vs. Noncancer Patients

	Cancer patients VTE, *n*/*N* (%)	Noncancer patients VTE, *n*/*N* (%)
Kakkar et al., 1970 (1)	24/59 (41%)	38/144 (26%)
Hills et al., 1972 (2)	8/16 (50%)	7/34 (21%)
Walsh et al., 1974 (3)	16/45 (35%)	22/217 (10%)
Rosenberg et al., 1975 (4)	28/66 (42%)	29/128 (23%)
Rem et al., 1975 (5)	16/30 (53%)	16/65 (28%)
Gallus et al., 1976 (6)	17/76 (22%)	49/306 (16%)
Allan et al., 1983 (7)	31/100 (31%)	21/100 (21%)
Multicenter Trial Committee 1984 (8)	62/304 (20%)	113/707 (16%)
Kakkar and Murray 1985 (9)	21/310 (6.7%)	10/597 (1.6%)
Sue-Ling et al., 1986 (10)	12/23 (52%)	16/62 (26%)
Kakkar et al., 1993 (11)	25/1407 (1.8%)	16/2402 (0.7%)
Total	260/2436 (10.7%)	337/4762 (7.1%)

Abbreviation: VTE, venous thromboembolism.

confirming that VTE is a clinically relevant disease in cancer patients and that its significance should not be underestimated (12). If clinically apparent thrombosis does occur, cancer patients experience poorer outcome after VTE treatment and tend to have more extensive thrombus and higher rates of recurrence and bleeding (13–15). Thus, guidelines recommend primary VTE prevention strategies for the cancer surgical population (12).

FACTORS DRIVING THE RISK FOR VTE

Surgery is one of the oldest known risk factors for VTE, with the trauma and postoperative immobility associated with surgery exposing patients to the risk of VTE. There are a number of other recognized risk factors for VTE that have been characterized across all patient groups, including increasing age, medical illness, hospitalization, and congenital thrombophilic states (12), but for cancer patients, additional factors drive the increased VTE risk.

The pathogenesis of VTE in cancer patients may be described according to the simple triad of factors first described by Virchow (16) in the nineteenth century. Virchow identified three key factors in thrombus formation: venous stasis, vascular trauma, and blood hypercoagulability. In the cancer patients, stasis can be due to external compression from the malignant mass or the immobility resulting from debilitation. Vascular trauma may occur from direct invasion of a vessel by the tumor itself, for example, as seen in thrombosis of the inferior vena cava in renal cell carcinoma invasion (17), through vascular catheterization, for example, when a central line is placed, which causes a direct mechanical insult (18–20), or by the treatment modalities used, including radiotherapy and chemotherapy. A generalized hypercoagulability in cancer patients is seen secondary to tumor elaboration of procoagulant factors, which directly affect the hemostatic balance and activate the coagulation system. A further factor in generating a hypercoagulable state is the response to the use of certain cytotoxic and biological anticancer agents. In particular, additional VTE risk has been reported with the use of a number of adjuvant treatments such as tamoxifen (21,22) and thalidomide (23,24). Finally, recent evidence suggests that the presence of congenital prothrombotic mutations, in particular *factor V Leiden* mutation and prothrombin 20210A mutation, appears to confer an even higher risk of VTE to cancer patients (25).

A recent prospective epidemiological study of 2373 patients undergoing abdominal, thoracic, urologic, or gynecologic cancer surgery offers important insight into which clinical and tumor-related factors are the most important in heightening VTE risk (26). The study identified five factors: age >60 years [odds ratio (OR) 2.63; 95% confidence interval (CI), 1.21–5.71], previous VTE (OR 5.98; 95% CI 2.13–16.80), advanced cancer (OR 2.68; 95% CI 1.37–5.24), anesthesia lasting more than two hours (OR 4.50; 95% CI 1.06–19.04), and bed rest longer than three days (OR 4.37; 95% CI 2.45–7.78).

The registry also provides insight into the natural history of VTE after cancer surgery (26). Although in-hospital thromboprophylaxis was provided in 82% of cases and continued after hospital discharge in 30%, 2.1% had symptomatic VTE. Interestingly, 40% of events occurred more than 21 days after surgery. The overall death rate was 1.72% and 46% of deaths were related to VTE, with VTE the most common cause of death at day 30.

METHODS OF THROMBOPROPHYLAXIS

There are two broad categories of methods for the prevention of venous thromboembolic disease: mechanical and pharmacological. Of the two, pharmacological methods have been most widely investigated and proven to be effective in prevention of both DVT and pulmonary embolism (PE). Mechanical methods have been less thoroughly evaluated and although effective in preventing DVT, have not been shown to offer protection against fatal PE.

Mechanical

Electrical Calf Stimulation

This method although beneficial in reducing venous stasis in a general surgical cohort did not appear to be effective in patients with malignancy (4).

Intermittent Pneumatic Compression

In a small study of cancer patients the frequency of DVT was reduced to 9% (2/23) from 40% (8/20) in the control group, but with a wide CI (27).

Graduated Static Compression Stockings

Stockings are used commonly in postoperative surgical patients, usually in combination with pharmacological methods of prophylaxis, to reduce the incidence of postoperative DVT (7). They have not been proven to reduce the risk of fatal PE when used as monotherapy against VTE and may be less effective in the oncological setting.

Inferior Vena Caval Filters

This prophylaxis method has been primarily evaluated in the setting of established VTE disease, with placement to prevent PE (28). There is no convincing evidence for filter use in primary prophylaxis unless pharmacological methods are contraindicated. They also do not appear as effective in protecting against fatal PE in cancer patients (29,30).

Pharmacological

Aspirin

This common agent works by inactivating platelet cyclo-oxygenase. Despite some advantages, including low cost and oral bioavailability, aspirin is generally regarded as ineffective in preventing VTE in surgical patients.

Oral Anticoagulants

These agents, such as warfarin, act as vitamin K antagonists, preventing posttranslational carboxylation of clotting factors II, VII, IX, and X in the liver. A limitation is that regular monitoring of the anticoagulant activity is required using the international normalized ratio (INR) and consequent dose adjustment. Controlling anticoagulation with oral anticoagulant (OAC) can be difficult because of the potential for drug interactions and the impact nutritional status can have on their action, making them unattractive for use in the postoperative period, especially if oral intake is contraindicated. The difficulty in achieving a safe and therapeutic INR can also be problematic in preventing postoperative VTE (31). Achieving therapeutic anticoagulation with OAC is more difficult in cancer patients than in noncancer patients (56.9% of the time vs. 43.3%; $P < 0.0001$) (32).

Unfractionated Heparin

The pentasaccharide sequence found on heparin species binds to the endogenous anticoagulant protein antithrombin with the effect of greatly increasing its ability to inhibit both thrombin and factor Xa. Low-dose unfractionated heparin (UFH) is given subcutaneously for VTE prophylaxis. The use of UFH may be complicated by the development of heparin-induced thrombocytopenia (HIT) (33). The effect of UFH may be rapidly reversed with protamine sulfate (34).

Low-Molecular-Weight Heparin

The mechanism of action is similar to UFH, but with diminished inhibition of thrombin. Prepared by chemical or enzymatic degradation of UFH, low-molecular-weight heparin (LMWH) has a lower average molecular weight than UFH, allowing effective absorption from the subcutaneous tissue. Its affinity for plasma proteins, platelets, macrophages, and endothelium is reduced, increasing the predictability of its anticoagulant response, with a longer plasma half-life (3.5–4.5 hours) and increased bioavailability (>85%). Subcutaneous administration is therefore facilitated on a once daily basis allowing for outpatient use. In addition, LMWH has a lower incidence of HIT (33,35), lower risk of bleeding (36–40), and has not been associated with osteoporosis (41–44).

PRIMARY SURGICAL THROMBOPROPHYLAXIS

Low-dose UFH is widely used in surgical thromboprophylaxis. It is commonly administered subcutaneously at a dose of 5000 units, starting two hours prior to surgery, and continued twice or three times a day. Early evidence supported the use of heparin (Table 2), and further evidence of a reduced incidence of VTE in cancer surgery patients who are given

Table 2 VTE Rates in Cancer and Noncancer Patients Receiving UFH Compared with Control

	Status	UFH	Control	Relative risk reduction
Rem et al., 1975 (5)	Benign	4/59 (7%)	18/65 (28%)	25%
	Malignant	7/24 (30%)	16/30 (53%)	55%
Gallus et al., 1976 (6)	Benign	8/304 (3%)	49/306 (16%)	18%
	Malignant	5/58 (9%)	17/76 (22%)	39%

Abbreviations: UFH, unfractionated heparin; VTE, venous thromboembolism.

Table 3 LMWH Vs. UFH: DVT Rates in Cancer Surgical Patients

	LMWH	Cancer patients (%)	VTE rates (%)	
			LMWH	UFH
Bergqvist et al., 1986 (47)	Dalteparin	45	6.4	4.3
Bergqvist et al., 1988 (48)	Dalteparin	63.3	5.5	8.3
Samama et al., 1988 (49)	Enoxaparin	30	3.2	5.0
Liezorovicz et al., 1991 (50)	Tinzaparin	38.5	5.8	4.2
Kakkar et al., 1993 (11)	Dalteparin	37.6	1.26	1.30
Boneu 1993 (51)	Reviparin	52.3	4.6	4.2
EFS group 1988 (52)	Nadroparin	100	4.2	5.4
Gallus et al., 1993 (53)	Danapariod	100	10.4	14.9
Nurmohamed et al., 1995 (54)	Enoxaparin	100	13.6	8.7
ENOXACAN Study Group 1997 (55)	Enoxaparin	100	14.7	18.2

Abbreviations: LMWH, low-molecular-weight heparin; UFH, unfractionated heparin; VTE, venous thromboembolism; DVT, deep vein thrombosis.
Source: Modified from Ref. 25.

thromboprophylaxis was provided by a meta-analysis conducted in 1988 which evaluated 29 trials in which surgical patients received UFH. Ten of the trials described findings in a total of 919 cancer patients. The study showed a significant reduction in the incidence of VTE from 30.6% in the absence of thromboprophylaxis to 13.6% in patients receiving UFH ($p < 0.001$) (45). UFH was also shown to reduce mortality due to PE from 1.6% to 0.4% in one randomized trial (46).

LMWH has been extensively investigated in surgery and has been proven to be at least as safe as, and at times more effective than, UFH in studies containing a high proportion of cancer patients (Table 3). In a study of patients undergoing elective, curative abdominal, or pelvic surgery for cancer, once daily LMWH was shown to be as effective as UFH given three times daily; of 631 evaluable patients, a total of 104 (16.5%) developed VTE of which 18.2% were patients receiving UFH and 14.7% received enoxaparin (55). There was no difference in bleeding events, other complications, or mortality at either 30 days or at three months. A recent systematic review described pooled findings from 26 randomized controlled trials of surgical oncology patients with a total of 7639 patients (56). The analysis showed a DVT rate without prophylaxis of 35.2%, which was reduced to 12.7% with heparin (UFH or LMWH) and the combination of heparin and mechanical prophylaxis further decreased the rate to 5%.

LMWH at higher doses (5000 units vs. 2500 units) may improve thromboprophylaxis efficacy without resulting in an increased risk of bleeding. In a study of 2097 surgical cancer patients, VTE rates were improved at the higher dose from 14.9% to 8.5% ($P = 0.001$) with no detrimental effect on bleeding rates (57). A systematic review found similar results, with significantly reduced rates of DVT apparent with higher dose LMWH and UFH in pooled analyses from 17 randomized controlled trials (Table 4) (56).

The optimal duration of thromboprophylaxis remains controversial for patients undergoing laparotomy for cancer. Prophylaxis should be administered for at least the duration of hospital stay. A recent well-designed clinical trial in over 300 patients undergoing laparotomy for cancer evaluated the benefits of continuing thromboprophylaxis for up to four weeks after operation. Patients received LWMH for 6 to 10 days and then received either LMWH or placebo for another 21 days. A total of 322 patients were followed for three months. Compared with patients receiving prophylaxis with LMWH for one week during

Table 4 High vs. Low-Dose Heparin: VTE Rates in Cancer Surgical Patients (56)

Agent	LMWH		UFH	
Dose level	High	Low	High	Low
Patients (n)	1025	954	363	486
DVT (%)	7.9	14.5	8	13.4
P value	$P < 0.0001$		$P = 0.0132$	

Abbreviations: LMWH, low-molecular-weight heparin; VTE, venous thromboembolism; DVT, deep vein thrombosis; UFH, unfractionated heparin.

hospital stay, those receiving the same for a further three weeks after hospital discharge had lower rates of VTE at four weeks after abdominal or pelvic surgical procedures for cancer (12% vs. 4.8.0%, $P = 0.02$) and at three months (13.8% vs. 5.5%, $P = 0.01$) (58).

LMWH has also been shown to be safe and effective in neurosurgery, despite the risk of intracranial bleeding. In a study in which about 85% of the subjects had malignancy of the central nervous system, thromboprophylaxis with LMWH achieved a 50% risk reduction in VTE rates ($p = 0.004$) (59), without increasing bleeding rates, when compared with compression stockings alone. Similar results were published in a large meta-analysis, showing a 48% VTE risk reduction (60).

CONCLUSIONS

Cancer is an important risk factor for thrombosis. Planning surgical intervention in this high-risk population where there may also be a bleeding risk requires careful consideration of the most appropriate prophylactic regimen. For the majority of cancer surgical patients this will be with either UFH or LMWH. In patients with active bleeding or a clear contraindication to pharmacological methods of thromboprophylaxis, the use of mechanical methods such as intermittent pneumatic compression and/or graduated compression stockings may be considered. The prophylaxis should be administered for at least the duration of hospital stay, and where additional risk factors for VTE persist, extended thromboprophylaxis with LMWH for up to four weeks after operation may be considered.

REFERENCES

1. Kakkar VV, Howe CT, Nicolaides AN, Renney JT, Clarke MB. Deep vein thrombosis of the leg. Is there a "high risk" group? Am J Surg 1970; 120(4):527–530.
2. Hills NH, Pflug JJ, Jeyasingh K, Boardman L, Calnan JS. Prevention of deep vein thrombosis by intermittent pneumatic compression of calf. Br Med J 1972; 1(793):131–135.
3. Walsh JJ, Bonnar J, Wright FW. A study of pulmonary embolism and deep leg vein thrombosis after major gynaecological surgery using labelled fibrinogen-phlebography and lung scanning. J Obstet Gynaecol Br Commonw 1974; 81(4):311–316.
4. Rosenberg IL, Evans M, Pollock AV. Letter: prophylaxis of postoperative deep vein thrombosis. Br Med J 1975; 3(5977):228.
5. Rem J, Duckert F, Fridrich R, Gruber UF. Subcutaneous small heparin doses for the prevention of thrombosis in general surgery and urology. Schweizerische Medizinische Wochenschrift. J Suisse Med 1975; 105(26):827–835.
6. Gallus AS, Hirsh J, O'Brien SE, McBride JA, Tuttle RJ, Gent M. Prevention of venous thrombosis with small, subcutaneous doses of heparin. JAMA 1976; 235(18):1980–1982.

7. Allan A, Williams JT, Bolton JP, Le Quesne LP. The use of graduated compression stockings in the prevention of postoperative deep vein thrombosis. Br J Surg 1983; 70(3):172–174.
8. Dihydroergotamine-heparin prophylaxis of postoperative deep vein thrombosis. A multicenter trial. The Multicenter Trial Committee. JAMA 1984; 251(22):2960–2966.
9. Kakkar VV, Murray WJ. Efficacy and safety of low-molecular-weight heparin (CY216) in preventing postoperative venous thrombo-embolism: a co-operative study. Br J Surg 1985; 72(10):786–791.
10. Sue-Ling HM, Johnston D, McMahon MJ, Philips PR, Davies JA. Pre-operative identification of patients at high risk of deep venous thrombosis after elective major abdominal surgery. Lancet 1986; 1(8491):1173–1176.
11. Kakkar VV, Cohen AT, Edmonson RA, et al. Low molecular weight versus standard heparin for prevention of venous thromboembolism after major abdominal surgery. The Thromboprophylaxis Collaborative Group [see comment]. Lancet 1993; 341(8840):259–265.
12. Geerts WH, Pineo GF, Heit JA, et al. Prevention of venous thromboembolism: the Seventh ACCP Conference on Antithrombotic and Thrombolytic Therapy. Chest 2004; 126(3 suppl):338S–400S.
13. Levitan N, Dowlati A, Remick SC, et al. Rates of initial and recurrent thromboembolic disease among patients with malignancy versus those without malignancy. Risk analysis using Medicare claims data. Medicine (Baltimore) 1999; 78:285–291.
14. Hutten BA, Prins MH, Gent M, Ginsberg J, Tijssen JG, Buller HR. Incidence of recurrent thromboembolic and bleeding complications among patients with venous thromboembolism in relation to both malignancy and achieved international normalized ratio: a retrospective analysis. J Clin Oncol 2000; 18(17):3078–3083.
15. Prandoni P. Cancer and thromboembolic disease: how important is the risk of thrombosis? Cancer Treat Rev 2002; 28(3):133–136.
16. Virchow R. Collected articles on scientific medicine. (Gesammalte abhandlungen zurwissenschaftlichen medtzin). Frankfurt, 1856.
17. Letai A, Kuter DJ. Cancer, coagulation, and anticoagulation. Oncologist 1999; 4(6):443–449.
18. Boraks P, Seale J, Price J, et al. Prevention of central venous catheter associated thrombosis using minidose warfarin in patients with haematological malignancies. Br J Haematol 1998; 101(3):483–486.
19. Monreal M, Alastrue A, Rull M, et al. Upper extremity deep venous thrombosis in cancer patients with venous access devices—prophylaxis with a low molecular weight heparin (Fragmin). Thromb Haemost 1996; 75(2):251–253.
20. De Cicco M, Matovic M, Balestreri L, et al. Central venous thrombosis: an early and frequent complication in cancer patients bearing long-term silastic catheter. A prospective study. Thromb Res 1997; 86(2):101–113.
21. Saphner T, Tormey DC, Gray R. Venous and arterial thrombosis in patients who received adjuvant therapy for breast cancer. J Clin Oncol 1991; 9:286–294.
22. Pritchard KI, Paterson AH, Paul NA, Zee B, Fine S, Pater J. Increased thromboembolic complications with concurrent tamoxifen and chemotherapy in a randomized trial of adjuvant therapy for women with breast cancer. National Cancer Institute of Canada Clinical Trials Group Breast Cancer Site Group. J Clin Oncol 1996; 14:2731–2737.
23. Zangari M, Anaissie E, Barlogie B, et al. Increased risk of deep-vein thrombosis in patients with multiple myeloma receiving thalidomide and chemotherapy. Blood 2001; 98:1614–1615.
24. Rus C, Bazzan M, Palumbo A, Bringhen S, Boccadoro M. Thalidomide in front line treatment in multiple myeloma: serious risk of venous thromboembolism and evidence for thromboprophylaxis. J Thromb Haemost 2004; 2:2063–2065.
25. Blom JW, Doggen CJ, Osanto S, Rosendaal FR. Malignancies, prothrombotic mutations, and the risk of venous thrombosis. JAMA 2005; 293:715–722.
26. Agnelli G, Bolis G, Capussotti L, et al. A clinical outcome-based prospective study on venous thromboembolism after cancer surgery: the @RISTOS project. Ann Surg 2006; 243(1):89–95.
27. Roberts VC, Cotton LT. Prevention of postoperative deep vein thrombosis in patients with malignant disease. Br Med J 1974; 1(904):358–360.

28. Decousus H, Leizorovicz A, Parent F, et al. A clinical trial of vena caval filters in the prevention of pulmonary embolism in patients with proximal deep-vein thrombosis. Prevention du Risque d'Embolie Pulmonaire par Interruption Cave Study Group [see comment]. N Engl J Med 1998; 338(7):409–415.
29. Athanasoulis CA, Kaufman JA, Halpern EF, Waltman AC, Geller SC, Fan CM. Inferior vena caval filters: review of a 26-year single-center clinical experience. Radiology 2000; 216(1):54–66.
30. Millward SF, Peterson RA, Moher D, et al. LGM (Vena Tech) vena caval filter: experience at a single institution. J Vasc Intervent Radiol 1994; 5(2):351–356.
31. Harrison L, Johnston M, Massicotte MP, Crowther M, Moffat K, Hirsh J. Comparison of 5-mg and 10-mg loading doses in initiation of warfarin therapy. Ann Intern Med 1997; 126(2):133–136.
32. Bona RD, Sivjee KY, Hickey AD, Wallace DM, Wajcs SB. The efficacy and safety of oral anticoagulation in patients with cancer. Thromb Haemost 1995; 74(4):1055–1058.
33. Hirsh J, Warkentin T, Raschke R, Granger C, Ohman E, Dalen J. Heparin and low-molecular-weight heparin: mechanisms of action, pharmacokinetics, dosing considerations, monitoring, efficacy, and safety. Chest 1998; 114(5):489S–510S.
34. Lee AY. Management of thrombosis in cancer: primary prevention and secondary prophylaxis. Br J Haematol 2004; 128(3):291–302.
35. Warkentin TE, Levine MN, Hirsh J, et al. Heparin-induced thrombocytopenia in patients treated with low-molecular-weight heparin or unfractionated heparin [see comment]. N Engl J Med 1995; 332(20):1330–1335.
36. Siragusa S, Cosmi B, Piovella F, Hirsh J, Ginsberg JS. Low-molecular-weight heparins and unfractionated heparin in the treatment of patients with acute venous thromboembolism: results of a meta-analysis [see comment]. Am J Med 1996; 100(3):269–277.
37. Lensing AW, Prins MH, Davidson BL, Hirsh J. Treatment of deep venous thrombosis with low-molecular-weight heparins. A meta-analysis [see comment]. Arch Intern Med 1995; 155(6):601–607.
38. Leizorovicz A, Simonneau G, Decousus H, Boissel JP. Comparison of efficacy and safety of low molecular weight heparins and unfractionated heparin in initial treatment of deep venous thrombosis: a meta-analysis. BMJ 1994; 309(6950):299–304.
39. Dolovich LR, Ginsberg JS, Douketis JD, Holbrook AM, Cheah G. A meta-analysis comparing low-molecular-weight heparins with unfractionated heparin in the treatment of venous thromboembolism: examining some unanswered questions regarding location of treatment, product type, and dosing frequency. Arch Intern Med 2000; 160(2):181–188.
40. Gould MK, Dembitzer AD, Doyle RL, Hastie TJ, Garber AM. Low-molecular-weight heparins compared with unfractionated heparin for treatment of acute deep venous thrombosis. A meta-analysis of randomized, controlled trials. Ann Intern Med 1999; 130(10):800–809.
41. Kakkar AK, Williamson RC. Prevention of venous thromboembolism in cancer using low-molecular-weight heparins. Haemostasis 1997; 27(suppl 1):32–37.
42. Muir JM, Hirsh J, Weitz JI, Andrew M, Young E, Shaughnessy SG. A histomorphometric comparison of the effects of heparin and low-molecular-weight heparin on cancellous bone in rats. Blood 1997; 89(9):3236–3242.
43. Shaughnessy SG, Young E, Deschamps P, Hirsh J. The effects of low molecular weight and standard heparin on calcium loss from fetal rat calvaria. Blood 1995; 86(4):1368–1373.
44. Monreal M, Lafoz E, Olive A, del Rio L, Vedia C. Comparison of subcutaneous unfractionated heparin with a low molecular weight heparin (Fragmin) in patients with venous thromboembolism and contraindications to coumarin. Thromb Haemost 1994; 71(1):7–11.
45. Clagett GP, Reisch JS. Prevention of venous thromboembolism in general surgical patients. Results of meta-analysis. Ann Surg 1988; 208(2):227–240.
46. Anonymous. Prevention of fatal postoperative pulmonary embolism by low doses of heparin. An international multicentre trial. Lancet 1975; 2(7924):45–51.

47. Bergqvist D, Burmark US, Frisell J, et al. Low molecular weight heparin once daily compared with conventional low-dose heparin twice daily. A prospective double-blind multicentre trial on prevention of postoperative thrombosis. Br J Surg 1986; 73(3):204–208.
48. Bergqvist D, Matzsch T, Burmark US, et al. Low molecular weight heparin given the evening before surgery compared with conventional low-dose heparin in prevention of thrombosis [erratum appears in Br J Surg 1988; 75(11):1077]. Br J Surg 1988; 75(9):888–891.
49. Samama M, Bernard P, Bonnardot JP, Combe-Tamzali S, Lanson Y, Tissot E. Low molecular weight heparin compared with unfractionated heparin in prevention of postoperative thrombosis. Br J Surg 1988; 75(2):128–131.
50. Liezorovicz A, Picolet H, Peyrieux JC, Boissel JP. Prevention of perioperative deep vein thrombosis in general surgery: a multicentre double blind study comparing two doses of Logiparin and standard heparin. H. B. P. M. Research Group. Br J Surg 1991; 78(4):412–416.
51. Boneu B. An international multicentre study: Clivarin in the prevention of venous thromboembolism in patients undergoing general surgery. Report of the International Clivarin Assessment Group. Blood Coagul Fibrinolysis 1993; 4(suppl 1):S21–S22.
52. Anonymous. Comparison of a low molecular weight heparin and unfractionated heparin for the prevention of deep vein thrombosis in patients undergoing abdominal surgery. The European Fraxiparin Study (EFS) Group. Br J Surg 1988; 75(11):1058–1063.
53. Gallus A, Cade J, Ockelford P, et al. Orgaran (Org 10172) or heparin for preventing venous thrombosis after elective surgery for malignant disease? A double-blind, randomised, multicentre comparison. ANZ-Organon Investigators' Group. Thromb Haemost 1993; 70(4):562–567.
54. Nurmohamed MT, Verhaeghe R, Haas S, et al. A comparative trial of a low molecular weight heparin (enoxaparin) versus standard heparin for the prophylaxis of postoperative deep vein thrombosis in general surgery. Am J Surg 1995; 169(6):567–571.
55. ENOXACAN Study Group. Efficacy and safety of enoxaparin versus unfractionated heparin for prevention of deep vein thrombosis in elective cancer surgery: a double-blind randomized multicentre trial with venographic assessment. Br J Surg 1997; 84:1099–1103.
56. Leonardi MJ, McGory ML, Ko CY. A systematic review of deep venous thrombosis prophylaxis in cancer patients: implications for improving quality. Ann Surg Oncol 2007; 14:929–936.
57. Bergqvist D, Burmark US, Flordal PA, et al. Low molecular weight heparin started before surgery as prophylaxis against deep vein thrombosis: 2500 versus 5000 XaI units in 2070 patients [see comment]. Br J Surg 1995; 82(4):496–501.
58. Bergqvist D, Agnelli G, Cohen AT, et al. Duration of prophylaxis against venous thromboembolism with enoxaparin after surgery for cancer. N Engl J Med 2002; 346(13):975–980.
59. Agnelli G, Piovella F, Buoncristiani P, et al. Enoxaparin plus compression stockings compared with compression stockings alone in the prevention of venous thromboembolism after elective neurosurgery. N Engl J Med 1998; 339(2):80–85.
60. Iorio A, Agnelli G. Low-molecular-weight and unfractionated heparin for prevention of venous thromboembolism in neurosurgery: a meta-analysis. Arch Intern Med 2000; 160(15):2327–2332.

14

Preventing Venous Thromboembolism in the Medical Cancer Patient

Sylvia Haas
Institut für Experimentelle Onkologie und Therapieforschung, Technische Universität München, Munich, Germany

- Cancer patients, particularly those with advanced disease or receiving active therapy, are at significant risk for venous thromboembolism (VTE) but also for fatal bleeding; careful risk–benefit assessments are necessary when evaluating for prophylaxis.
- For ambulatory cancer patients receiving chemotherapy, only a few prophylaxis studies have been conducted, and the value of routine primary thromboprophylaxis is not yet established.
- For hospitalized cancer patients, data derived from studies of prophylaxis in acutely ill medical patients may be extrapolated to the cancer population. Cancer patients are considered high risk and should receive anticoagulant prophylaxis, using either low-molecular-weight heparin (LMWH), Unfractionated heparin (UFH), or fondaparinux.
- In hospitalized cancer patients with a contraindication for anticoagulant prophylaxis, the use of mechanical prophylaxis is recommended.
- Compliance with prophylaxis recommendations continues to be suboptimal; use of computerized order entry alerts to health-care providers represents a novel way to improve rates of thromboprophylaxis in the hospital setting.

INTRODUCTION

Cancer is an important risk factor for venous thromboembolism (VTE) and is associated with at least a two- to fourfold increased risk compared with estimates for the normal population (1–3). High rates of fatal pulmonary embolism (PE) as well as fatal bleeding in cancer patients have been reported by Monreal et al. on behalf of the Riete investigators (4). Since both fatal PE and fatal hemorrhagic complications are more common in cancer patients with VTE than in those patients without cancer, a careful benefit/risk assessment regarding anticoagulation-based prophylaxis is necessary.

A literature review shows that certain tumor types are particularly associated with VTE, including pancreatic, prostatic, and colorectal carcinomas, and interestingly, this has been known since a long time (5–8). These findings suggest that adenocarcinomas are particularly associated with VTE. A recent study has confirmed that lung cancer, in particular, lung adenocarcinoma, is associated with a high risk of VTE. A 20-fold higher rate than the general population, with a symptomatic rate of about 6%, was seen in a large cohort study of non–small cell lung cancer (9).

Metastatic cancer is thought to carry a high risk of thrombosis, which is supported by a recent case–control study showing an approximately 20-fold increased risk in patients with metastatic disease compared with those without metastases. The authors also describe that the VTE risk is especially high in the first few months after diagnosis (10).

This chapter will address the issue of VTE prophylaxis in nonsurgical cancer patients and provide evidence-based recommendations or expert suggestions where the evidence is lacking.

CHEMOTHERAPY OR HORMONE THERAPY INCREASES THE RISK OF VTE

Nonsurgical cancer therapies can increase the risk of thromboembolic disease. The relation between VTE and chemotherapy has been most extensively investigated in patients with breast cancer. Levine et al. demonstrated that chemotherapy contributes to thrombosis in patients with breast cancer (11). They performed a randomized trial comparing 12 weeks of chemohormone therapy (using cyclophosphamide, methotrexate, fluorouracil, vincristine, prednisone, doxorubicin, and tamoxifen) with 36 weeks of chemotherapy (using cyclophosphamide, methotrexate, fluorouracil, vincristine, and prednisone) in patients with stage II breast cancer. Among 205 patients randomly assigned to treatment, there were 14 episodes of thrombosis (6.8%). These 14 episodes occurred during 979 patient-months of chemotherapy; in comparison, there were no events during 2413 patient-months without therapy.

Hormone therapy also affects the thrombotic risk. For example, tamoxifen raises the risk of developing a thromboembolism regardless of the presence of a neoplasm or use of chemotherapy. An editorial published by Goldhaber summarized four trials on the use of tamoxifen as prophylaxis against breast cancer. All tamoxifen-prevention trials compared tamoxifen 20 mg daily with placebo for at least five years. Overall, 14,192 patients were randomized to tamoxifen, and 14,214 patients received placebo. Of these, 289 breast cancers developed among women receiving tamoxifen as compared with 465 in the placebo group. The number of new breast cancers was 38% lower in tamoxifen-treated patients, with 95% confidence intervals (CIs) of 28% to 46% ($P < 0.0001$). Thus, all four studies trended in favor of tamoxifen; however, the most frequent side effect in patients treated with tamoxifen versus placebo was a doubling of the rate of VTE: 118 versus 62 cases. A similar increase in superficial phlebitis (68 vs. 30 cases) also occurred (12). The Italian Tamoxifen Study Group assessed the effect of tamoxifen on VTE in a breast cancer prevention trial and studied its association with risk factors for VTE. The incidence of VTE was studied in 5408 hysterectomized women randomly assigned to tamoxifen 20 mg/day or placebo for five years. There were 28 VTEs on placebo and 44 on tamoxifen therapy [hazard ratio (HR) = 1.63; 95% CI, 1.02 – 2.63), 80% of which were superficial phlebitis, accounting for all of the excess due to tamoxifen within 18 months from randomization. Compared with placebo, the risk of VTE on tamoxifen was higher in women aged 55 years or older, women with a body mass index ≥25 kg/m^2, elevated blood pressure, total cholesterol ≥250 mg/dL, current smoking, and a family history of coronary heart disease (CHD). Of the 685 women with a CHD risk score ≥5 who entered the trial, one in the placebo arm and 13 in the tamoxifen arm developed VTE (log-rank $P = 0.0013$). In multivariate regression analysis, age ≥60 years, height ≥165 cm, and diastolic blood pressure ≥90 mmHg had independent detrimental effects on VTE risk during tamoxifen therapy, whereas transdermal estrogen therapy concomitant with tamoxifen was not associated with any excess of VTE (HR = 0.64; 95% CI, 0.23–1.82). The authors conclude that women with conventional risk factors for atherosclerosis have a higher risk of VTE during tamoxifen therapy. This information should be incorporated into counseling women on its risk–benefit ratio, particularly in the prevention setting (13).

PROPHYLAXIS OF VTE

Placebo-Controlled Prophylaxis Trials in Nonsurgical Cancer and General Medical Patients

Metastatic Breast Cancer

Levine et al. have assessed the safety and efficacy of warfarin in very low doses as prophylaxis. Women receiving chemotherapy for metastatic breast cancer were randomly assigned either very-low-dose warfarin (152 patients) or placebo. The warfarin dose was 1 mg daily for six weeks and was then adjusted to maintain the prothrombin time at an international normalized ratio (INR) of 1.3 to 1.9. Study treatment continued until one week after the end of chemotherapy. The average daily dose from initiation of titration was 2.6 mg (SD 1.2) for the warfarin group, and the mean INR was 1.52. There were seven thromboembolic events [six deep-vein thrombosis (DVT), one PE] in the placebo group and one (PE) in the warfarin group, a relative risk reduction of about 85% ($p = 0.031$). Major bleeding occurred in two placebo recipients and one warfarin-treated patient. Very-low-dose warfarin was found to be a safe and effective method for prevention of thromboembolism in patients with metastatic breast cancer who were receiving chemotherapy (14). However, despite these interesting findings, additional studies are required before recommendations can be made regarding thromboprophylaxis use in cancer patients receiving chemotherapy.

A recent double-blind trial (TOPIC-I) focused on a similar patient population. Patients with objectively proven primary or secondary metastatic breast carcinoma and treated with chemotherapy were randomly assigned to receive the low-molecular-weight heparin (LMWH) certoparin at a dose of 3000 antiXa-IU, or placebo, subcutaneously once daily, for six months. All patients were routinely screened for DVT by compression ultrasound once per month. The primary efficacy outcome was any VTE (symptomatic and asymptomatic). Safety outcomes were major and minor bleeding and thrombocytopenia. VTE occurred in 7 (4%) of 174 patients on certoparin and 7 (4%) of 177 patients on placebo [odds ratio (OR), 1.02; 95% CI, 0.30–3.48]. The overall rate of thrombosis was not different between groups. The two treatment groups did not differ in the number of patients who experienced major and minor bleeding (nine events in certoparin-treated patients vs. three in the placebo group; OR, 3.18; 95% CI, 0.88–18.53). There was no difference in the incidence of thrombocytopenia. Since the incidence of VTE in ambulant patients with metastatic breast cancer was lower than expected (4%) and there was no risk reduction apparent after six months of LMWH, it can be concluded that routine prophylaxis is not appropriate for this patient group (15).

Non–Small Cell Lung Carcinoma

Adult patients with objectively proven, inoperable, disseminated primary non–small cell lung carcinoma of stage IIIa, IIIb, or IV, were eligible for inclusion in the TOPIC-II study.

The following chemotherapy regimens were permitted: platinum-containing compounds in combination with etoposide, vinca alkaloids, gemcitabine or any taxane; mitomycin, ifosfamide, cisplatin (MIC); mitomycin, vindesine, cisplatin (MVP); monotherapy with mitomycin, gemcitabine, or vinorelbine. Patients were assigned to receive single daily subcutaneous injections of placebo or certoparin sodium 3000 antiXa-IU for six months.

During the six-month treatment period, patients were screened monthly by compression ultrasound for DVT, an assessment of any symptoms of VTE, recording of any adverse event, such as bleeding episodes, the provision of study drug, and a review of concomitant medications and blood biochemistry. The primary efficacy outcome was the first incidence of objectively confirmed VTE during the six-month treatment period, either symptomatic or asymptomatic, including: DVT (proximal or distal) confirmed by venography and/or ultrasonography; PE confirmed by computerized tomography or ventilation-perfusion scintigraphy, or shown at autopsy; thrombosis of the jugular or subclavian veins confirmed by ultrasonography; and femoral thrombophlebitis (if heparin-based treatment was required).

In this study, the incidence of VTE in placebo-treated patients with inoperable cancer was 8.3% versus 4.5% in the certoparin group. Although the risk reduction seen with LMWH prophylaxis given for six months was not significant, the study was underpowered because of higher expected rates of VTE used in the sample size calculation. A post hoc analysis suggested that the risk of VTE may correlate with histologic stage, with stage IV patients experiencing the highest risk of an event (10.2%) and, distinct from the whole study population, a significant risk reduction with LMWH prophylaxis of around 65% was shown. The results are summarized in Table 1.

The patients enrolled in this study were newly diagnosed with cancer, with a mean time between diagnosis and study treatment initiation of 0.3 years. Given the view that patients with cancer have a highly increased risk of thrombosis in the first few months after cancer diagnosis (10) and the poor outlook for patients with inoperable lung cancer, the timing of the prophylaxis would appear to have been optimal to give patients the best hope of benefiting from LMWH. Although there was no risk reduction apparent, considering symptomatic VTE alone, the incidence was much higher in the placebo arm (3.4%). This risk of a symptomatic event is markedly higher than that associated with common orthopaedic procedures—rates of around 1.5% after one month of thromboprophylaxis have been reported (16). This suggests that late-stage lung cancer patients are at high risk, according to accepted definitions of risk (17). The higher risk of VTE in stage IV lung

Table 1 Efficacy Outcome Events TOPIC-II study

	Intervention	
	Certoparin	**Placebo**
Number of patients, *n* (%)	268 (100)	264 (100)
Venous thromboembolism (primary endpoint)	12 (4.5)	22 (8.3)
Symptomatic deep vein thrombosis	4 (1.5)	9 (3.4)
Asymptomatic pulmonary embolism	2 (0.8)	4 (1.5)
Asymptomatic deep vein thrombosis	4 (1.5)	7 (2.7)
Subclavian vein thrombosis	4 (1.5)	2 (0.8)
Femoral thrombophlebitis (heparin-treated)	0	2 (0.8)
Venous thromboembolism (according to stage)		
Stage IIIa and IIIb	7/124 (5.7)	8/125 (6.4)
Stage IV	5/144 (3.5)	14/139 (10.2)

cancer patients versus stage III may reflect higher levels of coagulopathy. These findings should help in the design of future studies in this higher-risk patient group.

Bleeding complications in medically unwell cancer patients with extensive disease are a particular concern. Although not significant, there were markedly more bleeding events in the LMWH treatment arm, including major bleeding events. Again, the study was underpowered to determine the significance of these findings.

Strengths of the study include the randomized, double-blind, placebo-controlled design, and the objective confirmation of VTE events. This study provides initial insight that extended prophylaxis may benefit patients with late-stage disease, but additional clinical trials are warranted to characterize the natural history of lung cancer–related VTE and to define better VTE prevention strategies for this cancer type (15).

Medical Patients

Medically ill patients are at increased risk for developing VTE while being hospitalized (17), and many studies indicate that such patients often do not receive VTE prophylaxis (18). As an example, in one study, 75% of patients admitted to a medical service were characterized as being at increased risk for VTE, yet only 43% received prophylaxis of any type (19).

Much more evidence has become available for routine use of prophylaxis in hospitalized general medical patients than for nonsurgical cancer patients. Patients with a broad variety of acute medical illnesses had been included in these trials and only some of these had cancer. Nevertheless, malignancy has been defined as an independent risk factor for VTE (20). However, the total number of cancer patients was too low to differentiate between patients with a history of cancer and those suffering from active malignancies requiring treatment. Furthermore, no detailed data could be obtained from these trials regarding various cancer types. In comparison to placebo, pharmacological methods of VTE prevention are highly efficacious and anticoagulant prevention with low-dose UFH, LMWH, and fondaparinux have been shown to be effective agents in the prevention of VTE in this setting (21–25). There is little, poor-quality data or no data on other methods such as aspirin and other antiplatelet agents, oral anticoagulants, or mechanical methods. A meta-analysis of heparin studies has shown an overall two-thirds reduction in VTE events. This benefit must be balanced against an increased risk of major bleeding, and the meta-analysis provided by Mismetti et al. indicates that risk is less when LMWH is compared to UFH (21). Current consensus statements recommend UFH or LMWH. Despite this, thromboprophylactic therapy utilization is sporadic and often infrequent, even in high-risk patients. This may in part be due to the failure to identify patients at risk of VTE. Risk assessment models are being further refined based on evidence from the recent data, and cancer has become an accepted risk factor. It should be mentioned that cancer may contribute to both an increase of exposing and predisposing risk. Active malignancy, in particular with concomitant risk-increasing treatment modalities such as chemotherapy or hormone therapy, may be assessed as an exposing (disease related) risk factor, whereas history of malignancy may be assessed as a permanent predisposing risk factor.

Important placebo controlled trials on general medical patients

Dahan et al. studied the antithrombotic efficacy of single daily doses of enoxaparin 60 mg in 270 medical patients over 65 years of age under placebo-controlled, double-blind conditions. The patients were screened for DVT by ^{125}I fibrinogen scanning. LMWH significantly reduced the frequency of DVT from 9% to 3% ($p = 0.03$). Adverse drug reactions did not differ significantly between the two groups, except for the injection site hematomas that were more frequent in the LMWH group. The authors concluded that LMWH appears to be of value in preventing the occurrence of DVT in an unselected elderly in-patient population (22).

Three recent placebo-controlled studies have confirmed the evidence on the efficacy and safety of pharmacologic prophylaxis in acutely ill medical patients treated in hospital. The Prophylaxis in Medical patients with Enoxaparin trial (MEDENOX) study blindly randomized 1102 hospitalized medical patients to receive either enoxaparin 40 mg subcutaneously daily, enoxaparin 20 mg subcutaneously daily, or placebo for 6 to 14 days. A total of 866 patients had bilateral venograms done; 5.5% of the enoxaparin 40 mg group developed VTE at that stage, as compared to 14.9% in the placebo group (relative risk of 0.37; $P < 0.001$). There were no significant differences in rates of VTE between the placebo group and the enoxaparin 20 mg group. The benefits of the higher dose were maintained throughout the three-month follow-up period, while the risk of major hemorrhage was not significantly increased. This study confirmed that medical patients are at considerable risk of VTE. Proximal and distal DVT rates were 4.9% and 9.4%, respectively, in the placebo arm (23).

The PRospective Evaluation of Dalteparin Efficacy for Prevention of VTE in immobilized patieNts Trial (PREVENT) blindly randomized 3706 hospitalized medical patients, with similar inclusion criteria to those used in the MEDENOX study. They received either dalteparin 5000 antiXa-IU daily or placebo for 14 days, and were evaluated by compression ultrasound after 21 days. The medication offered a relative risk reduction of 45% ($P = 0.0015$), reducing the rate of VTE from 4.96% to 2.77%. This benefit extended throughout the 90-day follow-up period, with a low associated risk of major bleeding. Despite this, there was no significant difference in overall all-cause mortality (24).

Fondaparinux is a chemical synthetic agent that specifically inhibits factor Xa with no platelet interaction, thus theoretically resulting in no heparin-induced thrombocytopenia.

The Arixtra for ThromboEmbolism prevention in a Medical Indications Study (ARTEMIS) blindly randomized 849 hospitalized medical patients over 60 years old to 6 to 14 days of either fondaparinux 2.5 mg subcutaneously daily or placebo. Venography showed a relative risk reduction for DVT of 46.7% ($P = 0.029$) (5.6% vs. 10.5%) in those receiving fondaparinux in this moderate-to-high-risk group. During the treatment period, five fatal PEs occurred in the placebo group only ($P = 0.029$), and the risk of major bleeding complications was minimal, being 1% in each group (25).

The efficacy results of these three recent studies are summarized in Table 2.

DISCUSSION

When considering the prevention of VTE in the medical cancer patient, two settings need to be discussed: the ambulatory patient who is receiving chemotherapy, radiation, and/or hormone therapy, and the patient who is bedridden for prolonged periods of time. Compared to data on patients undergoing cancer surgery, much less data are available on the primary prevention of thrombosis in ambulatory nonsurgical cancer patients. Despite first evidence on the effectiveness of low-intensity warfarin prophylaxis in patients with metastatic breast cancer and of LMWH in patients with advanced non–small cell lung cancer, no routine prophylaxis can be recommended for these patients. In particular for LMWH, the questions of optimal dose and duration of prophylaxis are still open.

The evidence for prophylaxis is much better for hospitalized medical patients than for specific cancer populations. The beneficial effects of UFH, LMWH, and fondaparinux

Table 2 Prevention of VTE in Medical Patients—Recent Placebo Controlled Trials

Results (%)		MEDENOX (23)			ARTEMIS (25)		PREVENT (24)	
		Enoxaparin 40 mg	Enoxaparin 20 mg	Placebo	Fondaparinux	Placebo	Dalteparin	Placebo
DVT	Distal	3.78	10.45	9.37	4.05	6.81	0.17	0.23
	Proximal	1.72	4.53	4.86	1.56	2.17	1.65	3.45
PE	Symptom	0	0	0.69	0	0	0.28	0.22
	Fatal	0	0	0	0	1.55	0	0.11

Abbreviations: MEDENOX, The Prophylaxis in Medical patients with Enoxaparin trial; ARTEMIS, Arixtra for Thromboembolism prevention in a Medical Indications Study; PREVENT, Prospective Evaluation of Dalteparin Efficacy for Prevention of VTE in Immobilized Patients Trial; VTE, venous thromboembolism; DVT, deep-vein thrombosis; PE, pulmonary embolism.

have been shown in various placebo-controlled trials where a broad variety of medical patients had been included of whom a few also had cancer. Thus, based on these considerations, it would seem reasonable that patients with advanced malignancy who are bedridden would benefit from prophylaxis with low-dose UFH or LMWH. Further research is required to evaluate prolonged antithrombotic prophylaxis in the medical cancer population. All hospitalized medical patients should be assessed for risk of VTE, and those at moderate (immobilized patients with active disease) or high risk (stroke, age >70 years, cardiac failure, shock, history of previous VTE, malignancy, or thrombophilia) should receive prophylaxis. Prospectively evaluated risk assessment models could help to define patients who may get most benefit from prophylaxis, and electronic alerts should be considered for hospitals with computerized order entry systems. Kucher et al. hypothesized that the use of a computer-alert program to encourage prophylaxis might reduce the frequency of DVT among high-risk hospitalized patients. The authors developed a computer program linked to the patient database to identify consecutive hospitalized patients at risk for DVT in the absence of prophylaxis. The computer program used eight common risk factors to determine each hospitalized patient's risk profile for VTE. Each risk factor was weighted according to a point scale: the major risk factors of cancer, prior VTE, and hypercoagulability were assigned a score of 3; the intermediate risk factor of major surgery was assigned a score of 2; and the minor risk factors of advanced age, obesity, bed rest, and the use of hormone-replacement therapy or oral contraceptives were assigned a score of 1. An increased risk of VTE was defined as a cumulative risk score of at least 4, so that patients who had at least one major risk factor and at least one intermediate risk factor or minor risk factor were eligible for the study. In the absence of a major risk factor, patients who had at least one intermediate risk factor and at least two minor risk factors were also eligible. Daily screening of the computer-alert program permitted them to identify and enroll patients who initially had a VTE risk score of less than four but whose score increased to four or higher during hospitalization. The program used medical record numbers to randomly assign 1255 eligible patients to an intervention group, in which the physician responsible was alerted to a patient's risk of DVT, and 1251 patients to a control group, in which no alert was issued. The physician was required to acknowledge the alert and could then withhold or order prophylaxis, including graduated compression stockings (GCS), pneumatic compression boots, UFH, LMWH, or warfarin. The primary end point was clinically diagnosed, objectively confirmed DVT or PE at 90 days. The authors were able to show that more patients in the intervention group than in the control group received mechanical prophylaxis (10.0% vs. 1.5%, $P < 0.001$) or pharmacologic prophylaxis (23.6% vs. 13.0%, $P < 0.001$). The primary end point occurred in 61 patients (4.9%) in the intervention group, as compared with

103 (8.2%) in the control group; the Kaplan-Meier estimates of the likelihood of freedom from DVT or PE at 90 days were 94.1% (95% CI, 92.5–95.4%) and 90.6% (95 CI, 88.7–92.2%), respectively ($P < 0.001$). The computer alert significantly reduced the risk of DVT or PE at 90 days by 41%. Thus, it can be concluded that the institution of a computer-alert program increased physicians' use of prophylaxis and markedly reduced the rates of DVT and PE among hospitalized patients at risk (26).

RECOMMENDATIONS OF VTE PREVENTION FOR NONSURGICAL CANCER PATIENTS

Medical patients can be classified as low-, moderate-, or high-risk for VTE depending upon their underlying medical condition and other comorbid factors, and should be treated as follows:

- In acutely ill medical patients who have been admitted to the hospital with congestive heart failure or severe respiratory disease, or who are confined to bed and have one or more additional risk factors, including active cancer, previous VTE, sepsis, acute neurologic disease, or inflammatory bowel disease, prophylaxis with UFH (Grade 1A) or LMWH (Grade 1A) is recommended (17).
- In medical patients with risk factors for VTE, and in whom there is a contraindication for anticoagulant prophylaxis, the use of mechanical prophylaxis with graduated compression stockings or intermittent pneumatic compression (Grade 1C+) is recommended (17).
- The optimal duration of thromboprophylaxis in medical patients is unknown.
- For ambulatory cancer patients receiving therapy out of hospital, only a few prospective trials have evaluated antithrombotic intervention. The value of routine primary thromboprophylaxis for these patients receiving chemotherapy is not yet established.
- For bed-ridden hospitalized cancer patients, there are no specific studies that have evaluated potential benefits from thromboprophylaxis. Therefore, data derived from contemporary trials assessing the value of LMWH in the prevention of thromboembolic disease in acutely ill medical patients may be extrapolated to the cancer population.
- For cancer patients hospitalized with acute medical illness, thromboprophylaxis should be based on the risk for VTE determined by the acute medical comorbidity. LMWH (initiated and dosed according to manufacturer's recommendations), fondaparinux, or UFH (5000 IU eight-hourly) should be used.
- According to available evidence, high-risk prophylactic doses of LMWH and fondaparinux have proven to be most effective in general medical patients. Therefore, no lower prophylactic doses should be given to cancer patients.

REFERENCES

1. Heit JA, Silverstein MD, Mohr DN, Petterson TM, O'Fallon WM, Melton LJ III. Risk factors for deep vein thrombosis and pulmonary embolism: a population-based case-control study. Arch Intern Med 2000; 160:809–815.
2. Samama MM. An epidemiologic study of risk factors for deep vein thrombosis in medical outpatients: the Sirius study. Arch Intern Med 2000; 160:3415–3420.

3. Ambrus JL, Ambrus CM, Mink IB, Pickren JW. Causes of death in cancer patients. J Med 1975; 6:61–64.
4. Monreal M, Falga C, Valdes M, et al. Fatal pulmonary embolism and fatal bleeding in cancer patients with venous thromboembolism: findings from the RIETE registry. J Thromb Haemost 2006; 4:1950–1956.
5. Thompson CM, Rodgers LR. Analysis of the autopsy records of 157 cases of carcinoma of the pancreas with particular reference to the incidence of thromboembolism. Am J Med Sci 1952; 223:469–478.
6. Mikal S, Campbell AJA. Carcinoma of the pancreas. Diagnostic and operative criteria based on one hundred consecutive autopsies. Surgery 1950; 28:963–969.
7. Miller JR, Baggenstoss AH, Comfort MW. Carcinoma of the pancreas. Effect of histological type and grade of malignancy on its behaviour. Cancer 1951; 4:233–241.
8. Monreal M, Fernandez-Llamazares J, Perandreu J, Urrutia A, Sahuquillo JC, Contel E. Occult cancer in patients with venous thromboembolism: which patients, which cancers. Thromb Haemost 1997; 78:1316–1318.
9. Blom JW, Osanto S, Rosendaal FR. The risk of a venous thrombotic event in lung cancer patients: higher risk for adenocarcinoma than squamous cell carcinoma. J Thromb Haemost 2004; 2:1760–1765.
10. Blom JW, Doggen CJ, Osanto S, et al. Malignancies, prothrombotic mutations, and the risk of venous thrombosis. JAMA 2005; 293:715–722.
11. Levine MN, Gent M, Hirsh J, et al. The thrombogenic effect of anticancer drug therapy in women with stage II breast cancer. N Engl J Med 1988; 318:404–407.
12. Goldhaber SZ. Tamoxifen: preventing breast cancer and placing the risk of deep vein thrombosis in perspective. Circulation 2005; 111:539–541.
13. Decensi A, Maisonneuve P, Rotmensz N, et al. Effect of tamoxifen on venous thromboembolic events in a breast cancer prevention trial. Circulation 2005; 111:650–656.
14. Levine M, Hirsh J, Gent M, et al. Double-blind randomized trial of a very-low-dose warfarin for prevention of thromboembolism in stage IV breast cancer. Lancet 1994; 343:886–889.
15. Haas SK, Kakkar AK, Kemkes-Matthes B, et al. Prevention of venous thromboembolism with low molecular weight heparin in patients with metastatic breast of lung cancer. Results of the TOPIC studies. J Thromb Haemost 2005; 3(suppl 1), abstr OR059.
16. Eikelboom JW, Quinlan DJ, Douketis JD. Extended-duration prophylaxis against venous thromboembolism after total hip or knee replacement: a meta-analysis of the randomized trials. Lancet 2001; 358:9–15.
17. Geerts WH, Pineo GF, Heit JA. Prevention of venous thromboembolism: the Seventh ACCP Conference on Antithrombotic and Thrombolytic Therapy. Chest 2004; 126(3 suppl):338S–400S.
18. Tapson VF, Hyers TM, Waldo AL, et al. Antithrombotic therapy practices in US hospitals in an era of practice guidelines. Arch Intern Med 2005; 165:1458–1464.
19. Stinnett JM, Pendleton R, Skordos L, et al. Venous thromboembolism prophylaxis in medically ill patients and the development of strategies to improve prophylaxis rates. Am J Hematol 2005; 78:167–172.
20. Alikhan R, Cohen AT, Combe S, et al. Risk factors for venous thromboembolism in hospitalized patients with acute medical illness: analysis of the MEDENOX Study. Arch Intern Med 2004; 164:963–968.
21. Mismetti P, Laporte-Simitsidis S, Tardy B, et al. Prevention of venous thromboembolism in internal medicine with unfractionated heparin or low-molecular-weight heparins: a meta-analysis of randomized clinical trials. Thromb Haemost 2000; 83:14–19.
22. Dahan R, Houlbert D, Caulin C, et al. Prevention of deep vein thrombosis in elderly medical in-patients by a low molecular weight heparin: a randomized double-blind trial. Haemostasis 1986; 16:159–164.
23. Samama MM, Cohen AT, Darmon J-Y, et al. A comparison of enoxaparin with placebo for the prevention of venous thromboembolism in acutely ill medical patients. N Engl J Med 1999; 341:793–800.

24. Leizorovicz A, Cohen AT, Turpie AGG, Olsson CG, Vaitkus PT, Goldhaber SZ. A randomized placebo controlled trial of dalteparin for the prevention of venous thromboembolism in acutely ill medical patients. Circulation 2004; 110:874–879.
25. Cohen AT, Davidson BL, Gallus AS, et al. Efficacy and safety of fondaparinux for the prevention of venous thromboembolism in older acute medical patients: randomized placebo controlled trial. BMJ 2006; 332:325–329.
26. Kucher N, Koo S, Quiroz R, et al. Electronic alerts to prevent venous thromboembolism among hospitalized patients. N Engl J Med 2005; 352:969–977.

15

Long-Term Central Vein Catheters and Venous Thromboembolism in Cancer Patients

Melina Verso and Giancarlo Agnelli
Division of Internal and Cardiovascular Medicine—Stroke Unit, Department of Internal Medicine, University of Perugia, Perugia, Italy

- Central venous catheter (CVC) increases four- to sixfold the risk of thrombosis in cancer patients.
- The incidence of symptomatic thromboembolic complications of CVCs has been reported to be up to 5%. Asymptomatic CVC-related thrombi are estimated to occur in about 20% of cancer patients.
- The nonocclusive nature of CVC-associated thrombi may partly explain the low rate of emerging symptomatic events.
- Analysis of the time course of CVC-associated venous thromboembolism (VTE) indicates that the risk of thromboembolic complications is maximum during the first six weeks after the CVC insertion.
- CVC-related thrombosis may be complicated by pulmonary embolism, CVC dysfunction, and postthrombotic syndrome.
- The results of the recent studies do not definitively establish the need and value of prophylaxis of CVC-related thrombosis in the general population of cancer patients.
- Treatment of CVC-related VTE requires a five- to seven-day course of adjusted-dose unfractionated heparin or low-molecular-weight heparin followed by oral anticoagulants or long-term low-molecular-weight heparin.
- In case of CVC-related deep vein thrombosis (DVT), removal of CVC is controversial and depends on the underlying disease and the need of vascular access for therapeutic options.

Venous thromboembolism (VTE) is a common complication of cancer, affecting approximately 1 in 150 cancer patients. Major risk factors include advanced disease, patient immobility, history of recent surgery, chemotherapy, and insertion of a CVC. The use of CVCs is commonly associated with upper-limb DVT. The incidence of symptomatic thromboembolic complications of CVCs has been reported to be up to 5%. Asymptomatic CVC-related thrombi are estimated to occur in about 20% of cancer patients, but their clinical significance is unclear. The incidence of clinically overt pulmonary embolism in cancer patients with CVC-related upper-limb DVT is reported to be between 15% and 25%. Moreover, in the same patients, an autopsy-proven pulmonary embolism rate of up to 50% has been reported. Pathogenic factors for CVC-related thrombosis include vessel injury caused by the CVC insertion procedure, venous stasis as a result of the indwelling CVC and hypercoagulability associated with cancer. Recent studies have provided conflicting conclusions regarding the efficacy of routine primary antithrombotic prophylaxis for CVC-related thrombosis in cancer patients. The most recent version of the guidelines of the American College of Chest Physicians does not recommend antithrombotic prophylaxis in the general cancer population with CVC. The recommended treatment for CVC-related thrombosis in patients with cancer is based on a sequential combination of unfractionated heparin or low-molecular-weight heparin, followed by long-term anticoagulant therapy with or without catheter removal.

INTRODUCTION

A variety of long-term, partially implantable central venous catheters (CVCs) has been introduced in clinical practice since the first long-term CVC was inserted by Broviac et al. in 1973 for parenteral nutrition (1). The Hickman catheter was the first long-term venous access device to be used for chemotherapy on a large scale (2). A substantial improvement in the management of cancer patients was achieved in the early 1980s with the introduction of the totally implantable port system (3). More recently, peripherally implanted central catheters (PICCs) have been developed to reduce the invasiveness of the procedure of CVC insertion (4). Currently, the use of partially implanted CVCs is reserved for short-term daily therapy in hospitalized patients, whereas totally implanted CVCs are preferred for long-term therapy in outpatients. The site of CVC insertion is generally the subclavian or internal jugular vein. PICCs can be inserted in the cephalic, basilic, or brachial veins (5). In the majority of cases, CVCs are inserted through direct puncture of the subclavian vein using the Seldinger method with fluoroscopic or ultrasonographic guidance.

CVCs have considerably improved the management of patients with cancer by facilitating long-term chemotherapy and supportive therapy. The benefit of long-term CVCs may be offset by major complications that may occur either early during the insertion procedure or later during the catheter dwell. Among the early complications, the reported rate of catheter misplacement or breakage, pneumothorax, hemothorax, air embolism or injury to adjacent anatomical structures ranges from 0.3% to 12% (6). Compared with the subclavian access, the internal jugular vein access is considered at lower risk of immediate complications such as pneumothorax, arterial puncture, nervous structures lesions, and arrhythmias. Late complications include catheter occlusion by catheter-related "sleeve," CVC-related thrombosis, and local or systemic infection.

Catheter-related sleeve, an adherent coat of fibrin and collagen that develops inside and outside the CVC, has been reported to occur in up to 47% of patients with CVC (7,8). The formation of this fibrin coat is in itself a benign event, but it may cause catheter malfunction and may become a substrate for the development of local infection or mural thrombosis or both (9).

In this chapter, we have reviewed the published literature regarding the epidemiology, pathogenesis, diagnosis, treatment, and prophylaxis of VTE in cancer patients with long-term CVC.

EPIDEMIOLOGY OF CVC-RELATED THROMBOSIS

The incidence of VTE associated with long-term CVC in cancer patients has been assessed in several studies, but lack of uniformity in the definition of VTE and diagnostic methods of CVC related deep vein thrombosis (DVT) across these studies has made this estimation difficult. Initial studies reported a rate of symptomatic CVC-related DVT of up to about 30% (see Table 1) (10–46) and of asymptomatic CVC-related DVT, screened by venography, of 27% to 66% (see Table 2) (47–57). In contemporary studies, the incidence of

Table 1 Incidence of Clinically Overt CVC-Related DVT in Cancer Patients: Results from Prospective Studies

Reference	Population	Number of CVC	CVC-related DVT (%)
Blackett, 1978 (10)	Adults	178	4.5
Di Costanzo, 1980 (11)	Adults	250	4.4
Lokich, 1983 (12)	Adults	53	28.3
Wagman, 1984 (13)	Adults	55	10.0
Raaf, 1985 (14)	Adults	826	0.7
Cassidy, 1987 (15)	Adults	416	2.6
Moss, 1989 (16)	Adults	190	3.7
Wenke, 1990 (17)	Adults	82	3.6
Jansen, 1990 (18)	Adults	123	4.1
Haire, 1990 (19)	Adults	162	12.9
Mertz, 1990 (20)	Children[a]	52	1.9
Rau, 1991 (21)	Adults	78	3.2
Mueller et al., 1992 (22)	Adults	92	6.0
Gould, 1993 (23)	Adults	255	14.5
Torromade, 1993 (24)	Adults	234	10.0
Wesenberg, 1993 (25)	Children	77	0
Soh, 1993 (26)	Adults	22	5.0
Anderson, 1995 (27)	Adults	168	17.0
Eastridge and Lefor, 1995 (28)	Adults	322	10.0
Horne, 1995 (29)	Adults	50	21.0
Cunningham, 1996 (30)	Adults	18	26.0
Dobois, 1997 (31)	Children	285	0.3
Nightingale, 1997 (32)	Adults	949	4.7
McBride et al., 1997 (33)	Adults	253	3.5
Wilimas, 1998 (34)	Children	23	12.0
Martin et al., 1999 (35)	Adults[b]	60	11.6
Knofler, 1999 (36)	Children	77	14
Schwartz, 2000 (37)	Adults	923	3.1
Lagro, 2000 (38)	Adults	390	6.9
Grove and Pevec, 2000 (39)	Adults	813	4.5
Hartkamp, 2000 (40)	Adults	126	7.3
Povoski, 2000 (41)	Adults	100	5.0
Biffi et al., 2001 (42)	Adults	304	6.6
Coccaro, 2001 (43)	Adults	98	2.1
Fijnheer et al., 2002 (44)	Adults	277	4.7
Harter, 2002 (45)	Adults	233	1.5
Kuriakose, 2002 (46)	Adults	422	7.1

[a]Critically ill children.
[b]Intensive care unit patients.
Abbreviations: CVC, central venous catheter; DVT, deep vein thrombosis.

Table 2 Incidence of Venographic CVC-Related DVT in Cancer Patients: Results from Prospective Studies

Reference	Population	Number of CVC	CVC-related DVT (%)
Stoney, 1976 (47)	Adults	203	31.0
Burt et al., 1981 (48)	Adults	21	33.3
Valerio, 1981 (49)	Adults	22	27.3
Brismar et al., 1982 (50)	Adults	53	35.8
Bozetti, 1983 (51)	Adults	52	28.8
Lokich, 1983 (12)	Adults	53	41.5
Pottecher et al., 1984 (52)	Adults	52	38.5
Bern et al., 1990 (53)[a]	Adults	42	37.5
Balestrieri et al., 1995 (54)	Adults	57	56.0
Monreal et al., 1996 (55)[a]	Adults	29	62.0
De Cicco et al., 1997(56)	Adults	127	66.0
Martin et al., 1999 (35)	Adults[b]	60	58.3
Glaser, 2001 (57)	Children	24	50.0

Note: the majority of CVC-related DVT in these studies were asymptomatic.
[a]In the control group.
[b]Intensive care unit patients.
Abbreviations: CVC, central venous catheter; DVT, deep vein thrombosis.

symptomatic catheter-related DVT has been found to be not higher than 5% (58–59), and a recent study reported a rate of 18% for asymptomatic CVC-related DVT in the absence of prophylaxis (18). The incidence of CVC-related DVT seems to be similar regardless of whether the CVC access is via the subclavian or the jugular vein (35).

The localization of upper-limb DVT was prospectively assessed in several studies (42, 56–66, 35). The axillosubclavian veins are involved more often than the innominate or superior caval veins (97%, 60%, and 13%, respectively; $P < 0.001$). In cancer patients with long-term CVC, the CVC-related upper-limb thrombosis has been reported to be completely occlusive in about 20% to 30% of cases (14,20). These findings have been recently confirmed by a prospective study with venography evaluation that showed an occlusive thrombus in 28% of patients with CVC-related thrombosis (58).

Patients receiving chemotherapy through a PICC are also at increased risk of thrombosis. The reported incidence of symptomatic DVT using PICCs ranges from 2% to 4% (61–62). Symptomatic thrombosis occurred in 7% of patients with PICCs inserted for chemotherapy compared with 1% of PICCs inserted for other reasons. The use of PICC lines has been linked to a high rate of clinically detectable thrombophlebitis of the cephalic and basilic veins (63–64). The rate of venography-detected DVT associated with PICCs has been reported to be about 20% to 25% (62).

A lower incidence of CVC-related DVT has been seen in patients with subcutaneous ports, according to an indirect comparison with patients who had partially implantable catheters (63). Few prospective (65) or randomized (66,42) studies have been performed to clarify this issue but their results do not allow any definitive conclusion.

The risk of upper-limb DVT in cancer patients is highest in the first few weeks following CVC insertion (67). Incidence of thrombosis at day 8 and day 30 after CVC insertion has been reported to be 64% and 98%, respectively (56). A mean interval of 42.2 days was found between CVC insertion and detection of thrombosis (67).

In summary, CVC insertion increases the risk of thrombosis in cancer patients by four- to sixfold compared with the general population (68). The incidence of CVC-associated VTE has probably been reduced by the introduction of more modern devices (i.e., Port-A-Cath model). There is inconclusive evidence that totally implantable CVCs are less thrombogenic than partially implantable CVCs (22). Most of the thrombi that develop are nonocclusive. Analysis of the time course of CVC-associated VTE indicates that the risk of thromboembolic complications is maximum during the first six weeks after the CVC introduction.

PATHOGENESIS AND RISK FACTORS FOR CVC-RELATED THROMBOSIS

CVC-related DVT of upper limb in cancer patients has a multifactorial pathogenesis. CVC as well as patient features may play an important role in the occurrence of CVC-related DVT in patients with cancer.

Some CVC features have been associated with the increased risk of CVC-related thrombosis. The type of CVC is an important determinant for this complication. Catheters made of both silicone and polyurethane have been shown to be less thrombogenic than CVCs made of polyvinylchloride and polyethylene (69). In addition, the risk of thrombosis tends to increase with multiple-lumen catheters (28), with catheters with large diameters (39), and with incorrect positioning of the catheter tip (70). A significantly lower rate of CVC-related upper-limb DVT (28,34) and a 2.6-fold reduced risk of need of CVC removal ($P = 0.003$) (71) have been observed when the catheter tip has been appropriately positioned at the junction between the superior vena cava and the right atrium (33). Multivariate analysis of data from a randomized prospective study in 385 cancer patients with CVCs confirmed that incorrect positioning of the CVC tip (CVC tip above the upper half of the superior vena cava as shown by venography) is an independent risk factor for CVC-related DVT [odds ratio (OR) 4.05, 95% confidence interval (CI) 1.64–10.02] (72).

A left insertion side has been reported as an independent risk factor for thrombotic complications of the upper limb in cancer patients (56,65). In a recent study, left-sided insertion was associated with an OR of 2.29 (95% CI 1.01–5.51) in comparison with right-sided insertion (72). This finding could be explained by the anatomical difference between the venous systems of the upper limbs.

Vessel injury caused by CVC insertion and venous stasis caused by indwelling CVC contribute to the occurrence of thrombotic complications in both adult (73,74) and pediatric (75) cancer patients. Additional risks have been reported including prior CVC insertion at the same puncture side or blinded, percutaneous landmark-guided, insertion technique, or multiple insertion attempts in positioning CVC (76). Screening with ultrasonography found a thrombosis in one or more central veins in approximately 40% of patients who had previously undergone long-term central venous catheterization (77). In addition, the use of the fluoroscopic- or ultrasonography-assisted cannulation instead of the external landmark-guided technique reduced the thrombotic rate in patients with CVC in the internal jugular vein (13.3% vs. 2.3%, respectively) (76).

Catheter-related infection and CVC-related thromboembolic complications are linked by a two-way relationship (9,78). The pathogenesis of CVC-related infection seems to depend on the development of fibrin sheath around the external surface of CVC. On the other hand, the presence of CVC-related infection may predispose to development of thrombosis. A direct correlation was found between mural thrombosis on catheterized veins found at autopsy and premortem microbiological data (9). Colonization of catheters or sepsis was found in 7 out of 31 patients who were then found to have mural thrombi on postmortem but had not been detected in any of the 41 patients without evidence of mural thrombi on postmortem ($P < 0.01$). More recently, a prospective study reported an increased risk of CVC-related thrombosis in patients with catheter-related infection in comparison to those without infection [relative risk (RR) 17.6; 95% CI 4.1–74.1] (79).

Heparin-bonded CVCs have been showed to be associated with a reduced rate of thrombotic and infective complications in critically ill children (symptomatic DVT rate: 0% vs. 8%; $P = 0.006$, infection rate: 4% vs. 33%; $P < 0.0005$) (23).

Over 80% of indwelling CVCs are associated with measurable thrombin activity at the time of removal (80). This suggests that physiologic anticoagulant mechanisms cannot break down surface-bound thrombin, which is relatively resistant to antithrombin inhibition.

Abnormalities in blood coagulation associated with cancer, especially in the advanced stages, and with different type and dose of chemotherapy (i.e., cisplatinum-based chemotherapy) may contribute to venous thromboembolic events (81). An increased risk for thrombosis was found in patients with metastatic cancer (OR 19.8, 95% CI 2.6–149.1) (67). The presence of active cancer therapy was significantly associated with PICC-associated DVT (OR 3.5, 95% CI 1.3–9.8) (82). No clear differences in CVC-related thrombosis have been demonstrated between different methods of administration (push/bolus vs. infusional regimens) or between home-based versus hospital-based administration of chemotherapy (83). In addition, a high platelet count at the time of CVC insertion was reported to be associated with an increased risk of thrombosis (65).

Reports on prevalence of thrombophilic molecular abnormalities in cancer patients with CVC-related DVT have provided conflicting results (60,84–88,44). Reduced levels of antithrombin might be a risk factor for CVC-related DVT (84). In contrast, a low prevalence of *factor V Leiden* gene mutation was reported in cancer patients with CVC-related DVT (7% of patients had a heterozygous mutation), leading the authors to suggest this mutation is unlikely to account for development of DVT (85). In a group of patients with acute lymphoblastic leukemia, DVT was found in 67% who had a genetic mutation (factor V G1691A, prothrombin G20210A, and homozygous MTHFR variant) versus 21% who did not have a genetic mutation (86). A CVC-related DVT was found in 54% of patients with heterozygous *factor V Leiden* genetic mutation, who were catheterized for bone marrow transplantation, suggesting that this genetic mutation is an independent risk factor for DVT occurring among cancer patients (44).

A recent publication reports that elevated plasma levels of D-dimer and fragment 1 + 2 after CVC insertion could identify patients at high risk of CVC-related thrombosis after bone marrow transplantation. Although these abnormalities were associated with a five- to sevenfold increased risk of CVC-related thrombosis, the positive predictive value was about 80% and the negative predictive value was only 40% (88). Further studies are required to support these findings, particularly in cancer patients.

In summary, the pathogenesis of upper-limb DVT in patients with CVC is probably multifactorial. Early thromboembolic events are essentially related to the loss of vessel integrity caused by CVC placement. Late thromboembolic events are probably related to CVC features and patient characteristics. The role of thrombophilic molecular abnormalities in the pathogenesis of CVC-related DVT in cancer patients remains to be defined.

CLINICAL PRESENTATION AND DIAGNOSIS OF CVC-RELATED THROMBOSIS

CVC-related DVT is less frequently associated with symptoms than upper-limb DVT not associated with CVC. This may be explained by the fact that thrombosis related to CVC develops more slowly and is less commonly occlusive. In the most recent study that used venography to screen for CVC-related DVT, only 3.1% of patients in the placebo group were symptomatic (18). The clinical significance of asymptomatic CVC-related thrombi is unclear. The incidence of clinically overt pulmonary embolism in cancer patients with CVC-related DVT varies between 15% and 25% (89,90).

A diagnostic workup, including imaging, is mandatory in patients with clinically suspected CVC-related DVT. The presence of a CVC almost doubles the incidence of upper-limb DVT in symptomatic patients. In about a third to one-half of all patients in whom thrombosis is clinically suspected, the diagnosis is confirmed. In the case of clinical suspicion of CVC-related DVT, color Doppler ultrasonography is commonly used to confirm the diagnosis. Color Doppler ultra sonography is the modality of choice for the diagnosis of CVC-related upper-limb DVT in symptomatic cancer patients and for screening for asymptomatic thrombosis in this population (91). Color Doppler ultrasonography can accurately detect CVC-related thrombi involving the jugular, axillary, distal subclavian, and arm veins (58,92). Contrast venographic imaging is restricted to cases where ultrasonography is not conclusive or to evaluate the deep central veins and pulmonary arteries (see Figure 1 and 2). A sensitivity of 94% and a specificity of 96% for color Doppler ultrasonography were observed in the only venography-controlled study available in symptomatic patients with CVC (86). Recently, promising results using magnetic resonance venography and spiral computed tomography (CT) in the diagnosis of CVC-related DVT have been published (93,94). These diagnostic methods can provide a global visualization of the central venous system and can be used in confirming or excluding the clinical suspicion of central venous thrombosis.

In summary, the nonocclusive nature of CVC-associated thrombi may partly explain the low rate of emerging symptomatic events. In the presence of symptoms and signs of CVC-related DVT, color Doppler ultrasonography should be used to rule in or rule out the diagnosis. Contrast venography is reserved for doubtful cases. Magnetic resonance venography and spiral CT represent potential alternatives in the diagnosis of CVC-related DVT.

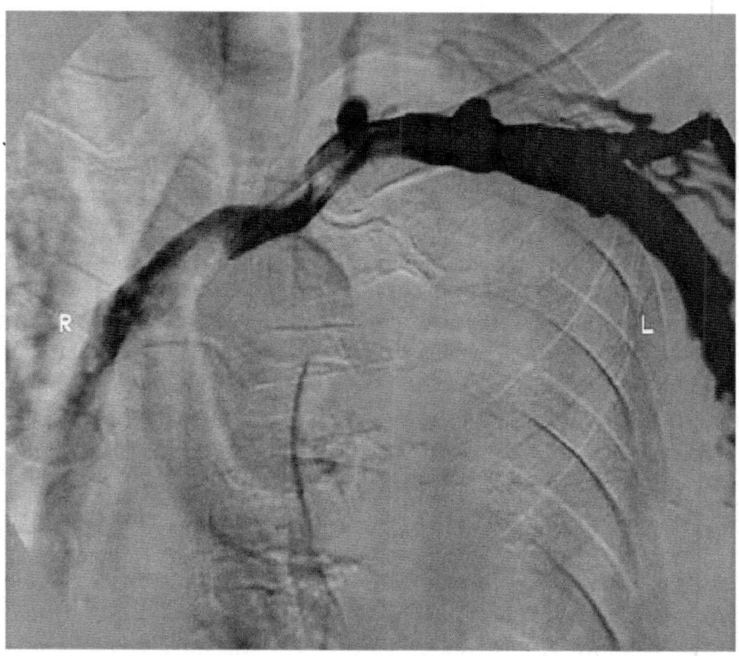

Figure 1 Partial thrombotic occlusion of subclavian and anonymous veins in cancer patient with a CVC for chemotherapy. *Abbreviations*: CVC, central venous catheter.

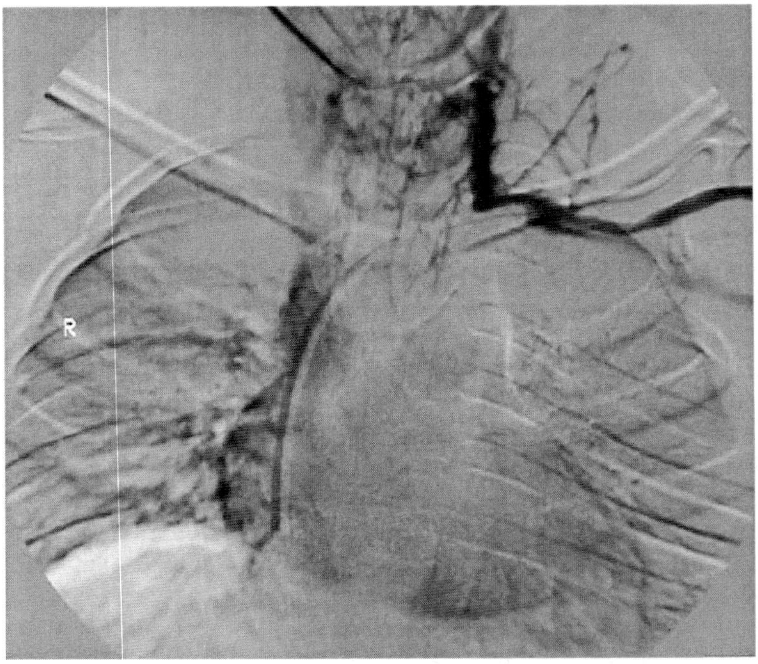

Figure 2 Complete thrombotic occlusion of subclavian vein in cancer patient with a CVC for chemotherapy. *Abbreviations*: CVC, central venous catheter.

COMPLICATIONS OF CVC-RELATED DVT

CVC-related thrombosis may be associated with several complications including pulmonary embolism, CVC dysfunction, and post-thrombotic syndrome. These complications of CVC-related DVT can lead to significant morbidity and mortality (95). The incidence of clinically overt pulmonary embolism in cancer patients with CVC-related DVT is estimated to be between 15% and 25% (89). During routine CT scan for cancer staging, unsuspected pulmonary emboli are frequently found (96). In about 60% of these patients, pulmonary embolism is clinically occult. Screening for pulmonary embolism in cancer patients with CVC is not usually mandatory, since in most patients, anticoagulant treatment is initiated.

CVC dysfunction is generally due to clot occlusion either of the CVC lumen or of the catheter tip by fibrin sheath. CVC dysfunction, if untreated, requires the CVC removal. Usually this complication causes difficulties in drawing blood sample or infusing solution through the CVC.

Post-thrombotic syndrome is a chronic, potentially serious complication after upper-limb DVT. The frequency of post-thrombotic syndrome after upper-limb DVT ranges from 7% to 46% (weighted mean 15%) (97). Residual thrombosis and axillosubclavian vein thrombosis appear to be associated with an increased risk of post-thrombotic syndrome. There is not a currently validated, standardized scale to assess upper extremity post-thrombotic syndrome and little consensus regarding the optimal management of this condition is available. Patients with post-thrombotic syndrome have an increased risk of recurrent VTE. There is no statistically significant difference in mortality rate or incidence of pulmonary embolism among the patients with subclavian/axillary or internal jugular vein thrombosis (98).

In summary, CVC-related thrombosis may be complicated by pulmonary embolism, CVC dysfunction, and post-thrombotic syndrome. These complications may negatively influence the overall clinical course of cancer patients.

PROPHYLAXIS OF CVC-RELATED THROMBOSIS IN CANCER PATIENTS

The role of antithrombotic prophylaxis in the prevention of CVC-related thrombosis remains controversial. Some open-label studies (53,55,58,99,100) reported a benefit in the prevention of CVC-related complications with both low-molecular-weight heparins and warfarin, whereas some more recent studies with improved methodology did not confirm this benefit (see Table 3) (58,101,102).

In an open, prospective study in 82 patients, Bern et al. (53) evaluated a low, fixed dose of warfarin (1 mg/day) beginning three days before the CVC was inserted and continued for 90 days, as prophylaxis against CVC-related thrombosis. Forty patients did not receive warfarin and served as controls. Four patients (9.5%) receiving warfarin treatment had venography-confirmed upper-limb DVT compared with 15 patients (37.5%) not receiving warfarin ($P < 0.01$). In another open, prospective study, dalteparin (2500 IU once daily) administered for 90 days was found to be an effective and safe regimen for the prophylaxis of CVC-related DVT (55). Upper-limb DVT was confirmed by venography in 9 of the 29 patients (31%): 1 of the 16 patients (6%) who received dalteparin sodium injection and 8 of the 13 patients (62%) who did not receive such treatment. In addition, a meta-analysis of randomized controlled trials published in 1998 showed a benefit for heparin in the prevention of venous thromboembolic complications (RR 0.43; 95% CI 0.23–0.78) and catheter colonization (RR 0.18; 95% CI 0.06–0.60) (99).

Boraks et al. (100) reported an open, historically-controlled, study on the efficacy and safety of warfarin prophylaxis in 108 patients with CVC. In this study, patients with hematological malignancies received 1 mg of warfarin during the period of CVC dwell. The incidence of CVC-related DVT in treated patients was compared with that observed in a historical population with similar characteristics. Venography or ultrasonography was used to confirm the clinical suspicion of CVC-related DVT. The reported rate of CVC-related DVT was 5% in the study patients and 13% in the historical control, $p = 0.03$. The uncontrolled nature of this study is a major limitation for the evaluation of the intervention tested.

More recently, randomized, placebo-controlled trials have been performed, with either symptomatic or venography-detected thrombosis as study outcomes (58,101,102). A study evaluated the efficacy and safety of 5000 IU of dalteparin for 16 weeks in preventing catheter-related complications in cancer patients (101). No benefit in preventing CVC-related complications (including thrombotic events requiring anticoagulant or thrombolytic therapy or clinically overt pulmonary embolism and CVC obstruction requiring CVC removal) was demonstrated by this study for dalteparin treatment versus placebo (3.7% vs. 3.4%, $P = 0.9$).

Couban et al. (102) reported the results of a study that evaluated the efficacy and safety of low-dose warfarin (1 mg daily) in the prevention of symptomatic CVC-associated DVT in 255 patients with cancer. A clinically overt thromboembolic event occurred in 5 of the 125 (4%) patients of the placebo group and in 6 of the 130 (4.6%) patients of the warfarin group. There was no difference in the incidence of major or minor bleeding events in the two groups. In a large number of patients (191/255, 75%) the treatment was interrupted because of the occurrence of thrombocytopenia. A complete blood count was measured monthly in all patients, weekly in hospitalized patients, or more frequently if clinically indicated. The study treatment was interrupted in 102 patients (55 in the placebo

Table 3 Clinical Trials of VTE Prophylaxis in Cancer Patients with CVC

Reference	Study design[a]	Number of patients	Prophylactic regimens	Duration	Endpoint assessment	CVC-DVT(%)	*P* value
Bern et al., 1990 (53)	P, O, C	82	Warfarin 1 mg/day	90 dayv	Mandatory venography	9.5	<0.001
			No treatment			37.5	
Monreal et al., 1996 (55)	P, O, C	29	Dalteparin	90 day	Mandatory 6 venography	0.002	
			2500 U/day				
			No treatment			62	
			Dalteparin			3.7	0.9
Karthaus et al., 2006 (101)	R, D-B, C	439	5000 U/day	16 wk	Symptomatic events	3.4	
			Placebo				
			Warfarin 1 mg/day			4.6	
Couban et al., 2005 (102)	R, D-B, C	255		Variable	Symptomatic events		Ns
			Placebo			4.0	
			Enoxaparin			14.1	
Verso et al., 2005 (58)	R, D-B, C	385	40 mg/day	42 day	Mandatory venography		0.35
			Placebo			18	

[a]P, prospective; O, open-label; R, randomized; C, controlled; D-B, double-blind trial.
Abbreviations: CVC, central venous catheter; DVT, deep vein thrombosis.

group and 47 in the warfarin group) due to thrombocytopenia. The study protocol required the interruption of the study drug when the platelet count was 20×10^9/L or less.

More recently, the first randomized double-blind study to evaluate the efficacy and safety of prophylaxis of CVC-related venous thrombosis in patients with cancer by means of venography has been published. The Enoxaparin in the prevention of THromboembolism in Indwelling catheter in Cancer patients (ETHIC) study was a multicenter, randomized, double-blind, placebo-controlled study evaluating the efficacy and safety of enoxaparin for the prevention of CVC-associated VTE (58). In 385 cancer patients who had had a CVC inserted for chemotherapy, enoxaparin, at the dose of 40 mg daily, was associated with a non-significant 22% risk reduction in the rate of venography-detected DVT in comparison with placebo. The incidence of bleeding was low and similar in the two groups.

The PRophylaxis of ThromboEmbolism, in Kids Trial (PROTEKT) study (103) was an open-label, randomized controlled trial on the prevention of CVC-related thrombotic complications with reviparin-sodium in children affected by leukemia. The dose of reviparin was 30 IU/Kg/day for patients under three months and 50 IU/Kg/day for patients over three months. The efficacy endpoint was DVT detected by venography performed at day 30 (+ 14 days) or earlier in case of CVC removal and symptomatic VTE confirmed by objective testing. The study was prematurely closed after the inclusion of 188 patients, due to the slow patient accrual and the high rate of adverse events. A rate of VTE of 14.1% (11/78) was reported in the reviparin-sodium group as compared with 12.5% (10/80) rate in the control group. The negative results observed in this study could be explained by the low responsiveness of children to antithrombotic prophylaxis, by the high frequency of patients with leukemia in the study, or by the use of an ineffective prophylactic dose.

The efficacy and safety of the low-molecular-weight heparin nadroparin and low-dose warfarin were compared in an open, prospective, randomized, venography trial in 57 cancer patients with long-term CVC for chemotherapy (104). Warfarin was given at the fixed daily dose of 1 mg, and nadroparin was injected at fixed daily dose of 2850 IU for 90 days. Six out of the 21 patients in the nadroparin group (28.6%) and 4 out of 24 patients in the warfarin group (16.7%) had venography-proved CVC-related DVT at 90 days ($p = 0.48$). Safety was similar in both treatments. The authors concluded that prophylactic doses of warfarin and nadroparin had comparable benefit-to-risk ratios in the prevention of CVC-related DVT in cancer patients.

Although effective in preventing VTE during chemotherapy for breast cancer, the 1 mg regimen of warfarin could be suboptimal in the prophylaxis of upper-limb DVT in cancer patients with CVC. This could suggest the use of higher doses of warfarin. Indeed, doses of warfarin adjusted to international normalized ratio (INR) between 1.5 and 2.0 has been recently shown to be more effective than placebo but associated with unacceptable bleeding rate in a prophylaxis study (105).

Two recent multicenter observational studies have provided further interesting data in this setting. Cortellezzi et al. (59) reported that antithrombotic prophylaxis helped to prevent the thrombotic complications (a combination of VTE, superficial thrombophlebitis, and CVC occlusion or mulfunction) after CVC positioning in patients with hematological malignances. Cimminiello et al. (106) evaluated the attitude toward antithrombotic prophylaxis in current practice in Italian oncology centers and the clinical impact of this prophylaxis on the systemic VTE and survival in 1410 patients with solid or hematological tumor. They reported that continuous antithrombotic prophylaxis of CVC with minidose of warfarin, given in 32.4% of enrolled patients, is unable to prevent CVC-related DVT (2.8% vs. 2.2%) but appeared to be effective in reducing systemic VTE and mortality. This finding was not observed in previous studies.

The reasons for the inconsistency between older and more recent studies are unclear. Improvements in catheter biocompatibility, insertion techniques, and CVC management could have reduced the risk of thrombosis and influenced the risk reduction associated with prophylaxis (107). Improved clinical trial methodology over time may have played a role as well. Altogether, the results of the recent studies do not definitively establish the value of prophylaxis of CVC-related thrombosis in the general population of cancer patients. Further studies specifically designed to assess the efficacy of thromboprophylaxis in groups of patients at high risk are warranted. Pending the results of these studies, recent guidelines recommended against routine antithrombotic prophylaxis to prevent catheter-related DVT in cancer patients.

TREATMENT OF CVC-RELATED THROMBOSIS IN CANCER PATIENTS

Clinical management of cancer patients is more challenging when CVC-related DVT is present, and critical analysis and standardization of the treatments available for this condition are lacking. The aims of treatment for CVC-related DVT are to reduce the acute morbidity and mortality associated with the event and to reduce late complications. Management recommendations differ between various clinical settings and according to clinical presentation, risk of bleeding, CVC malfunction, and other considerations.

Anticoagulant therapy, with or without catheter removal, is the treatment of choice for patients with CVC-induced acute DVT or pulmonary embolism, even in absence of specific prospective, comparative studies on this clinical issue. At present, anticoagulation is generally given according to the current guidelines for lower-limb DVT: with adjusted-dose, unfractionated heparin or low-molecular-weight heparin initially administered for five to seven days and long-term oral anticoagulation with warfarin (108). Patients for whom oral anticoagulation is not practical usually receive long-term treatment with low-molecular-weight heparins (109–110). A recent prospective cohort study evaluated the efficacy and safety of the low-molecular-weight heparin dalteparin (200 antifactor Xa U/Kg) in the treatment of 46 outpatients with upper-limb DVT (111). The results of this study suggest the safety and efficacy of dalteparin in this clinical setting with potential cost savings from outpatient treatment.

Other, more aggressive, therapeutic options for DVT associated with CVC include thrombolysis and thrombectomy. Although there have been a number of studies of thrombolytic therapy in CVC-related DVT, no randomized comparison of thrombolytic therapy with heparin has been performed in patients with venography-proven upper-limb DVT. It is not known whether thrombolytic therapy can reduce VTE symptoms or prevent systemic infection or line infection and the resultant CVC malfunction.

The need to remove the CVC is controversial and depends on the underlying disease and the need of vascular access for therapeutic options. Generally, this decision is left to the discretion of the attending physician. Another CVC can be implanted, generally on the contralateral upper limb, but this is associated with considerable morbidity and cost. The effect of CVC removal on long-term outcome is unknown.

Optimal duration of anticoagulation for DVT associated with CVC in cancer patients has not been established. While the cancer is active, we recommend that patients who have a venous thromboembolic episode should receive anticoagulation for at least six months or indefinitely. A superior vena cava filter has been used in patients who have upper-limb DVT and in whom anticoagulant therapy is contraindicated (112–113). Approaches to managing catheter patency, including the use of thrombolytic agents, are limited by limited published experience. Local, low-dose thrombolytic therapy with single or repeated bolus doses of urokinase, streptokinase, or rt-PA is generally given for this indication. Treatment with rt-PA (alteplase) at a dose of 2 mg per 2 mL, allowed to dwell for two hours, has been shown to be effective in restoring flow to catheters patency in 85% to 90% of patients, providing the CVC is well positioned (114–115). This treatment is safe and effective in restoring function in occluded centrally and peripherally inserted catheters.

CONCLUSION

Recently, upper-limb DVT has emerged as a significant clinical problem. Until 10 to 15 years ago, upper-limb DVT represented about 2% of all DVT of the limbs, whereas upper-limb DVT currently represents about 8% to 10% of total DVT (116–117). The long-term CVCs represent a major cause of upper-limb DVT, especially in cancer patients. CVC-related DVT in cancer patients complicates the management of cancer, contributing to morbidity and mortality (118). In cancer patients, there is no clear benefit from routine antithrombotic prophylaxis. Recognition of risk factors associated with CVC-related DVT may help to define a subgroup of cancer patients with CVC who benefit from prophylaxis (107). Treatment of CVC-related VTE requires a five- to seven-day course of adjusted-dose unfractionated heparin or low-molecular-weight heparin followed by oral anticoagulants, or long-term low-molecular-weight heparin. The need to remove the CVC depends on the underlying disease and the need for vascular access. The optimal duration of anticoagulation remains undefined but patients with active cancer and CVC-related DVT should receive anticoagulation for at least six months or indefinitely. Thrombolysis is seldom required, and removal of the CVC in patients with CVC-related DVT is still controversial.

REFERENCES

1. Broviac JW, Cole JJ, Scribner BH. A silicone rubber atrial catheter for prolonged parenteral alimentation. Surg Gynecol Obstet 1973; 36:602–605.
2. Hickman RO, Buckner CD, Clift RA. A modified right atrial catheter for access to the venous system in marrow transplant recipient. Surg Gynecol Obstet 1979; 148:871–875.
3. Niederhuber JE, Ensminger W, Gyves JW, et al. Totally implanted venous and arterial access system to replace external catheter in cancer treatment. Surgery 1982; 92:706–712.
4. Bregenzer T, Dieter C, Sakmann P, et al. Is routine replacement of peripheral intravenous catheters necessary? Arch Intern Med 1998; 158:151–156.
5. Lam S, Scannell R, Roessler D, et al. Peripherally inserted central catheters in an acute-care hospital. Arch Intern Med 1994; 154:1833–1837.
6. Mansfield PF, Hohn DC, Fornage BD, et al. Complication and failure of subclavian-vein catheterization. N Engl J Med 1994; 331:1735–1738.
7. Hoch JR. Management of the complications of long-term venous access. Semin Vasc Surg 1997; 10:135–143.
8. Xiang DZ, Verbeken EK, Van Lommel AT, et al. Composition and formation of the sleeve enveloping a central venous catheter. J Vasc Surg Aug 1998; 28:260–271.
9. Raad II, Luna M, Khalil SAM, et al. The relationship between the thrombotic and infectious complications of central venous catheters. JAMA 1994; 271:1014–1016.
10. Blackett RL, Bakran A, Bradley JA, et al. A prospective study of subclavian vein catheters used exclusively for the purpose of intravenous feeding. Br J Surg 1978; 193:264–270
11. Di Costanzo J, Cano N, Martin J, et al. Venous thrombosis due to central venous catheters during total parenteral nutrition. JPEN 1980; 4:439–41.
12. Lokich JJ, Becker B. Subclavian vein thrombosis in patients treated with infusion chemotherapy for advanced malignancy, Cancer 1983; 52:1586–1589.

13. Wagman LD, Kirkemo A, Johnston MR. Venous access: a prospective, randomized study of the Hickman catheter. Surgery 1984; 95(3):303–308.
14. Raaf JH. Results from use of 826 vascular access devices in cancer patinets. Cancer 1985; 55:1312–1321.
15. Cassidy FP Jr, Zajko AB, Bron KM, et al. Noninfectious complications of long-term central venous catheters: radiologic evaluation and management. AJR Am J Roentgenol 1987; 149(4): 671–675.
16. Moss JF, Wagmen LD, Riihimaki DU, et al. Central venous thrombosis related to the silastic Hickman-Broviac catheter in an oncologic poulation. JPEN 1989; 13(4):397–400.
17. Wenke K, Markewitz A. Fully implantable catheter systems: long-term results-complications. Fortschr Med 1990; 108(14):276–279.
18. Jansen RF, Wiggers T, Van Geel BN, et al. Assessment of insertion techniques and complication rates of dual lumen central venous catheters in patients with hematological malignancies. World J Surg 1990; 14(1):100–104.
19. Haire WD, Leiberman RP, Edney J, et al. Hickman catheter-induced thoracic vein thrombosis. Frequency and long-term sequelae in patients receiving high-dose chemotherapy and marrow transplantation. Cancer 1990; 66:900–908.
20. Mertz RI, Lucking SE, Chaten FC, et al. Percutaneous catheterization of the axillary vein in infants and childern, Pediatrics 1990; 85(4):531–53.
21. Rau WS, Rauber K, Weimar B, et al. The implantation of Hickman catheters. A new function of interventional radiology. Radiologe 1991; 31(3):125–131.
22. Mueller BU, Skelton J, Callender DP, et al. A prospective randomized trial comparing the infectious and non infectious complications of an externalized catheter versus subcutaneously implanted device in cancer patients. J Clin Oncol 1992; 10:1943–1948.
23. Gould JR, Carloss HW, Skinner WL. Groshong catheter-associated subclavian venous thrombosis. Am J Med 1993; 95(4):419–423.
24. Torromade JR, Cienfuegos JA, Hernandez JL, et al. The complications of central venous access system: a study of 218 patinets. Eur J Surg 1993; 159, (6-7):323–32.
25. Wesenberg F, Flaatten H, Janssen CW, et al. Central venous catheter with subcutaneous injection port (port a cath): 8 years clinical follow up with children. Pediatr Hematol Oncol 1993; 10(3):233–239.
26. Soh LT, Ang PT. Implantable subcutaneous infusion ports. Support Care Cancer 1993; 1(2):108–110.
27. Anderson AJ, Krasnow SH, Boyer MW, et al. Thrombosis: the major Hickman catheter complication in patients with soild tumor. Chest 1995; 95(1):71–75.
28. Eastridge BJ, Lefor AT. Complications of indwelling venous access devices in cancer patients. J Clin Oncol 1995; 13:233–238.
29. Horne MK 3rd, May DJ, Alexander HR, et al. Venographic surveillance of tunneled venous access devices in adult oncology patients. Ann Surg Oncol 1995; 2(2):174–178.
30. Cunningham MJ, Collins MB, Kredentser DC, et al. Peripheral infusion ports for central venous access in patients with gynecologic malignancies. Gynecol Oncol 1996; 60(3):397–399.
31. Dobois J, Garel L, Tapiero B, et al. Peripherally inserted central catheters in infants and children. Radiology 1997; 204(3):622–626 (suppl).
32. Nightingale CE, Norman A, Cunningham D, et al. A prospective analysis of 949 long-term central venous catheters for ambulatory chemotherapy in patients with gastrointestinal malignancy. Eur J Cancer 1997; 33 (3):398–403.
33. McBride KD, Fisher R, Warnock N, et al. A comparative analysis of radiological and surgical placement of central venous catheters. Cardiovasc Intervent Radiol 1997; 20:17–22.
34. Wilimas JA, Hudson M, Rao B, et al. Late vascular occlusion of central lines in pediatric malignancies. Pediatrics 1998; 101(2): E7.
35. Martin C, Viviand X, Saux P, et al. Upper extremity deep vein thrombosis after central venous catheterization via the axillary vein. Crit Care Med 1999; 27:2626–2629.
36. Knofler R, Siegert E, Lauterbach I, et al. Clinical importance of prothrombotic risk factors in pediatric patients with malignancy-impact of central venous lines. Eur J Pediatr 1999; 158: S147–S150.

37. Schwarz RE, Coit DG, Groeger JS. Transcutaneously tunneled central venous lines in cancer patients: an analysis of device-related morbidity factors based on prospective data collection. Ann Surg Oncol 2000; 7(6):441–449.
38. Largro SW, Verdonck LF, Borel Rinkes IH, et al. No effect of nadroparin prophylaxis in the prevention of central catheter (CVC)-associated thrombosis in bone marrow transplant recipients. Bone Marrow Transplant 2000; 26(10):1103–1106.
39. Grove JR, Pevec WC. Venous thrombosis related to peripherally inserted central catheters. J Vasc Interv Radiol 2000; 11:837–840.
40. Hartkamp A, van Boxtel AJ, Zonnenberg BA, et al. Totally implantable venous access devices: evaluation of complications and a prospective comparative study of two different port systems. Neth J Med 2000: 57(6):215–223.
41. Povoski SP. A prospective analysis of the cephalic vein cutdown approach for chronic indwelling central venous access in 10 consecutive cancer patients. Ann Surg Oncol 2000; 7(7):496–502.
42. Biffi R, De Braud F, Orsi F, et al. A randomized, prospective trial of central venous ports connected to standard open-ended or Groshong catheters in adult oncology patients. Cancer 2001; 92:1204–1212.
43. Coccaro M, Bochicchio AM, Capobianco AM, et al. Long-term infusional systems: complications in cancer patients. Tumori 2001; 87(5):308–311.
44. Fijnheer R, Paijmans B, Verdonck LF, et al. Factor V Leiden in central venous catheter-associated thrombosis. Br J Haematol 2002; 118:267–270.
45. Harter C, Salwender HJ, Bach A, et al. Catheter-related infection and thrombosis of the internal jugular vein in hematologic-oncologic patients undergoing chemotherapy: a prospective comparison of silver coated and uncoated catheters. Cancer 2002; 94(1):245–251.
46. Kuriakose P, Colon-Otero G, Paz-Fumagalli R. Risk of deep venous thrombosis associated with chest versus arm central venous subcutaneous port catheters: a 5-year single-institution retrospective study. J Vasc Interv Radiol 2002; 13(2):179–184.
47. Stoney WS, Addlestone RB, Alford WC, et al. The incidence of venous thrombosis following long-term transvenous pacing. Ann Thorac Surg 1976; 22:166–170.
48. Burt ME, Dunnick NR, Krudy AG, et al. Prospective evaluation of subclavian vein thrombosis during total parenteral nutrition by contrast venography. Clin Res 1981; 29:264–267.
49. Valerio D, Hussey JK, Smith FW. Central vein thrombosis associated with intravenous feeding- a propective study. JPEN 1981; 5:240–242.
50. Brismar B, Hardsedt C, Jacobson S, et al. Reduction of catheter-associated thrombosis in parenteral nutrition by intravenous heparin therapy. Arch Surg 1982; 117:1196–1199.
51. Bozetti F, Scarpa D, Terno G, et al. Subclavian vein thrombosis due to indwelling catheters: a prospective study on 52 patients. JPEN 1983; 7:560–562.
52. Pottecher T, Forrler M, Picardat P, et al. Thrombogenicity of central venous catheters: prospective study of polyethylene, silicone and polyurethane catheters with phlebography or post-mortem examination. Eur J Anaesthesiol 1984; 1:361–365.
53. Bern HM, Lokich JJ, Wallach SR, et al. Very low dose of warfarin can prevent thrombosis in central venous catheters: a randomized, prospective trial. Ann Intern Med 1990; 112:423–428.
54. Balestrieri L, De Cicco M, Matovic M, et al. Central venous catheter-related thrombosis in clinically asymptomatic oncologic patients: a phlebographic study. Eur J Radiol 1995; 20:108–111.
55. Monreal M, Alastrue A, Rull M, et al. Upper extremity deep venous thrombosis in cancer patients with venous access devices. Prophylaxis with a low molecular weight heparin (Fragmin). Thromb Haemost 1996; 75:251–253.
56. De Cicco M, Matovic M, Balestrieri L, et al. Central venous thrombosis: an early and frequent complication in cancer patients bearing long term silastic catheter. A prospective study. Thromb Res 1997; 86:101–113.
57. Glaser DW, Mederios D, Rollins N, et al. Catheter-related thrombosis in children with cancer. J Pediatr 2001; 138(2):255–259.
58. Verso M, Agnelli G, Bertoglio S, et al. Enoxaparin for the prevention of venous thromboembolism associated with central vein catheter: a double-blind, placebo-controlled, randomized study in cancer patients. J Clin Oncol 2005; 23:4057–4062.

59. Cortellezzi A, Moia M, Falanga A, et al. Incidence of thrombotic complications in patients with haematological malignancies with central venous catheters: a prospective multicentre study. Br J Haem 2005; 129:811–817.
60. Frank DA, Meuse J, Hirsch D, et al. The treatment and outcome of cancer patients with thromboses on central venous catheters. J Thromb Thrombolysis 2000; 10:271–275.
61. Trerotola SO, Kuhn-Fulton J, Johnson MS, et al. Tunneled infusion catheters: increased incidence of symptomatic venous thrombosis after subclavian versus internal jugular venous access. Radiology 2000; 217:89–93.
62. Duerksen DR, Papineau N, Siemens J, et al. Peripherally inserted central catheters for parenteral nutrition: a comparison with centrally inserted catheters. J Parenter Enteral Nutr 1999; 23:85–89.
63. Cowl CT, Weinstock JV, Al-Jurf A, et al. Complications and cost associated with parenteral nutrition delivered to hospitalized patients through either subclavian or peripherally inserted central catheters. Clin Nutr 2000; 19:237–243.
64. Lersch C, Eckel F, Sader R, et al. Initial experience with Healthport miniMax and other peripheral arm port in patients with advanced gastrointestinal malignancy. Oncology 1999; 57:269–275.
65. Pierce CM, Wade A, Mok Q. Heparin-bonded central venous lines reduce thrombotic and infective complications in critically ill children. Intensive Care Med 2000; 26:967–972.
66. Gould JR, Carloss HW, Skinner WL. Groshong catheter-associated subclavian venous thrombosis. Am J Med 1999; 95:419–423.
67. Luciani A, et al. Catheter-related upper extremity deep venous thrombosis in cancer patients: a prospective study based on doppler US. Radiology 2001; 220:655–660.
68. Blom JW, Doggen CJM, Osanto S, Rosendaal FR. Malignancies, prothrombotic mutations and the risk of venous thrombosis. JAMA 2005; 293:715–722.
69. Borow M, Crowley JG. Evaluation of central venous catheter thrombogenicity. Acta Anest Scand 1985; 81:S59–S64.
70. Petersen J, Delaney JH, Brakstad MT, et al. Silicone venous access devices positioned with their tip high in the superior vena cava are more likely to malfunction. Am J Surg 2000; 178:78–79.
71. Puel V, Caudry M, Metayer P, et al. Superior vena cava thrombosis related to catheter malposition in cancer chemotherapy given through implanted ports. Cancer 1993; 72:2248–2252.
72. Verso M, Agnelli G, Kamphiusen PW, et al. Risk factors for CVC-associated thrombosis in cancer patients: analysis of ETHIC study. J Thromb Haemost 2005; 3(suppl 1):a2188.
73. McGee WT, Ackerman BL, Rouben LR, et al. Accurate placement of central venous catheters: a prospective, randomized, multicenter trial. Crit Care Med 1993; 21:1118–1123.
74. Lameris J, Post PJ, Zonderland HM, et al. Percutaneous placement of Hickman catheters: comparison of sonographically guided and blind techniques. Am J Roentgenol 1990; 155:1097–1099.
75. Lorenz JM, Funaki B, Van Ha T, et al. Radiologic placement of implantable chest ports in pediatric patients. Am J Roentgenol 2001; 176:991–994.
76. Denys BG, Uretsky BF, Reddy PS. Ultrasound-assisted cannulation of the internal jugular vein. A prospective comparison to the external landmark-guided technique. Circulation 1993; 87:1557–1562.
77. Kraybill WG, Allen BT. Preoperative duplex venous imaging in the assessment of patients with venous access. J Surg Oncol 1993; 5:244–248.
78. Timsit JF, Farkas JC, Boyer JM, et al. Central vein catheter-related thrombosis in intensive care patients. Incidence, risk factors and relationship with catheter-related sepsis. Chest 1998; 114:207–213.
79. Van Rooden CJ, Schippers EF, Barge RMY, et al. Infectious complications of central venous catheters increase the risk of catheter-related thrombosis in hematology patients: a prospective study. J Clin Oncol 2005; 23:2655–2660.
80. Francis CW, Felcher AH, White J, et al. Thrombin activity associated with indwelling central venous catheters. Thromb Haemost 1997; 77:48–52.
81. Koksoy C, Kuzu A, Erden I, et al. The risk factors in central venous catheter-related thrombosis. Aust N Z J Surg 1995; 65:796–798.

82. King MM, Rasnake MS, Rodriguez RG, Riley NJ, Stamm JA. Peripherally inserted central venous catheter-associated thrombosis: retrospective analysis of clinical risk factors in adult patients. South Med J 2006; 99(10):1073–1077.
83. Brown DF, Muirhead MJ, Travis PM, et al. Mode of chemotherapy does not affect complications with an implantable venous access device. Cancer 1997; 80:966–972.
84. De Cicco M, Matovic M, Balestrieri L, et al. Antithrombin III deficiency as a risk factor for catheter-related central vein thrombosis in cancer patients. Thromb Res 1995; 78:127–137.
85. Riordan M, Weiden PL. Factor V Leiden mutation does not account for central venous catheter-related thrombosis. Am J Hematol 1998; 58:150–152.
86. Wermes C, von Depka Prondzinski M, Lichtinghagen R, et al. Clinical relevance of genetic risk factors for thrombosis in paediatric oncology patients with central venous catheters. Eur J Pediatr 1999; 158:S143–S146.
87. Van Rooden CJ, Rosendaal FR, Meinders AE, et al. The contribution of factor V Leiden and prothrombin G20210A mutation to the risk of central venous catheter-related thrombosis. Haematologica 2004; 89:201–206.
88. Jansen FH, Wiggers T, van Geel BN, et al. Elevated levels of D-dimer and fragment 1+2 upon central venous catheter insertion and factor V Leiden predict subclavian vein thrombosis. Haematologica 2005; 90:499–504.
89. Verso M, Agnelli G. Venous thromboembolism associated with long-term use of central venous catheters in cancer patients. J Clin Oncol 2003; 21:3665–3675.
90. Agnelli G, Verso M. Therapy insight: venous catheter-related thrombosis in cancer patients. Nat Clin Pract Oncol 2006; 3(4):214–222.
91. Gaitini D, Beck-Razi N, Haim N, Brenner B. Prevalence of upper extremity deep venous thrombosis diagnosed by color Doppler duplex sonography in cancer patients with central venous catheters. J Ultrasound Med 2006; 25(10):1297–1303.
92. Koksoy C, Kuzu A, Kutlay J, et al. The diagnostic value of colour Doppler ultrasound in central venous catheter related thrombosis. Clin Radiol 1995; 50:687–689.
93. Shankar KR, Abernethy LJ, Das KS, et al. Magnetic resonance venography in assessing venous patency after multiple venous catheters. J Pediatr Surg 2002; 37:175–179.
94. Forneris G, Quarello F, Pozzato M, et al. Spiral x-ray computed tomography in the diagnosis of central venous catheterization complications. Nephrologie 2001; 22:495–499.
95. Monreal M, Raventos A, Lerma R, et al. Pulmonary embolism in patients with upper extremity DVT associated to venous central lines. A prospective study. Thromb Haemost 1994; 72(4):548–550.
96. O'Connell CL, Boswell WD, Duddalwar V, et al. Unsuspected pulmonary emboli in cancer patients: clinical correlates and relevance. J Clin Oncol 2006; 24(30):4928–4932.
97. Prandoni P, Lensing AW, Cogo A, et al. The long-term clinical course of acute deep venous thrombosis. Ann Intern Med 1996; 25:1–7.
98. Ascher E, Salles-Cunha S, Hingorani A. Morbidity and mortality associated with internal jugular vein thromboses. Vasc Endovascular Surg 2005; 39(4):335–339.
99. Randolph AG, Cook DJ, Gonzales CA, et al. Benefit of heparin in central venous and pulmonary artery catheters. A meta-analysis of randomized controlled trials. Chest 1998; 113:165–171.
100. Boraks P, Seale J, Price J, et al. Prevention of central venous catheter associated thrombosis using minidose warfarin in patients with haematological malignancies. Br J Haematol 1998; 101:483–486.
101. Karthaus M, Kretzschmar A, Kroning H, et al. Dalteparin for prevention of catheter-related complications in cancer patients with central venous catheters: final results of a double-blind, placebo-controlled phase III trial. Ann Oncol 2006; 17:289–296.
102 Couban S, Goodyear M, Burnell M, et al. Randomized placebo-controlled study of low-dose warfarin for the prevention of central venous catheter-associated thrombosis in patients with cancer. J Clin Oncol 2005; 23:4063–4069.
103. Massicotte P, Julian JA, Gent M, et al. An open-label, randomized controlled trial of low molecular weight heparin for the prevention of central venous line-related thrombotic for complications in children: the PROTECKT trial. Thromb Res 2003; 109:101–108.

104. Mismetti P, Mille D, Laporte S, et al. low-molecular-weight heparin (nadroparin) and very low doses of warfarin in the prevention of upper extremity thrombosis in cancer patients with indwelling long-term central venous catheters: a pilot randomized trial. Haematologica 2003; 88:67–73.
105. WARP—A multicentre prospective randomized controlled trial (RCT) of thrombosis prophylaxis with warfarin in cancer patients with central venous catheters (CVCs). Annual ASCO Meeting 2005: abstr n 8004.
106. Cimminiello C, Isa L, Vergani C, et al. Effect of antithrombotic prophylaxis on thrombosis-related complications and mortality in cancer patients carrying a central venous device. JCO 2006; ASCo AMP part I, 24(suppl):8596.
107. Agnelli G, Verso M. Is antithrombotic prophylaxis required in cancer patients with central venous catheters? No. J Thromb Haemost 2006; 4(1):14–15.
108. Buller HR, Agnelli G, Hull RD, et al. Antithrombotic therapy for venous thromboembolic disease. Chest 2004; 126:401S–428S.
109. Meyer G, Marjanovic Z, Valcke J, et al. Comparison of low-molecular-weight-heparin and warfarin for the secondary prevention of venous thromboembolism in patients with cancer: a randomized controlled study. Arch Intern Med 2002; 162:1729–1735.
110. Lee YYA, Levine M, Baker RI, et al. Low molecular weight heparin versus a coumarin for the prevention of the recurrent venous thromboembolism in patients with cancer. N Engl J Med 2003; 349:146–153.
111. Savage KJ, Wells PS, Schulz V, et al. Outpatient use of low molecular weight heparin (dalteparin) for the treatment of deep vein thrombosis of the upper extremity. Thromb Haemost 1999; 82:1008–1010.
112. Spence LD, Gironta MG, Malde HM, et al. Acute upper extremity deep venous thrombosis: safety and effectiveness of superior vena caval filters. Radiology 1999; 210:53–58.
113. Ascher E, Hingorani A, Tsemekhin B, et al. Lesson learned from a 6-year clinical experience with superior vena cava Greenfield filters. J Vasc Surg 2000; 32:881–887.
114. Ponec D, Irwin D, Haire WD, Hill PA, Li X, McCluskey ER; COOL investigators. Recombinant tissue plasminogen activator (alteplase) for restoration of flow in occluded central venous access devices: a double-blind placebo-controlled trial—the Cardiovascular Thrombolytic to Open Occluded Lines (COOL) efficacy trial. J Vasc Interv Radiol 2001; 12(8):951–955.
115. Semba CP, Deitcher SR, Li X, Resnansky L, Tu T, McCluskey ER; Cardiovascular thrombolytic to Open Occluded Lines Investigators. Treatment of occluded central venous catheters with alteplase: results in 1,064 patients. J Vasc Interv Radiol 2002; 13(12):1199–205.
116. Horattas MC, Wright DJ, Fenton AH, et al. Changing concepts of deep venous thrombosis of the upper extremity- report of a series and review of the literature. Surgery 1988:561–567.
117. Hill SL, Berry RE. Subclavian vein thrombosis: a continuing challenge. Surgery 1990; 108:1–9.
118. Agnelli G, Verso M. Thrombosis and cancer: clinical relevance of a dangerous liaison. Haematologica 2005; 90(2):154–156.

16

Treating Venous Thromboembolism in Cancer Patients: The Case for Low-molecular-weight Heparin Therapy

Agnes Y. Y. Lee
Department of Medicine, McMaster University, Hamilton, Ontario, Canada

- Anticoagulant therapy remains the cornerstone of treatment for acute venous thromboembolism (VTE).
- Risks of recurrent VTE and major bleeding are substantially higher in patients with cancer than in patients without cancer.
- In contrast to unfractionated heparin and vitamin K antagonists, low-molecular-weight heparins (LMWHs) can be dosed according to the patient's weight without the need for routine laboratory monitoring.
- Level II evidence shows that LMWH is comparable to unfractionated heparin for the initial treatment of VTE in patients with cancer.
- Vitamin K antagonist therapy is difficult to mange in cancer patients because of the unpredictable anticoagulant effects from drug interaction, gastrointestinal disturbances, liver dysfunction, and borderline nutritional status. Frequent laboratory monitoring is also burdensome.
- Level I evidence from a single randomized control trial supports the use of once-daily injections of LMWH dalteparin for the treatment of deep vein thrombosis and/or PE in most cancer patients.
- Treatment duration must be individualized. It is recommended for a minimum of three months and until there are no ongoing risk factors that could increase the risk of recurrent VTE.
- Once- and twice-daily administrations of LMWH appear to be equally efficacious and safe, but comparison data are lacking.
- Treatment of recurrent VTE is best managed with LMWH; the use of inferior vena cava (IVC) filter is not recommended unless the patient is actively bleeding.

INTRODUCTION

Low-molecular-weight heparins (LMWHs) have improved and simplified the management of venous thromboembolic disorders. Supported by robust data from many randomized controlled trials conducted over the past two decades, these agents are now established as the agents of choice over standard unfractionated heparin for the initial treatment and the primary prevention of venous thromboembolism (VTE). More recently, a major advancement was made in the treatment of cancer patients with VTE when a LMWH was found to be significantly more efficacious than warfarin for reducing symptomatic, recurrent VTE in cancer patients with acute deep vein thrombosis (DVT) and/or pulmonary embolism (PE). This finding has led to new treatment recommendations in international and U.S. consensus guidelines and changes in practice worldwide. However, the limitations of LMWH still leave room for improvement, and many questions regarding the management of VTE in cancer patients remain unanswered.

TRADITIONAL THERAPY WITH HEPARIN AND WARFARIN

Anticoagulant therapy is the mainstay treatment for newly diagnosed VTE (1). It alleviates the acute symptoms of venous congestion, reduces the likelihood of embolism, and prevents the extension of established thrombi. However, in order to prevent recurrent thromboembolic events over the long term, continuous anticoagulant therapy for a minimum of three months is necessary. Hence, the treatment of VTE is usually considered as having two phases—initial and long term—that are aimed at different therapeutic goals. This classification is also reflective of the transition from the use of unfractionated heparin, a parenterally administered anticoagulant with a rapid onset of action, for initial therapy, to an oral vitamin K antagonist such as warfarin, which does not achieve an immediate therapeutic anticoagulant effect but is more convenient to use in the long term. Thus, heparin provides bridging anticoagulation when warfarin has not yet established a therapeutic effect, defined as an international normalized ratio (INR) between 2.0 to 3.0 (2).

Initial Therapy with Heparins

Although combination therapy with heparin and warfarin has been in use since the 1970s, the necessity of giving heparin initially was not firmly established until 1992 in a randomized, double-blind trial. In this landmark study by Brandjes et al., patients with proximal DVT were randomly allocated to receive a vitamin K antagonist acenocoumarol alone or intravenous heparin plus acenocoumarol (3). The study was terminated early by the data safety and monitoring committee after 12 of 60 (20%) patients in the acenocoumarol group developed symptomatic events compared with 4 of 60 (6.7%) patients in the combined therapy group. Following this study, the combined regimen of initial heparin and long-term warfarin became the gold standard, and this remained unchallenged until LMWHs were introduced. By the late 1990s, clinical trials had demonstrated that subcutaneous LMWHs and intravenous heparin therapy were equally efficacious and safe, but that LMWHs could be given on an outpatient basis without the need for routine laboratory monitoring of the anticoagulant effect (1,4). In all of these studies, the dose of LMWH was calculated based solely on the patient's weight whereas heparin was administered by continuous infusion with the dose adjusted according to the activated partial thromboplastin time (aPTT). The heparins were administered for a minimum of five days and until the INR value is therapeutic. For all of the LMWHs evaluated in phase III randomized trials, the three-month incidence of recurrent VTE was approximately 4% and the risk of major bleeding during the first week of LMWH therapy was less than 2% (5–7). Although none of the individual studies found any difference in efficacy and safety between each LMWH and unfractionated heparin, a meta-analysis of 22 randomized trials by Cochrane Systematic Reviews has shown that LMWH is associated with a lower risk of recurrent VTE [odds ratio (OR) 0.68; 95% confidence interval (CI) 0.55–0.84] and a lower risk of major bleeding (OR 0.57; 95% CI 0.39–0.83) (7). Furthermore, the meta-analysis found a survival benefit associated with the use of LMWH (OR 0.76; 95% CI 0.62–0.92) (Table 1). Presumably, the mortality reduction is due to fewer fatal PEs with LMWH, although other mechanisms cannot be excluded.

However, whether these results apply equally to patients with and without cancer is less certain (8,9). In the majority of these trials, patients with cancer represented about only 10% to 15% of the study population. Also, the vast majority of patients with cancer and VTE would not have been eligible because of their shortened life expectancy, thrombocytopenia, high risk for bleeding, or other relative contraindications to anticoagulant therapy. Consequently, the results from these randomized controlled trials may not apply to cancer patients with symptomatic VTE who have more advanced malignancy or serious comorbid conditions. To date, there is only limited data from randomized trials and cohort studies that show LMWH and heparin are equally effective in preventing symptomatic, recurrent VTE in cancer patients with VTE (10). As is the case in patients without cancer, the indisputable advantages of LMWHs over heparin are the convenience of outpatient treatment and the elimination of routine laboratory monitoring (11–14).

Long-Term Therapy with Vitamin K Antagonists

Once the INR has reached the therapeutic target, heparin or LMWH can be stopped and warfarin is continued for the remainder of the treatment period. During this time, fre-

Table 1 Summary of Meta-Analyses Comparing the Incidence of Recurrent VTE, Major Bleeding, and Morality During LMWH and UFH Treatment

Study	No. trials included	Recurrent VTE [OR ((%CI)]	Major bleeding [OR ((%CI)]	Mortality[a] [OR ((%CI)]
Leizorovicz, 1996 (61)	16	0.66 (0.41–1.07)	0.65 (0.36–1.16)	NA
Lensing et al., 1995 (62)	10	0.47 (0.27–0.82)	0.32 (0.15–0.69)	0.53 (0.31–0.90)
Sirgusa et al., 1996 (63)	13	0.39 (0.30–0.80)	0.42 (0.2–0.9)	0.33 (0.1–0.8)
Hettiarachchi et al., 1998 (64)	13	0.77 (0.56–1.04)	0.60 (0.38–0.95)	0.61 (0.40–0.93)
Gould et al., 1999 (6)	11	0.85 (0.63–1.14)	0.57 (0.33–0.99)	0.57 (0.31–1.03)
Dolovich et al., 2000 (5)	13	0.85 (0.65–1.12)	0.63 (0.37–1.05)	NA
Van Dongen et al., 2004 (7)	23	0.68 (0.55–0.84)	0.57 (0.39–0.83)	0.53 (0.33–0.85)

[a]In cancer patients.
Abbreviations: OR, odds ratio; CI, confidence interval; NA, not available; VTE, venous thromboembolism; LMWH, low-molecular-weight heparin; UFH, unfractionated heparin.

quent monitoring of the INR is required in order to adjust the dose of warfarin to maintain a therapeutic anticoagulant effect. For most patients without cancer, laboratory monitoring is a minor inconvenience that requires weekly to monthly venipunctures for blood sampling. But for cancer patients, this can be an onerous task because drug interactions, gastrointestinal disturbances, liver dysfunction, and borderline nutritional status all lead to unpredictable INR values (15). Lack of venous access further complicates blood monitoring and reduces patients' quality of life (16). The need for frequent visits to the laboratory or hospital can also add greater burden on family members or friends who are needed to provide transportation or other support. Another limitation of vitamin K antagonists is their delayed onset of action and prolonged clearance of the anticoagulant effect. For cancer patients who may require interruption of their anticoagulant therapy for invasive procedures or experience frequent episodes of chemotherapy-induced thrombocytopenia, balancing adequate anticoagulation with the risk of bleeding is very problematic using vitamin K antagonists.

In addition to these logistical challenges to warfarin therapy, patients with cancer frequently develop recurrent thrombosis while on anticoagulant therapy, even when therapeutic anticoagulant levels have been maintained. Strong evidence have now confirmed that patients with cancer have a two- to fourfold higher risk of recurrent thrombosis, including fatal PE, compared with patients without cancer (17–20). In a prospective cohort study of 181 cancer and 661 noncancer patients on warfarin, Prandoni et al. found that the 12-month cumulative incidence of recurrent VTE was 20.7% in cancer patients versus 6.8% in patients without cancer (17). The risk was highest during the first three months and it remained elevated compared to the risk in patients without cancer. Other studies have also reported that the *incidence* of recurrent VTE in cancer patients *is increased* even when the INR is maintained in the therapeutic range. In one study, the incidence of VTE recurrence for INRs within the therapeutic range is 18.9 per 100 patient-years in cancer patients versus 7.2 per 100 patient-years in patients without cancer (18) (Table 2).

Moreover, cancer patients have a high risk of anticoagulant-related bleeding. The source of bleeding is usually related to their underlying malignancy, such as hemoptysis in a patient with lung carcinoma or hematuria in a patient with bladder cancer. In the study by Prandoni et al., the 12-month cumulative incidence for major bleeding was 12.4% versus 4.9% for patients with and without cancer, respectively (17). The risk of major bleeding is high and accumulates while cancer patients are receiving warfarin, whereas the risk appears to plateau after the first month of anticoagulation in patients without cancer. This higher risk of anticoagulant-related bleeding in cancer patients is also evident in the study by Hutten et al., in which the incidence of major bleeding in these patient groups were 13.3 per 100 patient-years, compared with 2.1 per 100 patient-years in patients without cancer.

Table 2 The Incidence of Recurrent VTE and Major Bleeding in Relation to the INR (18)

	Recurrent VTE		Major bleeding	
	Cancer	No cancer	Cancer	No cancer
INR range	No. of events (per 100 pt-years)	No. of events (per 100 pt-years)	No. of events (per 100 pt-years)	No. of events (per 100 pt-years)
≤2.0	54.0	15.9	30.6	0.0
2.0–3.0	18.9	7.2	11.2	0.8
>3.0	18.4	6.4	0.0	6.3

Abbreviations: VTE, venous thromboembolism; INR, international normalized ratio.

In contrast to the INR-related increase in bleeding observed in patients without cancer, the incidence of bleeding in patients with malignancy did not follow a similar pattern (19).

In summary, treatment failure associated with warfarin therapy is considerable (21). The incidence of symptomatic, recurrent VTE is approximately 21% and incidence of major bleeding is approximately 12% in the first year of warfarin therapy. The rate of recurrent VTE is highest during the first one to three months after the index thrombotic event, but the incidence of serious bleeding continues to accumulate throughout the period of anticoagulation. Recurrent VTE occurs because of the heightened hypercoagulable state associated with the underlying malignancy and its treatments, whereas the high risk of bleeding is often attributed to the patients' comorbidities, the need for invasive procedures, disease-related or chemotherapy-induced thrombocytopenia, and tumor invasion (22).

LMWH AS AN ALTERNATIVE TO VITAMIN K ANTAGONISTS

LMWHs have a number of theoretical advantages over warfarin therapy. Compared to warfarin, LMWHs have more stable pharmacokinetic properties and fewer drug interactions, and they do not rely on gastrointestinal absorption (23). Consequently, weight-based dosing of these agents produces a predictable anticoagulant effect that does not require routine laboratory monitoring. However, LMWH therapy must be given once- or twice-daily subcutaneously, is relatively contraindicated in patients with renal insufficiency, and is associated with a low risk of heparin-induced thrombocytopenia (24,25).

Since the mid-1990s, a number of small studies have been conducted to compare the efficacy and safety of long-term LMWH with vitamin K antagonists for the secondary prophylaxis of VTE. The trials included primarily patients without cancer and used prophylactic doses of LMWH for extended treatment rather than full therapeutic doses that are used for initial treatment (26–33). Two meta-analyses of these studies found a statistically nonsignificant reduction of approximately 30% in the risk of recurrent VTE favoring LMWH, while one of these analyses found a significant reduction of 62% in the risk of bleeding with LMWH (34,35). A more recent and larger study (Long-term Innovations in TreatmEnt program (LITE) study) also failed to find a significant difference between LMWH tinzaparin given at a full therapeutic dose and warfarin adjusted to a target INR of 2.0 to 3.0. Symptomatic, recurrent VTE occurred in 3% in both groups (31). Overall, LMWHs do not appear to offer any measurable efficacy or safety advantage over standard treatment with vitamin K antagonists in patients without cancer.

LMWH in Patients with Cancer and VTE

To-date, several published clinical trials have examined the use of long-term LMWH as an alternative to warfarin therapy in cancer patients with acute VTE (36–39). The CANTHANOX trial compared three months of standard warfarin therapy with enoxaparin therapy in cancer patients with proximal DVT, PE, or both (36). All patients were treated initially for at least four days with therapeutic doses of enoxaparin at 1.5 mg/kg once daily. They were then randomized to either continue with enoxaparin at the same dose or warfarin therapy. After 147 patients were randomized, the study was terminated prematurely because of slow recruitment. A total of 75 patients in the warfarin group and 71 patients in the enoxaparin group were evaluable for the primary end point of treatment failure, defined as symptomatic, recurrent VTE and/or major bleeding within the three-month treatment period. About 52% of the study patients had metastatic malignancy at randomization, and these patients were equally distributed between the treatment groups. By three months, 15 patients had recurrent VTE or major bleeding in the warfarin group compared with 7 patients assigned to enoxaparin. The difference was not statistically significant ($P = 0.09$). The majority of the outcome events were major bleeding, reported in 12 and 5 patients, respectively. Of these, six patients in the warfarin group died of bleeding. At the six-month follow-up, 38.7% of the warfarin patients and 31.0% of the enoxaparin patients had died. Based on these results, the investigators concluded that warfarin is associated with a high bleeding risk in cancer patients with VTE and that prolonged treatment with LMWH may be as effective as and safer than warfarin therapy. Another study that also evaluated enoxaparin in cancer patients compared two different doses of enoxaparin (1.5 mg/kg once daily and 1.0 mg/kg twice daily) with warfarin therapy (38). Designed as a feasibility study, the three-arm ONCENOX trial included 101 cancer patients with VTE. Due to the small number of patients in each arm, differences in recurrent VTE, major bleeding, or death were not observed. The study did demonstrate a high level of compliance with self-administered subcutaneous injections.

The Randomized Comparison of Low-molecular-weight heparin versus Oral anticoagulant Therapy for the prevention of recurrent venous thromboembolism in patients with cancer (LOT) trial evaluated the use of long-term dalteparin in cancer patients with newly diagnosed proximal DVT, PE, or both (37). In this multicenter, randomized, open-label study, 676 cancer patients with proximal DVT, PE, or both were randomized to receive dalteparin alone or usual treatment with dalteparin initially followed by six months of therapy with a vitamin K antagonist (warfarin or acenocoumarol) dosed for a target INR of 2.5. All patients received dalteparin 200 IU/kg once daily for the first five to seven days. In the dalteparin group, patients continued with the therapeutic dose of 200 IU/kg once daily until the end of the first month and then received 75% to 80% of the full dose for the next five months. Prefilled syringes at fixed doses of dalteparin were used for the extended period. The primary outcome was symptomatic, recurrent VTE, and the secondary outcomes were bleeding and survival. A panel of experts who were masked to treatment allocation centrally adjudicated all outcome events. Over the six-month treatment period, a total of 80 patients had a confirmed, symptomatic recurrent thromboembolic event, 27 of 338 (8.0%) in the dalteparin group and 53 of 338 (15.7%) in the vitamin K antagonist group. The cumulative risk of recurrent VTE at six months was reduced from 17% in the vitamin K antagonist group to 9% in the dalteparin group, resulting in a statistically significant risk reduction of 52% (two-sided log-rank, $P = 0.002$). In the control group, the INR was therapeutic or higher for 70% of the total treatment time, and 25 of the 53 recurrences occurred while the INR was 2.0 or above. Accordingly, one episode of recurrent VTE is prevented for every 13 patients treated with dalteparin. Overall, there were no differences in major or any bleeding between the groups. Major bleeding was reported in 6% in the dalteparin group versus 4% in the control group (two-sided Fisher's exact, $P = 0.27$). By six months, 39% of the patients had died in each group; 90% were due to progressive cancer. At one year, about 60% of the patients were dead in each group. The poor prognosis is reflective of the high proportion (67%) of the patients with metastatic cancer. However, a post hoc analysis found that dalteparin was associated with a 50% reduction in overall mortality in patients who did not have metastatic disease at the time of randomization (40).

One study has evaluated LMWH tinzaparin for long-term use. The LITE study reported improved efficacy with tinzaparin over warfarin in 167 patients with cancer (39). Tinzaparin reduced the rate of recurrent VTE by half, but this was not statistically significant at the end of the 3-month treatment period. As in other studies, no difference in bleeding was observed.

In summary, there is strong evidence that long-term LMWH is more efficacious than warfarin for preventing symptomatic, recurrent VTE in cancer patients. Bleeding does not appear to be increased and daily self-injections are well tolerated. Studies have also shown that cancer patients prefer LMWH over warfarin therapy (41). Drug cost appears to be the main obstacle in using LMWH for the long term. However, when the cost of investigations and hospitalization that are needed for recurrent VTE and the practical burden of vitamin K antagonist treatment are taken into consideration, LMWH becomes a very attractive alternative. Based on the evidence to date, long-term treatment with LMWH dalteparin or tinzaparin for cancer patients with DVT has been given the highest recommendation by the 2004 American College of Chest Physicians Consensus Guidelines (Grade 1A) (1) and are also endorsed by the National Comprehensive Cancer Network Clinical Practice Guidelines in Oncology (Category 2A) published in 2006 (42). Dalteparin is the only LMWH with regulatory approval for this indication.

DURATION OF THERAPY

Based on the accepted concept that the risk of recurrent thrombosis is increased in the presence of any ongoing risk factor, it is generally recommended that patients with metastases continue with "indefinite" therapy because metastatic malignancy is a persistent risk factor for thrombosis (1,43). In those without metastases, anticoagulant treatment is recommended for as long as the cancer is "active" and while the patient is receiving antitumor therapy. In general, periodic evaluation of the risk–benefit ratio of continuing anticoagulant therapy in individual patients is recommended. The decision should take into consideration the patient's preference, the anticancer treatments, the comorbid conditions, and most importantly, the quality of life and life expectancy (41).

After six months of treatment with LMWH, there is also no evidence for or against continuing LMWH in those patients who would continue anticoagulant therapy. It is recommended that the risks and benefits of LMWH versus warfarin are discussed with the patient in order to individualize the treatment. Besides the ongoing risk of bleeding, there do not appear to be any significant side effects associated with long-term use of LMWH. Although animal studies suggest that LMWH exposure may reduce bone density, this has not been shown to be a concern in pregnant women or other patient populations that may need extended treatment with LMWH (44,45).

ONCE- OR TWICE-DAILY INJECTIONS

For several LMWHs, both once-daily and twice-daily injections are available and approved for use for the initial treatment of VTE. Theoretically, twice-daily injections may provide more steady anticoagulant levels and avoid high peaks and low troughs, but there is a paucity of data that have directly compared the efficacy and safety of the two administration regimens (46). In a study by Merli et al., intravenous UFH was compared with subcutaneous enoxaparin at 1.0 mg/kg of body weight given twice daily or 1.5 mg/kg injected once daily for the initial treatment of DVT (47). No difference in symptomatic recurrent VTE or bleeding was detected among the three treatment groups for all patients. However, among the subgroups of patients with cancer, patients receiving once-daily enoxaparin had a twofold risk of recurrent VTE compared with patients on twice-daily injections (12.2% vs. 6.4%). This difference was not statistically significant. It should be noted that patients in the once-daily enoxaparin group received only 75% of the total daily doses received by those in the twice-daily group, so that the observed difference in recurrent VTE in this study could have been related to dose rather than frequency of injections. Twice-daily administration of the LMWH reviparin also appeared to be more efficacious on reducing thrombus burden than once-daily injections in a randomized trial conducted by Breddin et al. (48). Results of patients with cancer were not reported separately in this study.

For long-term treatment, only once-daily regimens have been tested. It is certainly more convenient and less onerous than twice-daily injections. However, there may be a role for twice-daily injections that break through once-daily dosing with recurrent VTE.

TREATMENT OF RECURRENT VTE

Although recurrent VTE is frequent in cancer patients treated with warfarin therapy, optimal treatment in this setting has not been investigated in clinical trials. Traditionally, four options are available: continue with vitamin K antagonist therapy aiming for a higher target INR after initial retreatment with UFH or LMWH; switch to aPTT-adjusted, twice-daily injections of UFH; use once-daily, weight-adjusted LMWH; or insert an inferior vena caval filter. None of these alternatives has been compared directly or adequately evaluated.

Only one small study has looked at using long-term LMWH in this setting. This retrospective study evaluated the efficacy of dalteparin for the treatment of recurrent VTE that occurred while patients are on warfarin therapy (49). Using the databases of thrombosis clinics at three tertiary facilities, the investigators identified 32 patients who were treated with long-term dalteparin 200 U/kg once daily. Twenty (62.5%) of these patients had cancer. During follow-up, 3/32 (9%) patients experienced a subsequent recurrent thrombotic event and one of them had cancer; all responded to treatment with higher doses of dalteparin. Considering these results and the evidence from the CLOT study, switching to long-term LMWH dalteparin would seem a sensible approach to treat those with recurrent VTE while on warfarin therapy.

As for vena caval filters, a randomized, controlled trial has shown that filters can reduce the short-term risk of PE but they also increase the risk of recurrent DVT and post-phlebitic syndrome (50). A large retrospective study in 529 cancer patients with VTE also reported a high rate of recurrent VTE of 32% in those who received inferior vena caval filters (51). The recurrence rate reflects the heightened hypercoagulable state in cancer patients that is not treated by insertion of a vena caval filter. Overall, given the weak evidence for the use of filters in this population, their role in treating recurrent VTE is highly questionable. Filters should be used conservatively and primarily in situations where anticoagulant therapy cannot be used because of serious, active bleeding.

The management of patients who develop recurrent VTE while on LMWH also has not been investigated. Experts have recommended empirically increasing the dose of LMWH, dividing the daily dose in half to be given as twice-daily injections (perhaps to achieve more stable anticoagulant effects) or to be treated with aPTT-adjusted unfractionated heparin. Because fewer patients break through LMWH therapy, it will take some time to accumulate the experience and data necessary to generate recommendations. An international registry sponsored by the International Society on Thrombosis and Haemostasis is currently collecting this information (52).

SURVIVAL ADVANTAGE ASSOCIATED WITH LMWH

One of the most controversial topics concerning the use of LMWHs in cancer patients is the unexpected observation of a survival benefit. Since the original reports from meta-analyses of initial treatment studies that suggested LMWHs may have an antineoplastic effect, further data have emerged to support this finding. Four randomized trials have now been performed to investigate whether LMWHs can improve cancer patient survival (53–56). Two of the studies had positive results in favor of LMWH, and all of them provided evidence that patients with limited disease may enjoy a greater benefit than those with metastatic disease. The major criticism of most of these studies is the inclusion of patients with different tumor types and the lack of control over anticancer therapy. Therefore, potential imbalance in the prognosis of patients with different tumor types may have accounted for the observed difference in survival. The single study that included only patients with newly diagnosed small-cell lung cancer was small (53). Indirect evidence has also emerged in a post hoc analysis of the CLOT Trial, in which dalteparin was associated with a 50% reduction in mortality in patients with limited disease (39). Mechanisms of action have not been identified but multiple pathways, including inhibition of angiogenesis and induction of apoptosis, have been proposed (57–60). Certainly, protection against fatal PE alone cannot explain the observation since the difference in survival was noted only after the discontinuation of LMWH in all these studies. Nonetheless, the limited evidence to date is encouraging, but conclusions about the potential benefits of LMWH on long-term survival remain uncertain.

OTHER UNANSWERED QUESTIONS

The introduction of LMWHs has advanced the treatment of VTE, particularly in cancer patients. The CLOT trial presents compelling evidence that LMWHs should become the standard of care for monotherapy of VTE in cancer patients. Although LMWHs offer advantages over unfractionated heparin and vitamin K antagonist therapy, they also have undesirable limitations that fuel the ongoing search for the "ideal" anticoagulant.

To date, the studies evaluating new anticoagulants have included few or no patients with cancer. Given the differences in the natural history and response to anticoagulant therapy between patients with and without cancer, research is needed to study the efficacy and safety of these agents specifically in the various oncology settings. New oral agents are potentially the most attractive alternatives to traditional anticoagulants because of their route of administration and the elimination of laboratory monitoring. However, their efficacy and safety profiles must be evaluated carefully in patients with cancer before they can be used in this high risk and vulnerable population. In particular, concerns regarding hepatotoxicity, bioaccumulation, and drug interaction are very important.

Also, more studies are required to look at specific details of the antithrombotic regimen, especially regarding duration of therapy, predictors of recurrent VTE and bleeding, quality of life, cost-effectiveness, and the influence of anticoagulants on cancer survival. Whether novel anticoagulants will be superior to traditional agents including LMWHs awaits further study.

REFERENCES

1. Buller HR, Agnelli G, Hull RD, Hyers TM, Prins MH, Raskob GE. Antithrombotic therapy for venous thromboembolic disease: the Seventh ACCP Conference on Antithrombotic and Thrombolytic Therapy. Chest 2004; 126(3 suppl):401S–428S.
2. Ansell J, Hirsh J, Poller L, Bussey H, Jacobson A, Hylek E. The pharmacology and management of the vitamin K antagonists: the Seventh ACCP Conference on Antithrombotic and Thrombolytic Therapy. Chest 2004; 126(3 suppl):204S–233S.
3. Brandjes DP, Heijboer H, Buller HR, de Rijk M, Jagt H, ten Cate JW. Acenocoumarol and heparin compared with acenocoumarol alone in the initial treatment of proximal-vein thrombosis. N Engl J Med 1992; 327(21):1485–1489.
4. Hirsh J, Raschke R. Heparin and low-molecular-weight heparin: the Seventh ACCP Conference on Antithrombotic and Thrombolytic Therapy. Chest 2004; 126(3 suppl):188S–203S.

5. Dolovich LR, Ginsberg JS, Douketis JD, Holbrook AM, Cheah G. A meta-analysis comparing low-molecular-weight heparins with unfractionated heparin in the treatment of venous thromboembolism: examining some unanswered questions regarding location of treatment, product type, and dosing frequency. Arch Intern Med 2000; 160(2):181–188.
6. Gould MK, Dembitzer AD, Doyle RL, Hastie TJ, Garber AM. Low-molecular-weight heparins compared with unfractionated heparin for treatment of acute deep venous thrombosis. A meta-analysis of randomized, controlled trials. Ann Intern Med 1999; 130(10):800–809.
7. van Dongen CJ, van den Belt AG, Prins MH, Lensing AW. Fixed dose subcutaneous low molecular weight heparins versus adjusted dose unfractionated heparin for venous thromboembolism. Cochrane Database Syst Rev 2004; (4):CD001100.
8. Lee AY, Levine MN. Venous thromboembolism and cancer: risks and outcomes. Circulation 2003; 107(23 suppl 1):I17–I21.
9. Sutherland DE, Weitz IC, Liebman HA. Thromboembolic complications of cancer: epidemiology, pathogenesis, diagnosis, and treatment. Am J Hematol 2003; 72(1):43–52.
10. Lee AY. Management of thrombosis in cancer: primary prevention and secondary prophylaxis. Br J Haematol 2005; 128(3):291–302.
11. Wells PS, Kovacs MJ, Bormanis J, et al. Expanding eligibility for outpatient treatment of deep venous thrombosis and pulmonary embolism with low-molecular-weight heparin: a comparison of patient self-injection with homecare injection. Arch Intern Med 1998; 158(16):1809–1812.
12. Harrison L, McGinnis J, Crowther M, Ginsberg J, Hirsh J. Assessment of outpatient treatment of deep-vein thrombosis with low- molecular-weight heparin [see comments]. Arch Intern Med 1998; 158(18):2001–2003.
13. O'Shaughnessy D, Miles J, Wimperis J. UK patients with deep-vein thrombosis can be safely treated as out-patients. QJM 2000; 93(10):663–667.
14. Ageno W, Steidl L, Marchesi C, et al. Selecting patients for home treatment of deep vein thrombosis: the problem of cancer. Haematologica 2002; 87(3):286–291.
15. Wells PS, Holbrook AM, Crowther NR, Hirsh J. Interactions of warfarin with drugs and food. Ann Intern Med 1994; 121(9):676–683.
16. Johnson MJ, Sherry K. How do palliative physicians manage venous thromboembolism? Palliat Med 1997; 11(6):462–468.
17. Prandoni P, Lensing AW, Piccioli A, et al. Recurrent venous thromboembolism and bleeding complications during anticoagulant treatment in patients with cancer and venous thrombosis. Blood 2002; 100(10):3484–3488.
18. Hutten BA, Prins MH, Gent M, Ginsberg J, Tijssen JG, Buller HR. Incidence of recurrent thromboembolic and bleeding complications among patients with venous thromboembolism in relation to both malignancy and achieved international normalized ratio: a retrospective analysis. J Clin Oncol 2000; 18(17):3078–3083.
19. Palareti G, Legnani C, Lee A, et al. A comparison of the safety and efficacy of oral anticoagulation for the treatment of venous thromboembolic disease in patients with or without malignancy. Thromb Haemost 2000; 84(5):805–810.
20. Nieto JA, De Tuesta AD, Marchena PJ, et al. Clinical outcome of patients with venous thromboembolism and recent major bleeding: findings from a prospective registry (RIETE). J Thromb Haemost 2005; 3(4):703–709.
21. Prandoni P, Piccioli A, Pagnan A. Recurrent thromboembolism in cancer patients: incidence and risk factors. Semin Thromb Hemost 2003; 29(suppl 1):3–8.
22. Prandoni P, Falanga A, Piccioli A. Cancer and venous thromboembolism. Lancet Oncol 2005; 6(6):401–410.
23. Weitz JI. Low-molecular-weight heparins. N Engl J Med 1997; 337(10):688–698.
24. Warkentin TE, Levine MN, Hirsh J, et al. Heparin-induced thrombocytopenia in patients treated with low-molecular- weight heparin or unfractionated heparin. N Engl J Med 1995; 332(20):1330–1335.
25. Warkentin TE, Greinacher A. Heparin-induced thrombocytopenia: recognition, treatment, and prevention: the Seventh ACCP Conference on Antithrombotic and Thrombolytic Therapy. Chest 2004; 126(3 suppl):311S–337S.

26. Gonzalez-Fajardo JA, Arreba E, Castrodeza J, et al. Venographic comparison of subcutaneous low-molecular weight heparin with oral anticoagulant therapy in the long-term treatment of deep venous thrombosis. J Vasc Surg 1999; 30(2):283–292.
27. Veiga F, Escriba A, Maluenda MP, et al. Low molecular weight heparin (enoxaparin) versus oral anticoagulant therapy (acenocoumarol) in the long-term treatment of deep venous thrombosis in the elderly: a randomized trial. Thromb Haemost 2000; 84(4):559–564.
28. Lopaciuk S, Bielska-Falda H, Noszczyk W, et al. Low molecular weight heparin versus acenocoumarol in the secondary prophylaxis of deep vein thrombosis. Thromb Haemost 1999; 81(1):26–31.
29. Das SK, Cohen AT, Edmondson RA, Melissari E, Kakkar VV. Low-molecular-weight heparin versus warfarin for prevention of recurrent venous thromboembolism: a randomized trial. World J Surg 1996; 20(5):521–526.
30. Pini M, Aiello S, Manotti C, et al. Low molecular weight heparin versus warfarin in the prevention of recurrences after deep vein thrombosis. Thromb Haemost 1994; 72(2):191–197.
31. Hull RD, Pineo GF, Mah AF, Brant RF, for the LITE Study Investigators. A randomized trial evaluating long-term low-molecular-weight heparin therapy for three months versus intravenous heparin followed by warfarin sodium. Blood 2002; 100:148a.
32. Lopez-Beret P, Orgaz A, Fontcuberta J, et al. Low molecular weight heparin versus oral anticoagulants in the long-term treatment of deep venous thrombosis. J Vasc Surg 2001; 33(1):77–90.1
33. Hamann H. Low molecular weight heparin versus coumarin in the prevention of recurrence after deep vein thrombosis. Rezidivprophylaxe nach Phlebothrombose—orale antikoagulation oder niedermolekulares heparin subkutan. Vasemed 1998; 10:133–136.
34. Iorio A, Guercini F, Pini M. Low-molecular-weight heparin for the long-term treatment of symptomatic venous thromboembolism: meta-analysis of the randomized comparisons with oral anticoagulants. J Thromb Haemost 2003; 1(9):1906–1913.
35. van der Heijden JF, Hutten BA, Buller HR, Prins MH. Vitamin K antagonists or low-molecular-weight heparin for the long term treatment of symptomatic venous thromboembolism. Cochrane Database Syst Rev 2003; (1):CD002001.
36. Meyer G, Marjanovic Z, Valcke J, et al. Comparison of low-molecular-weight heparin and warfarin for the secondary prevention of venous thromboembolism in patients with cancer: a randomized controlled study. Arch Intern Med 2002; 162(15):1729–1735.
37. Lee AY, Levine MN, Baker RI, et al. Low-molecular-weight heparin versus a coumarin for the prevention of recurrent venous thromboembolism in patients with cancer. N Engl J Med 2003; 349(2):146–153.
38. Deitcher SR, Kessler CM, Merli G, Rigas JR, Lyons RM, Fareed J. Secondary prevention of venous thromboembolic events in patients with active cancer: enoxaparin alone versus initial enoxaparin followed by warfarin for a 180-day period. Clin Appl Thromb Hemost 2006; 12(4):389–396.
39. Hull RD, Pineo GF, Brant RF, et al for the LITE Trial Investigators. Long-term low-molecular-weight heparin versus usual care in proximal-vein thrombosis patients with cancer. Am J Med 2006; 119:1062–1072.
40. Lee AY, Rickles FR, Julian JA, et al. Randomized comparison of low molecular weight heparin and coumarin derivatives on the survival of patients with cancer and venous thromboembolism. J Clin Oncol 2005; 23(10):2123–2129.
41. Noble SIR, Finlay IG. Is long-term low-molecular-weight heparin acceptable to palliative care patients in the treatment of cancer related venous thromboembolism? A qualitative study. Palliat Med 2005; 19(3):197–201.
42. Venous Thromboembolic Disease. NCCN clinical practice guidelines in oncology. 2006. http://www.nccn.org/professionals/physician_gls/PDF/vte.pdf. (accessed November 10, 2006).
43. Levine MN, Lee AY, Kakkar AK. From Trousseau to targeted therapy: new insights and innovations in thrombosis and cancer. J Thromb Haemost 2003; 1(7):1456–1463.
44. Casele HL, Laifer SA. Prospective evaluation of bone density in pregnant women receiving the low molecular weight heparin enoxaparin sodium. J Matern Fetal Med 2000; 9(2):122–125.
45. Pfeilschifter J, Diel IJ. Osteoporosis due to cancer treatment: pathogenesis and management. J Clin Oncol 2000; 18(7):1570–1593.

46. van Dongen CJ, Mac Gillavry MR, Prins MH. Once versus twice daily LMWH for the initial treatment of venous thromboembolism. Cochrane Database Syst Rev 2003; (1):CD003074.
47. Merli G, Spiro TE, Olsson CG, et al. Subcutaneous enoxaparin once or twice daily compared with intravenous unfractionated heparin for treatment of venous thromboembolic disease. Ann Intern Med 2001; 134(3):191–202.
48. Breddin HK, Hach-Wunderle V, Nakov R, Kakkar VV. Effects of a low-molecular-weight heparin on thrombus regression and recurrent thromboembolism in patients with deep-vein thrombosis. N Engl J Med 2001; 344(9):626–631.
49. Luk C, Wells PS, Anderson D, Kovacs MJ. Extended outpatient therapy with low molecular weight heparin for the treatment of recurrent venous thromboembolism despite warfarin therapy. Am J Med 2001; 111(4):270–273.
50. Decousus H, Leizorovicz A, Parent F, et al. A clinical trial of vena caval filters in the prevention of pulmonary embolism in patients with proximal deep-vein thrombosis. Prevention du Risque d'Embolie Pulmonaire par Interruption Cave Study Group. N Engl J Med 1998; 338(7):409–415.
51. Elting LS, Escalante CP, Cooksley C, et al. Outcomes and cost of deep venous thrombosis among patients with cancer. Arch Intern Med 2004; 164(15):1653–1661.
52. International Society on Thrombosis and Haemostasis website. 2006. http://www.med.unc.edu/isth/welcome. (accessed November 10, 2006).
53. Altinbas M, Coskun HS, Er O, et al. A randomized clinical trial of combination chemotherapy with and without low-molecular-weight heparin in small cell lung cancer. J Thromb Haemost 2004; 2(8):1266–1271.
54. Kakkar AK, Levine MN, Kadziola Z, et al. Low molecular weight heparin therapy with dalteparin and survival in advanced cancer: the Fragmin Advanced Malignancy Outcome Study (FAMOUS). J Clin Oncol 2004; 22(10):1944–1948.
55. Klerk CP, Smorenburg SM, Otten HM, et al. The effect of low molecular weight heparin on survival in patients with advanced malignancy. J Clin Oncol 2005; 23(10):2130–2135.
56. Sideras K, Schaefer PL, Okuno SH, et al. Low-molecular-weight heparin in patients with advanced cancer: a phase 3 clinical trial. Mayo Clin Proc 2006; 81(6):758–767.
57. Nash GF, Walsh DC, Kakkar AK. The role of the coagulation system in tumour angiogenesis. Lancet Oncol 2001; 2:608–613.
58. Nasir FA, Patel HK, Scully MF, Fareed J, Lemoine NR, Kakkar AK. The low molecular weight heparins dalteparin sodium inhibits angiogenesis and induces apoptosis in an experimental tumour model. Blood 2003; 102(11):808a, (abstract #2993).
59. Wojtukiewicz MZ, Sierko E, Klement P, Rak J. The hemostatic system and angiogenesis in malignancy. Neoplasia 2001; 3(5):371–384.
60. Zacharski LR, Ornstein DL. Heparin and cancer. Thromb Haemost 1998; 80(1):10–23.
61. Leizorovicz A. Comparison of the efficacy and safety of low molecular weight heparins and unfractionated heparin in the initial treatment of deep venous thrombosis. An updated meta-analysis. Drugs 1996; 52(suppl 7):30–37.
62. Lensing AW, Prins MH, Davidson BL, Hirsh J. Treatment of deep venous thrombosis with low-molecular-weight heparins. A meta-analysis. Arch Intern Med 1995; 155(6):601–607.
63. Siragusa S, Cosmi B, Piovella F, Hirsh J, Ginsberg JS. Low-molecular-weight heparins and unfractionated heparin in the treatment of patients with acute venous thromboembolism: results of a meta-analysis. Am J Med 1996; 100(3):269–277.
64. Hettiarachchi RJ, Prins MH, Lensing AW, Buller HR. Low molecular weight heparin versus unfractionated heparin in the initial treatment of venous thromboembolism. Curr Opin Pulm Med 1998; 4(4):220–225.

17

Antithrombotic Therapy and Survival in Cancer Patients

Gloria Petralia and Ajay Kakkar
Centre for Surgical Sciences, Institute of Cancer, Barts, and the London School of Medicine and Dentistry, and Thrombosis Research Institute, London, U.K.

- A complex relationship exists between the coagulation system and the tumor cells, with common mechanisms linking hemostasis and malignancy.
- Inhibiting hemostasis activation may therefore impact on outcomes from malignancy.
- Preclinical and some clinical data suggest that antithrombotic drugs, in particular low-molecular-weight heparins, may have potential antitumor effects.
- Although data from contemporary trials remain only partially convincing, further evaluation is warranted to determine if coagulation modulation prolongs survival in cancer patients.

INTRODUCTION

Treating a patient with cancer is a challenging clinical problem entailing a multidisciplinary approach, whether the intention is to cure or to palliate. Life expectancy may be improved in certain patients by aggressive intervention, but if a limited life span is expected, preserving quality of life becomes paramount. In both scenarios, the occurrence of venous thromboembolism (VTE) is an important clinical consideration. The association of VTE with malignant disease was first described in 1865 (1) by Trousseau lecturing about thrombophlebitis migrans; since then, a two-way relationship between VTE and cancer has been clearly established. Thromboembolic events may be the first clinical manifestation of undiagnosed malignancy (2–4); two large studies in the Danish and Swedish population showed an increased incidence of cancer of respectively 1.3- and 3.2-fold in patients with idiopathic VTE when compared to the native population (5,6). Patients with an established diagnosis of malignant disease are at high risk of developing VTE, with a wide range of clinical manifestations, ranging from asymptomatic deep vein thrombosis (DVT) at one extreme to fatal pulmonary embolism (PE) at the other. It is estimated that up to 60% of thromboembolic deaths occur at an otherwise favorable time in the history of the cancer (7). Cancer patients are often debilitated either by malignant cachexia or as a result of treatment toxicity, may be bed-bound for significant periods of time, and often require central venous access to dispense treatment or nutrients. These factors contribute to the increased risk of VTE and may be compounded by the hypercoagulable state associated with tumor activity, which has been described in patients with a variety of solid tumors (8).

The particular clinical challenge of preventing and treating VTE in cancer patients (9) has driven the formulation of specific guidelines (10,11), which recognize VTE as a clinically relevant disease in cancer patients with important implications for outcome. The systemic hypercoagulable state, its relationship to tumorigenesis, and the effects that antithrombotic agents such as the low-molecular-weight heparins (LMWHs) may have on cancer survival open interesting new perspectives on treatment planning.

PATHOPHYSIOLOGY OF BLOOD COAGULATION IN CANCER

The coagulation and fibrinolytic systems are in a constant and delicate balance, which ensures a prompt and regulated response to vascular injury and clot formation when required, without causing of intravascular thrombosis. A large number of circulating proteins, usually in inactive form, are involved in this process, forming a regulated cascade of proteolytic enzymes activated in sequence, with increasing quantity and culminating in fibrin formation. A balance is maintained with the fibrinolytic cascade, with activation resulting in thrombus degradation. Thus, intravascular occlusive thrombosis is avoided but hemostatic plug formation is facilitated, with subsequent repair and remodeling after the acute injury has been stabilized.

The mechanisms responsible for pathological thrombus formation in the venous systems were first identified by Virchow in 1856 (12). He described a triad of venous stasis, vascular trauma, and increased blood coagulability. For cancer patients, this results from a complex interplay between tumor and patient- and therapy-related factors. The genesis of Virchow's triad in cancer patients may be considered as follows:

- Alteration in blood flow (venous stasis): increased viscosity, mechanical blockage (tumor extrinsic compression or invasion), and patient immobility (due to cancer complication/therapy)
- Alteration in blood vessels (vascular trauma): mechanical endothelial trauma (tumor invasion/therapy), dysfunctional endothelium (loss of antithrombotic properties), and angiogenic stimuli
- Alteration in blood components (blood hypercoagulability): increase in procoagulant activities, decrease in anticoagulant activities, and increase in overall platelet activity

PROCOAGULANT ACTIVITY IN CANCER

A variety of procoagulant molecules, including tissue factor (TF) and the cysteine protease growth factor, cancer procoagulant (CP), are known to be expressed by tumor cells; and increased plasma levels of procoagulant markers, such as TF, activated factor VII (FVIIa), prothrombin-activation peptide, and thrombin-antithrombin complexes, have been observed in a wide variety of cancers.

TF and CP

TF is a transmembrane glycoprotein, cell-surface bound, with a strong structural homology with the class II cytokine receptor family. It interacts with factor VII and FVIIa to form the TF/VIIa complex that is the major activator of coagulation in vivo. On formation of that complex, filamin A, an intracellular protein implicated in cell motility, is recruited to the cytoplasmic end of TF (13). TF is expressed by endothelial cells and therefore becomes exposed to the circulating blood in circumstances of vascular damage and endothelium disruption. It is also expressed on activated circulating monocytes, thus playing a role in the inflammatory response and wound healing. TF is expressed on a variety of epithelial derived tumors; in pancreatic adenocarcinoma, it is expressed in ductal epithelial elements, and its expression correlates with histological grade. TF is not expressed in benign ductal epithelium (14). TF is also expressed in tumor cell lines including sarcoma, melanoma, neuroblastoma, lymphoma, and acute promyelocytic leukemia (15). Systemic activation of blood coagulation in cancer patients appears to be TF dependent with resulting activation of the extrinsic and common pathways of blood coagulation.

CP is a calcium-dependant cysteine protease, which is expressed by a variety of tumors (16,17). CP exerts a procoagulant effect by directly activating factor X independently of TF: VIIa complex (18), but the precise contribution of this procoagulant mechanism for cancer patients remains unclear.

Tumor Cytokines

Malignant cells can also promote coagulation indirectly by releasing inflammatory mediators such as tumor necrosis factor (TNF) and interleukin proteins [such as interleukin (IL)-1] (2). These act on endothelial and mononuclear cells, stimulating the secretion of procoagulant molecules that may also have a role in platelet activation (19).

COAGULATION PROTEASES AND TUMOR BIOLOGY

Beyond its role as the physiological initiator of blood coagulation, TF expression may also be associated with changes in tumor phenotypic behavior. It is well recognized that for certain tumor types (e.g., pancreatic adenocarcinoma), TF expression correlates with histological grade and that the appearance of TF results from transformation from benign to malignant phenotype (14). In experimental models, manipulation of TF expression by tumor cells is associated with a change in behavior. Using techniques of gene transfer, overexpression of TF in pancreatic adenocarcinoma is associated with enhanced primary tumor growth in vivo and invasion in vitro (20). An enhancement of tumor growth has similarly been identified as a result of TF overexpression in an experimental sarcoma model (21) in which manipulation of TF levels were associated with a corresponding increase in tumor production of vascular endothelial growth factor (VEGF) and decrease in the antiangiogenic regulatory protein thrombospondin. There also appears to be a complex relationship between tumor and endothelial TF and VEGF production: overexpression of TF in the tumor results in increased VEGF expression, which promotes TF expression in adjacent endothelial cells.

The relationship between TF expression and invasive breast cancer has also been well established (22). Interestingly, the expression of TF in human hepatocellular carcinoma may be associated with poor prognosis. In a recent study, reviewing 58 resection specimens, TF expression correlated significantly with tumor microvessel density and TF content in tumor cytosols with VEGF levels. High tumor content of TF was associated with increased venous invasion and advanced tumor stage and was an independent predictor of poor survival (23). There is also increasing evidence that cross talk between the integrin αIII βI and TF is responsible for the regulation of cell migration. As is seen with angiogenesis, the phosphorylation status of the cytoplasmic domain of TF will influence integrin-mediated migration dependent on αIII βI integrin (24).

Recognizing the role that TF plays in embryonic vascular development (25), it is conceivable that TF plays a predominant role in tumor angiogenesis. A recent observation has identified a pivotal role for TF in control of pathological angiogenesis. Belting et al. (26), have identified a regulatory function for the cytoplasmic tail of TF in protease activated receptor 2 (PAR-2)-dependent angiogenesis. PAR-2 is expressed in endothelial cells and promotes angiogenesis, this being regulated by intracellular cross talk between the cytoplasmic tails of TF and PAR-2. TF cytoplasmic tail deletion results in uncontrolled PAR-2 dependent angiogenesis. This feature is absent in PAR-2 knockout mice.

Circulating endothelial cells do not express TF, but do so if stimulated and may, therefore, have a role in intratumoral coagulation and angiogenesis (27). The TF/VIIa complex (28) and tumor hypoxia (29) also upregulate the expression of VEGF (30). Its ability to promote megakaryocyte maturation may explain increased platelet turnover in cancer patients (31) and cancer-related thrombocythemia (32). TF expression in tumor cells is associated with downregulation of thrombospondin, which is an antiangiogenic factor (21). Thus, TF appears to be an important regulator of angiogenesis influencing tumor levels of both pro- and antiangiogenic factors.

Constitutive expression of TF in cancer cells may have a profound effect on tumor cell phenotype. Using the technique of short hairpin RNA-mediated RNA interference to knock down TF expression in a human metastatic melanoma cell line, Wang et al. (33) were able to identify 44 human genes that were significantly upregulated and 228 genes significantly downregulated compared to control cells that had not had their constitutive TF expression altered. A variety of cellular pathways including transcription, translation cell communication, and cell growth/death were affected. These gene expression changes were associated with a reduction in pulmonary metastasis.

Interestingly, FVIIa/TF interaction appears to inhibit cell death and caspase III activation induced by serum deprivation and loss of adhesion. For TF overexpressing cells, this may represent an important mechanism of protection against apoptosis, increasing cell survival and thus might be related to the mechanism by which TF is able to promote successful metastasis (34). More recently, attention has turned to trying to find an explanation by which tumor expression of TF is controlled. It appears that the activation of the *K-ras* oncogene and inactivation of the *p53* tumor suppressor gene, both major transforming genetic events in colorectal cancer, and which result in progressive disease, are both involved in the control of TF expression (35). Using RNA interference techniques, Yu et al. were able to demonstrate that TF expression was an important determinant of K-ras-dependent phenotype in vivo, for colorectal cancer (35).

DOWNSTREAM GENERATION OF ACTIVATED PROTEASES INCLUDE FACTOR XA

Specific receptors have been identified that regulate cellular responses to the coagulation proteases. A receptor for activated factor II—thrombin, a member of the G-protein-coupled receptor family, is PAR-1. Originally shown to mediate the effects of thrombin on platelets (36), it is now known to mediate other cellular biological functions of thrombin. Thrombin interacts with PAR-1, which is overexpressed in a number of tumor lines, and especially in highly metastatic cell lines (37). Thrombin/PAR signaling results in upregulation of TF expression, and urokinase plasminogen in prostatic carcinoma cell lines, enhanced procoagulant activity in colonic cancer lines, and invasiveness of breast (38) and pancreatic (39–41) cancer lines. Thrombin induces neoangiogenesis in the chick chorioallantoic membrane via PAR-1 activation, with subsequent upregulation of VEGF and angiopoietin 2 (42). This effect is mediated by the endothelial receptors KDR-Fc and Tie-2-Fc. Interestingly, in this model, the direct thrombin inhibitor hirudin inhibited the proangiogenic effects of thrombin.

RISK OF VTE

In patients with malignant disease, VTE is estimated to be the second most common cause of death (43) and its treatment accounts for 6% of in-patient day usage on medical oncology wards (44). Up to 15% of cancer patients will experiences a symptomatic thromboembolic event (44). Risk of PE seems to be dependent on tumor histology. In a necroscopy study, the highest rates were found in ovarian cancer (34.6%), followed by malignancies of the extrahepatic biliary system (31.7%) and of the stomach (15.2%); whereas the lowest rates (0–5%–6%) were in cancer of the esophagus and larynx, myelomatosis, and lymphoma.

The risk of VTE associated with the use of chemotherapeutic agents has been well documented in trials relating to the treatment of breast cancer; the incidence of thrombotic events ranges from 1.7% to 17.6%. Furthermore, Levine's review of 205 women with breast cancer (stage II) showed an increased risk of DVT when combination chemotherapy was administered (45). Clahsen et al. compared postmenopausal women with breast cancer (stages I and II) undergoing surgery alone with those receiving postoperative chemotherapy and showed an increased risk associated with adjuvant therapy (0.7% vs. 2.3%, $p = 0.001$) (46). Tamoxifen increases DVT risk both in premenopausal (2.3% vs. 0.8%, $p = 0.003$) and postmenopausal (8.0% vs. 2.3%, $p = 0.003$) women (47). Chemotherapy associated with tamoxifen increased DVT risk when compared to tamoxifen alone in a group of stage II breast cancer from 1.4% to 9.6% ($p = 0.0001$) (48). Radiotherapy similarly increases VTE risk. A study in patients receiving neoadjuvant radiotherapy for rectal carcinoma reported an increased rate of thromboembolic events in the first 30 days following surgery (49). Comparable results were found on a five-year follow-up study in similar patients (7.5% vs. 3.6%, $p = 0.001$) (50).

ANTITHROMBOTIC THERAPY WITH LMWH AND SURVIVAL IN CANCER

Evidence from clinical trials of antithrombotic agents suggests their administration to cancer patients may influence survival. The Veterans Administration (VA) Cooperative trial evaluated the potential benefit of warfarin therapy in cancer; they first reported enrolled patients with lung, colon, head and neck, and prostate cancer. They randomized patients to either warfarin in addition to standard treatment or standard treatment alone, the randomization period lasting for an average of 26 weeks. The main outcome showed no significant difference between the two study arms. However, among the 50 patients with small-cell lung cancer, there were significant improvements in time to disease progression and in overall survival (51). They proceeded to target small-cell lung cancer (SCLC) patients and enrolled 328 subjects undergoing two different regimens of standardized chemotherapy. They were randomized to receive additional warfarin therapy or not. In this study, they were able to show a statistically significant advantage in the proportion of patients receiving warfarin in achieving complete or partial responses. In addition, they highlighted trends toward improved failure-free survival and overall survival in the active treatment arm, which came with comparable toxicities among the three regimens (52).

In a separate multicenter study, Lebeau et al. (53) randomized 277 patients with SCLC to either receive or not receive subcutaneous heparin injections for five weeks in addition to one of two chemotherapy regimens. The group that received heparin obtained better complete response rates (37% vs. 23%, $p = 0.04$), better median survival (317 days vs. 261 days, $P = 0.01$), and better survival rates at one, two, and three years. A subgroup analysis suggested that the benefit was greater in patients with less extensive disease.

More recently, a study evaluated the effect warfarin with chemotherapy and radiation therapy in patients with limited-stage small-cell lung cancer (54). The analysis included 347 patients and showed no significant differences in response rates, survival, failure-free survival, disease-free survival, or patterns of relapse between the two groups.

Studies comparing LMWH with unfractionated heparin (UFH) for DVT treatment have provided interesting retrospective data that suggest a potential survival advantage for cancer patients with an acute thrombosis having received LMWH for the initial treatment of their thrombosis (55–58).

Comparison of the initial treatment of patients with proximal DVT by Prandoni et al. (59) evaluated LMWH versus UFH. There was an advantage toward the LMWH arm versus the UFH in terms of six months survival for cancer patients (8/18, 44% vs. 1/15, 7%, $p = 0.02$).

Meta-analyses of these DVT treatment studies suggest an improved three-month survival of about 10% to 20% for such patients (58). For example, Hettiarachchi et al. (57) compared mortality rates in cancer patients receiving initial treatment for DVT with LMWH versus UFH in nine randomized trials. They analyzed data from 581/6293 (17.6%) patients with cancer that had been enrolled in those studies. In all cases, initial treatment with heparin was given for a short time of five to 10 days, following which both groups received the same treatment with a vitamin K antagonist. Of those, 46 patients in the LMWH group and 71 in the UFH group died in the first three months of followup [odds ratio (OR) 0.61, 95% confidence interval (CI), 0.40–0.93] in favor of LMWH. The excluded that the difference in mortality could be attributed to either fatal bleeding or PE but could not establish the mechanism by which such a brief treatment with a LMWH could favorably influence outcomes in cancer patients.

However, one must be cautious in overinterpretation of these data, since the original DVT treatment studies upon which the survival meta-analyses are based did not include cancer-associated mortality as a study endpoint, and little is known about the distribution of prognostic variables that might influence cancer outcome.

The Fragmin Advanced Malignancy Outcome study (FAMOUS) trial was the first randomized, placebo-controlled, double-blind evaluation designed to address the question of whether LMWH could prolong survival in patients with advanced malignant disease (60). Three hundred and eighty five patients with a variety of advanced cancers were randomized to receive either the LMWH dalteparin sodium at a dose of 5000 units once daily or a normal saline placebo injection for one year or until death, whichever event occurred sooner. At 12 months, the authors were not able to detect the 15% difference in survival between groups, for which the study was powered (Fig. 1). A 5% absolute increase in survival for patients randomized to receive LMWH was observed (41% placebo, 46% dalteparin). A post-hoc analysis of patients with good prognosis, surviving beyond 17 months (Fig. 2), revealed an increase in median survival from 24 months with placebo to approximately 43 months with dalteparin.

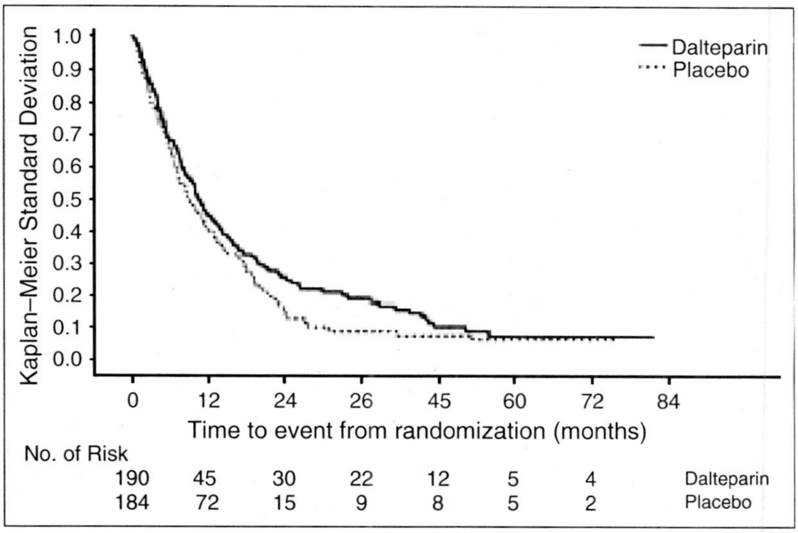

Figure 1 Kaplan–Meier survival curves for all intent-to-treat population patients in the dalteparin and placebo groups. Source: From Ref. 60.

The comparison of LMWH versus oral anticoagulant therapy for the prevention of recurrent VTE in patients with cancer trial (CLOT) assessed whether six months of LMWH therapy were more effective at preventing recurrent thromboembolic disease in cancer patients who presented with acute symptomatic VTE, compared with the standard treatment of six months with oral anticoagulant vitamin-K antagonists (61). Patients received five to seven days of dalteparin in full-treatment doses. Thereafter, the dalteparin arm continued to receive dalteparin at full doses for one month followed by 75% of the full treatment dose for the remaining five months. The oral anticoagulant group, after its short course of dalteparin, received six months of vitamin-K antagonist therapy with a target

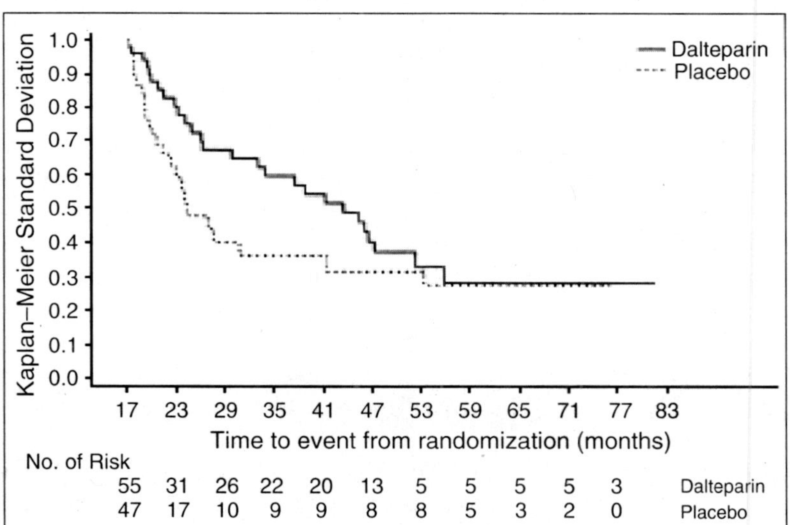

Figure 2 Kaplan–Meier survival curves for the subgroup of patients with a better prognosis who survived beyond 17 months after randomization. Source: From Ref. 60.

international normalized ratio of between 2 and 3 (61). There was no benefit associated with dalteparin therapy for the overall population at one year. However, for a subgroup of patients without metastasis at randomization, who received up to six months of LMWH, survival rates were 80% compared to 64% for vitamin K antagonist (62).

A trial of 84 patients with small cell lung cancer (SCLC) randomized to receive a standard chemotherapy alone or in combination with dalteparin at a dose of 5000 units once daily, demonstrated a modest but significant survival advantage for patients receiving the combination. Patients with a good prognosis with only limited disease had an even greater survival advantage (63). Patients with SCLC showed an improvement in survival when LMWH was administered in addition to chemotherapy, with a median survival increase especially marked in patients with a better prognosis (median survival 8 month vs. 13 month).

Klerk et al. conducted a trial in which patients with metastasized or locally advanced solid tumors were randomly assigned to receive a six-week course of a LMWH nadroparin or placebo (64). Nadroparin was administered in a weight-based dose with a higher dose during the first two weeks followed by a reduction to half the initial dose for the remaining four weeks. There was a mean followup of one year for the 148 patients in the nadroparin and 154 in the placebo groups. The overall hazard ratio of mortality was 0.75 (95% CI, 0.59–0.96) with a median survival of eight months in the nadroparin patients and 6.6 months in the placebo group ($P = 0.021$). Bleeding complications did not differ significantly in the two groups.

Sideras et al. recently reported the results of a small trial of 141 patients with breast, colon, lung, or prostate cancer that were randomized to receive standard therapy alone or in combination with dalteparin daily (65). All patients had advanced disease. Because of slow accrual, the study design was changed during enrollment from double-blind to open label. No differences in outcome measures were observed between the two groups.

The results of these studies suggest that LMWH does not improve outcomes in patients with advanced cancer, but there may be a benefit in patients with nonmetastatic disease.

Proposed mechanisms by which LMWH therapy exerts a beneficial survival effect in patients with malignant disease include (*i*) an effect on the prevention of fatal thromboembolic disease, (*ii*) interference with the coagulation proteases that have been shown to influence tumor phenotype and which are neutralized through the effect of LMWH:antithrombin III complex or through the release of tissue factor pathway inhibitor (TFPI), and (*iii*) a potential direct antitumor cell effect of heparin itself. It appears unlikely that all the benefits demonstrated through long-term administration of LMWH in the four contemporary studies of survival are attributable to the prevention of PE alone as the benefit appears to be seen beyond the period of active LMWH administration.

Either through potentiation of the activity of antithrombin III and the ability to neutralize activated factor X and thrombin or through the release of TFPI with the resultant ability to neutralize the TF/VIIa; Xa complex, LMWH may have a neutralizing effect on activated coagulation proteases, potentially altering tumor phenotype in a dramatic way. Direct antitumor effects of heparin, independent from its antithrombotic properties include (66) antiangiogenesis, inhibition of heparanase (67), interference with P-selectin-mediated adhesion, apoptosis induction, and modification of oncogene expression. In an experimental model, heparin treatment attenuated metastasis formation by inhibiting P-selectin-mediated aggregation of tumor cell with platelets via cell-surface mucin ligands (68).

LMWH, such as those that have been treated by periodate-oxidization or borohydride-reduction, can also inhibit lung colonization in the Lewis lung carcinoma model (69). This may be due to the ability of those heparins to competitively inhibit cell surface heparan sulphate functions, which in turn are responsible for tumor cell ability to attach to the subendothelial matrix in the lung capillary beds. UFH is able to bind platelet integrin $\alpha_{IIb}\beta_3$, thus enhancing ligand binding and differentially modulating adhesion of cancer cells to vitronectin, a process potentially interfering with tumor cells invasion and metastasis. It has been shown that LMWH and chondroitin sulfate induce a significantly reduced enhancement of this adhesion in a way that is dependent on the integrin β-chain (70). Experimental models (71,72) have shown that the antiangiogenic effect of LMWH may be in part mediated through release of TFPI.

Folkman et al. (73) demonstrated that heparin administered with cortisone had an antiangiogenic effect. More recently, Fareed et al. (74) have demonstrated that administration of LMWH to tumor-bearing mice in the NDST-2 knockout model where cells are unable to synthesize endogenous heparin, was able to induce tumor apoptosis. This observation suggests a potential role for administration of LMWH in induction of an unfavorable tumor phenotype. In the same model assessing primary growth of murine melanoma (75), in the NDST-2 knockout or wild-type mice, tumors were larger in NDST-2 knockout animals, suggesting a role for endogenous heparin production in the regulation of primary tumor growth.

REFERENCES

1. Trousseau A. Plegmasia Alba dolens. London: The New Syndeham Society, 1872:282–332.
2. Prandoni P, Piccioli A. Venous thromboembolism and cancer: a two-way clinical association. Front Biosci 19971 2:e12–e20.
3. Kakkar AK, Williamson RC. Antithrombotic therapy in cancer [see comment]. BMJ 1999; 318:1571–1572.
4. Di Carlo V et al. Dermatan sulphate for the prevention of postoperative venous thromboembolism in patients with cancer. DOS (Dermatan sulphate in Oncologic Surgery) Study Group. Thromb Haemost 1999; 82:30–34.
5. Sorensen HT, Mellemkjaer L, Steffensen FH, Olsen JH, Nielsen GL. The risk of a diagnosis of cancer after primary deep venous thrombosis or pulmonary embolism [see comment]. N Engl J Med 1998; 338:1169–1173.
6. Baron JA, Gridley G, Weiderpass E, Nyren O, Linet M. Venous thromboembolism and cancer. Lancet 1998; 351:1077–1080.
7. Shen VS, Pollak EW. Fatal pulmonary embolism in cancer patients: is heparin prophylaxis justified? South Med J 1980; 73:841–843.
8. Kakkar AK, DeRuvo N, Chinswangwatanakul V, Tebbutt S, Williamson RC. Extrinsic-pathway activation in cancer with high factor VIIa and tissue factor. Lancet 1995; 346:1004–1005.
9. Kakkar V. The diagnosis of deep vein thrombosis using the 125 I fibrinogen test. Arch Surg 1972; 104:152–159.
10. Geerts WH et al. Prevention of venous thromboembolism: the Seventh ACCP Conference on Antithrombotic and Thrombolytic Therapy. Chest 2004; 126.
11. Buller HR et al. Antithrombotic therapy for venous thromboembolic disease: the Seventh ACCP Conference on Antithrombotic and Thrombolytic Therapy. [erratum appears in Chest 2005; 127(1):416]. Chest 2004; 126.
12. Virchow R. Collected articles on scientific medicine. Gesammalte abhandlungen zur wissenschaftlichen medizin. Frankfurt: Medinger Sohn & Co, 1856:219–732.
13. Ott I, Fischer EG, Miyagi Y, Mueller BM, Ruf W. A role for tissue factor in cell adhesion and migration mediated by interaction with actin-binding protein 280. J Cell Biol 1998; 140:1241–1253.
14. Kakkar AK, Lemoine NR, Scully MF, Tebbutt S, Williamson RC. Tissue factor expression correlates with histological grade in human pancreatic cancer. Br J Surg 1995; 82:1101–1104.

15. Rickles FR, Hair GA, Zeff RA, Lee E, Bona RD. Tissue factor expression in human leukocytes and tumor cells. J Thromb Haemost 1995; 74:391–395.
16. Tallman MS, Kwaan HC. Reassessing the hemostatic disorder associated with acute promyelocytic leukemia [see comment]. Blood 1992; 79:543–553.
17. Donati MB et al. Cancer procoagulant in human tumor cells: evidence from melanoma patients. Cancer Res 1986; 46:6471–6474.
18. Letai A, Kuter DJ. Cancer, coagulation, and anticoagulation. Oncologist 1999; 4:443–449.
19. Lee AY. Cancer and thromboembolic disease: pathogenic mechanisms. Cancer Treat Rev 2002; 28:137–140.
20. Kakkar AK, Chinswangwatanakul V, Lemoine NR, Tebbutt S, Williamson RC. Role of tissue factor expression on tumour cell invasion and growth of experimental pancreatic adenocarcinoma. Br J Surg 1999; 86:890–894.
21. Zhang Y et al. Tissue factor controls the balance of angiogenic and antiangiogenic properties of tumor cells in mice. J Clin Invest 1994; 94:1320–1327.
22. Contrino J, Hair G, Kreutzer DL, Rickles FR. In situ detection of tissue factor in vascular endothelial cells: correlation with the malignant phenotype of human breast disease [see comment]. Nat Med 1996; 2:209–215.
23. Poon RT-P et al. Tissue factor expression correlates with tumor angiogenesis and invasiveness in human hepatocellular carcinoma. Clin Cancer Res 2003; 9:5339–5345.
24. Dorfleutner A, Hintermann E, Tarui T, Takada Y, Ruf W. Cross-talk of integrin (alpha)3(beta)1 and tissue factor in cell migration. Mol Biol Cell 2004; 15:4416–4425.
25. Carmeliet P et al. Role of tissue factor in embryonic blood vessel development. Nature 1996; 383:73–75.
26. Belting M et al. Regulation of angiogenesis by tissue factor cytoplasmic domain signaling. Nat Med 2004; 10:502–509.
27. Beerepoot LV et al. Circulating endothelial cells in cancer patients do not express tissue factor. Cancer Lett 2004; 213:241–248.
28. Rickles FR, Shoji M, Abe K. The role of the hemostatic system in tumor growth, metastasis, and angiogenesis: tissue factor is a bifunctional molecule capable of inducing both fibrin deposition and angiogenesis in cancer. Int J Hemotol 2001; 73:145–150.
29. Shweiki D, Itin A, Soffer D, Keshet E. Vascular endothelial growth factor induced by hypoxia may mediate hypoxia-initiated angiogenesis. Nature 1992; 359:843–845.
30. Poon RT, Fan ST, Wong J. Clinical implications of circulating angiogenic factors in cancer patients. J Clin Oncol 2001:1207–1225.
31. Mohle R, Green D, Moore MA, Nachman RL, Rafii S. Constitutive production and thrombin-induced release of vascular endothelial growth factor by human megakaryocytes and platelets. Proc Natl Acad Sci 1997; 94:663–668.
32. Edwards RL et al. Abnormalities of blood coagulation tests in patients with cancer. Am J Clin Path 1987; 88:596–602.
33. Wang X et al. Downregulation of tissue factor by RNA interference in human melanoma LOX-L cells reduces pulmonary metastasis in nude mice. Int J Cancer 2004; 112:994–1002.
34. Versteeg HH, Spek CA, Richel DJ, Peppelenbosch MP. Coagulation factors VIIa and Xa inhibit apoptosis and anoikis. Oncogene 2004; 23:410–417.
35. Yu JL et al. Oncogenic events regulate tissue factor expression in colorectal cancer cells: implications for tumor progression and angiogenesis. Blood 2005; 105:1734–1741.
36. Coughlin SR. Thrombin signalling and protease-activated receptors. Nature 2000; 407:258–264.
37. Even-Ram S et al. Thrombin receptor overexpression in malignant and physiological invasion processes. Nat Med 1998; 4:909–914.
38. Levine MN, Lee AY, Kakkar AK. From Trousseau to targeted therapy: new insights and innovations in thrombosis and cancer. J Thromb Haemost 2003; 1:1456–1463.
39. Taniguchi T, Kakkar AK, Tuddenham EG, Williamson RC, Lemoine NR. Enhanced expression of urokinase receptor induced through the tissue factor-factor VIIa pathway in human pancreatic cancer. Cancer Res 1998; 58:4461–4467.
40. Wojtukiewicz MZ et al. Localization of blood coagulation factors in situ in pancreatic carcinoma. Thromb Haemost 2001; 86:1416–1420.

41. Kakkar AK, Chinswangwatanakul V, Tebbutt S, Lemoine NR, Williamson RC. A characterization of the coagulant and fibrinolytic profile of human pancreatic carcinoma cells. Haemostasis 1998; 28:1–6.
42. Caunt M, Huang Y-Q, Brooks PC, Karpatkin S. Thrombin induces neoangiogenesis in the chick chorioallantoic membrane. J Thromb Haemost 2003; 1:2097–2102.
43. Rickles FR, Edwards RL. Activation of blood coagulation in cancer: Trousseau's syndrome revisited. Blood 1983; 62:14–31.
44. Harrington KJ et al. Cancer-related thromboembolic disease in patients with solid tumours: a retrospective analysis. Ann Oncol 1997; 8:669–673.
45. Levine M et al. The thrombogenic effect of anticancer drug therapy in women with stage II breast cancer. N Engl J Med 1988; 318:404–407.
46. Clahsen PC, van de Velde CJ, Julien JP, Floiras JL, Mignolet FY. Thromboembolic complications after perioperative chemotherapy in women with early breast cancer: a European Organization for Research and Treatment of Cancer Breast Cancer Cooperative Group study. J Clin Oncol 1994; 12:1266–1271.
47. Saphner T, Tormey DC, Gray R. Venous and arterial thrombosis in patients who received adjuvant therapy for breast cancer. J Clin Oncol 1991; 9:286–294.
48. Pritchard KI et al. Increased thromboembolic complications with concurrent tamoxifen and chemotherapy in a randomized trial of adjuvant therapy for women with breast cancer. National Cancer Institute of Canada Clinical Trials Group Breast Cancer Site Group. J Clin Oncol 1996; 14:2731–2737.
49. Goldberg PA, Nicholls RJ, Porter NH, Love S, Grimsey JE. Long-term results of a randomised trial of short-course low-dose adjuvant pre-operative radiotherapy for rectal cancer: reduction in local treatment failure [see comment]. Eur J Cancer 1994; 30A:1602–1606.
50. Holm T, Singnomklao T, Rutqvist LE, Cedermark B. Adjuvant preoperative radiotherapy in patients with rectal carcinoma. Adverse effects during long term follow-up of two randomized trials. Cancer 1996; 78:968–976.
51. Zacharski LR et al. Effect of warfarin anticoagulation on survival in carcinoma of the lung, colon, head and neck, and prostate. Final report of VA Cooperative Study #75. Cancer 1984; 53:2046–2052.
52. Chahinian AP et al. A randomized trial of anticoagulation with warfarin and of alternating chemotherapy in extensive small-cell lung cancer by the Cancer and Leukemia Group B. J Clin Oncol 1989; 7:993–1002.
53. Lebeau B et al. Subcutaneous heparin treatment increases survival in small cell lung cancer. "Petites Cellules" Group. Cancer 1994; 74:38–45.
54. Maurer LH et al. Randomized trial of chemotherapy and radiation therapy with or without warfarin for limited state small-cell lung cancer: a Cancer and Leukemia Group B study. J Clin Oncol 1997; 15(11):3378–3387.
55. Green D, Hull RD, Brant R, Pineo GF. Lower mortality in cancer patients treated with low-molecular-weight versus standard heparin. Lancet 1992; 339:1476.
56. Siragusa S, Cosmi B, Piovella F, Hirsh J, Ginsberg JS. Low-molecular-weight heparins and unfractionated heparin in the treatment of patients with acute venous thromboembolism: results of a meta-analysis [see comment]. Am J Med 1996; 100:269–277.
57. Hettiarachchi RJ et al. Do heparins do more than just treat thrombosis? The influence of heparins on cancer spread. Thromb Haemost 1999; 82:947–952.
58. Gould MK, Dembitzer AD, Doyle RL, Hastie TJ, Garber AM. Low-molecular-weight heparins compared with unfractionated heparin for treatment of acute deep venous thrombosis. A meta-analysis of randomized, controlled trials. Ann Intern Med 1999; 130:800–809.
59. Prandoni P et al. Comparison of subcutaneous low-molecular-weight heparin with intravenous standard heparin in proximal deep-vein thrombosis. Lancet 1992; 339:441–445.
60. Kakkar AK et al. Low molecular weight heparin, therapy with dalteparin, and survival in advanced cancer: the fragmin advanced malignancy outcome study (FAMOUS). J Clin Oncol 2004; 22:1944–1948.
61. Lee AY et al. Low-molecular-weight heparin versus a coumarin for the prevention of recurrent venous thromboembolism in patients with cancer [see comment]. N Engl J Med 2003; 349:146–153.

62. Lee AYY, Rickles FR, Julian JA, et al. Randomized comparison of low molecular weight heparin and coumarin derivatives on the survival of outpatients with cancer and venous thromboembolism. J Clin Oncol 2005; 23:1–7.
63. Altinbas M et al. A randomized clinical trial of combination chemotherapy with and without low-molecular-weight heparin in small cell lung cancer [see comment]. J Thromb Haemost 2004; 2:1266–1271.
64. Klerk CP, Smorenburg SM, Otten HM, et al. The effect of low molecular weight heparin on survival in patients with advanced malignancy. J Clin Oncol 2005; 23:2130–2135.
65. Sideras K et al. Low-molecular-weight-heparin in patients with advanced cancer: a phase 3 clinical trial. Mayo Clin Proc 2006; 81(6):758–767.
66. Smorenburg SM, Van Noorden CJ. The complex effects of heparins on cancer progression and metastasis in experimental studies [Review]. Pharmacological Rev 2001; 53:93–105.
67. Vlodavsky I et al. Mammalian heparanase: gene cloning, expression and function in tumor progression and metastasis [see comment]. Nat Med 1999; 5:793–802.
68. Borsig L et al. Heparin and cancer revisited: mechanistic connections involving platelets, P-selectin, carcinoma mucins, and tumor metastasis. Proc Natl Acad Sci U S A 2001; 98:3352–3357.
69. Yoshitomi Y et al. Inhibition of experimental lung metastases of Lewis lung carcinoma cells by chemically modified heparin with reduced anticoagulant activity. Cancer Lett 2004; 207:165–174.
70. Da Silva MS et al. Heparin modulates integrin-mediated cellular adhesion: specificity of interactions with alpha and beta integrin subunits. Cell Commun Adhes 2003; 10:59–67.
71. Mousa SA, Mohamed S. Anti-angiogenic mechanisms and efficacy of the low molecular weight heparin, tinzaparin: anti-cancer efficacy. Oncol Rep 2004; 12:683–688.
72. Mousa SA, Mohamed S. Inhibition of endothelial cell tube formation by the low molecular weight heparin, tinzaparin, is mediated by tissue factor pathway inhibitor [see comment]. Thromb Haemost 2004; 92:627–633.
73. Folkman J, Langer R, Linhardt RJ, Haudenschild C, Taylor S. Angiogenesis inhibition and tumor regression caused by heparin or a heparin fragment in the presence of cortisone. Science 1983; 221:719–725.
74. Fareed A, Patel HK, Scully MF, Fareed J, Lemoine NR, Kakkar AK. The low molecular weight heparins dalteparin sodium inhibits angiogenesis and induces apoptosis in an experimental tumour model. Blood 2003; 102, Abstract #2993 .
75. Samoszuk M et al. Inhibition of thrombosis in melanoma allografts in mice by endogenous mast cell heparin. Thromb Haemost 2003; 90:351–360.

18

Improving Outcomes with Prophylactic Anticoagulation in Patients with Cancer: Lessons from the American Society of Clinical Oncology Guidelines

Gary H. Lyman and Nicole M. Kuderer
Department of Medicine, Duke University and the Duke Comprehensive Cancer Center, Durham, North Carolina, U.S.A.

- Important venous thromboembolism (VTE) clinical outcomes in cancer patients include the risk of VTE and the morbidity, mortality, and costs associated with VTE and bleeding.
- Randomized controlled trials of anticoagulant treatment include studies of both primary and secondary prevention as well as studies of overall survival.
- The American Society of Clinical Oncology (ASCO) has developed more than 20 clinical practice guidelines and technology assessments on a variety of important oncology issues following a rigorous evidence-based approach based on a formal systematic review of the world's literature.
- In 2006, an ASCO VTE Guideline process was initiated, a systematic review commissioned, and a panel of methodological and content experts assembled.
- The Panel reviewed the evidence provided by the systematic review and developed guidelines addressing the following questions:
  Should hospitalized cancer patients receive anticoagulation for prophylaxis?
  Should ambulatory cancer patients receive anticoagulation for VTE prophylaxis during systemic chemotherapy?
  Should cancer patients undergoing surgery receive VTE prophylaxis?
  What is the best method for treatment of cancer patients with established VTE to prevent recurrence?
  Should cancer patients receive anticoagulants in the absence of established VTE to improve survival?

INTRODUCTION

Risk of Venous Thromboembolism in Cancer Patients

The risk of venous thromboembolism (VTE) is substantially increased in cancer patients, most notably those with cancers of gastrointestinal origin (1–3). Risk factors for VTE in cancer patients also include hospitalization, systemic chemotherapy with subsequent neutropenia, and presumed infection, older age, and several comorbidities including obesity, pulmonary disease, and renal failure (4). Additional risk factors for VTE in cancer patients include the stage of disease, the type of treatment including hormonal therapy and surgery, and the use of a central venous catheter. More recent studies have also demonstrated a considerable risk of VTE in patients with malignant lymphoma (4,5). The risk of VTE in hospitalized cancer patients appears to be increasing at a concerning rate (4). Although the reason for the apparent rise in the rate of VTE is unknown, increased acuity in hospitalized cancer patients, an increased awareness of diagnosing VTE, and broad use of better, high-resolution computed tomography (CT) imaging methods may all play a role (6–8). A number of new cancer therapies also appear to be associated with an increased risk of VTE (9–11). Likewise, Erythroid-stimulating proteins appear to place patients at increased risk of VTE (3,12).

Consequences of VTE in Cancer Patients:

VTE is associated with a variety of adverse consequences including increased mortality. Thromboembolism represents a leading cause of death in cancer patients (2,13). Cancer patients hospitalized with neutropenia and presumed infection with documented thromboembolism have a greater in-hospital mortality [odds ratio (OR) = 2.01; 95% confidence interval (CI): 1.83–2.22, $p < 0.0001$] than those without VTE (3). In a recent study of ambulatory cancer patients receiving chemotherapy, of the 3.2% of patients who died over the first three to four cycles of treatment, 13 (9.2%) died of thromboembolic-related causes (14). In a recent study of over 100,000 breast cancer patients, VTE was a significant predictor of decreased two-year survival [hazard ratio (HR) = 2.3; 95% CI: 2.1–2.6] including patients with localized disease (HR = 5.1; 95% CI: 3.6–7.1) (15). Additional serious clinical consequences include recurrent VTE as well as serious bleeding complications–associated anticoagulation (16).

Outcomes of Interest in Cancer Patients at Risk for VTE

Traditional clinical outcomes of interest in the study of VTE in cancer patients include the occurence of VTE and its consequences as well as the impact and complications of treatment or prevention strategies. Often, these outcomes depend critically upon their definition and the methods of monitoring and identification, e.g., clinical, imaging, frequency of followup, etc. Additional important outcomes of interest include mortality, morbidity, the delivery of cancer therapy, and the use of health-care resources (17). In fact, the impact of anticoagulation on the overall survival of patients with chemotherapy has been the focus of a number of prospective clinical trials (18–21). VTE also has significant economic consequences related to the direct costs of hospitalization (22). Unfortunately, almost no data are available on the impact of VTE and its treatment on health-related quality of life.

Randomized Clinical Trials of Anticoagulation in Cancer Patients

Efforts to prevent VTE are premised on the potential benefits and harms associated with treating established VTE and potential life-threatening complications including pulmonary embolism and the bleeding risk of full-dose anticoagulation. Evidence on the benefit and safety of anticoagulation in patients with cancer comes from many sources including retrospective and prospective population studies and both uncontrolled and controlled clinical trials. Randomized controlled trials (RCTs) of the role of anticoagulant treatment in cancer patients may be categorized on the basis of the study hypothesis or the primary objectives of the study including (*i*) to prevent VTE and its complications in patients without a prior occurrence (primary prophylaxis) in the medical setting; (*ii*) to prevent VTE and its complications in patients without a prior occurrence in the perioperative setting (primary prophylaxis); (*iii*) to prevent a recurrence of VTE or its complications in patients with a recent occurrence of VTE (secondary prophylaxis), and (*iv*) to reduce mortality or improve overall survival in cancer patients without VTE (antineoplastic therapy). By consensus, the strongest evidence in support of treatment efficacy comes from RCTs or meta-analyses of RCTs. Even within RCTs, the treatment effect size will vary. This variation may be due to limited power generally due to small sample size (random error), poor study design resulting in bias (systematic error), or true differences between the studies or the study populations (heterogeneity).

Meta-analyses of Prophylactic Anticoagulation in Cancer Patients

Methodological Challenges

Meta-analyses of individual clinical trial may, in part, address concerns related to random variation and between study heterogeneity. However, the conclusions from a meta-analysis are only as valid as the quality reflected in the study design of the individual RCTs along with efforts made to obtain the totality of evidence from publications, presentations, and other completed studies in an effort to minimize the risk of a publication bias. Global efforts to improve the quality of published meta-analyses have resulted in a set of guidelines known as the Quality of Reporting of Meta-analyses (QUOROM) statement similar to the Consolidated Standards of Reporting Track (CONSORT) statement for assessing the quality of RCTs (23). The issues addressed by the QUOROM statement are summarized in Table 1, emphasizing the search strategy, inclusion and exclusion criteria, quality appraisal, independent data abstraction, assessment of heterogeneity, appropriate statistical analysis and assessment for publication/selection bias, and proper presentation of results including a summary of trial flow (Fig. 1), descriptive data for each trial, appropriate summary measures, and a discussion of the strengths and weaknesses of the study. Although the ideal for meta-analyses remains access to individual patient data, this is rarely achievable and very costly. The vast majority of meta-analyses reported in oncology including those utilized by the U.S. Preventive Services Task Force, the Cochrane Collaboration and American Society of Clinical Oncology (ASCO) to support clinical practice guidelines are based on aggregate patient data largely derived from the published literature (24). Many, meta-analyses however, are of poor quality with many that are used to support guidelines failing to meet criteria for being truly systematic or of reasonable quality based on QUOROM criteria (25). The American College of Chest Physicians (ACCP) Conference on Antithrombotic and Thrombolytic Therapy employs a grading system to reflect the may strength or certainty of the recommendations (26). Such formal grading schemes that create a somewhat unrealistic perception of objectivity and have have largely been replaced by more reflective assessments of the individual factors related to study quality (27). Although a small number of meta-analyses of the value of anticoagulation in patients with cancer have been conducted, they are all limited in their study methodology including incomplete

Table 1 Improving the Quality of Reports of Meta-analyses of Randomized Controlled Trials: The QUOROM Statement Checklist

Heading	Subheading	Descriptor	Reported? (Y/N)	Page number
Title		Identify the report as a meta-analysis [or systematic review] of RCTs		
Abstract		Use a structured format		
		Describe		
	Objectives	The clinical question explicitly		
	Data sources	The databases (ie, list) and other information sources		
	Review methods	The selection criteria (ie, population, intervention, outcome, and study design); methods for validity assessment, data abstraction, and study characteristics, and quantitative data synthesis in sufficient detail to permit replication		
	Results	Characteristics of the RCTs included and excluded; qualitative and quantitative findings (ie, point estimates and confidence intervals); and subgroup analyses		
	Conclusion	The main results		
		Describe		
Introduction		The explicit clinical problem, biological rationale for the intervention, and rationale for review		
Methods	Searching	The information sources, in detail (eg, databases, registers, personal (line, expert informants, agencies, hand-searching), and any restrictions (years considered, publication status, language of publication)		
	Selection	The inclusion and exclusion criteria (defining population, intervention, principal outcomes, and study design)		
	Validity assessment	The criteria and process used (e.g, masked conditions, quality assessment, and their findings)		

	Data abstraction	The process or processes used (eg, completed independently, in duplicate)
	Study characteristics	The type of study design, participants' characteristics, details of intervention, outcome definitions, and now clinical heterogeneity was assessed
	Quantitative data synthesis	The principal measures of effect (eg, relative risk), method of combining results (statistical testing and confidence intervals), handling of missing data; how statistical heterogeneity was assessed; a rationale for any a-priori sensitivity and subgroup analyses; and any assessment of publication bias''
Results	Trial flow	Provide a meta-analysis profile summarising trial flow (see figure)
	Study characteristics	Present descriptive data for each trial (eg, age, sample size, intervention, dose, duration, follow-up period)
	Quantitative data synthesis	Report agreement on the selection and validity assessment; present simple summary results (for each treatment group in each trial, for each primary outcome); present data needed to calculate effect sizes and confidence intervals in intention-to-treat analyses (eg 2 X 2 tables of counts, means and SDs, proportions)
Discussion		Summarise key findings; discuss clinical inferences based on internal and external validity; interpret the results in light of the totality of available evidence; describe potential biases in the review process (eg, publication bias); and suggest a future research agenda.

Quality of reporting of meta-analyses

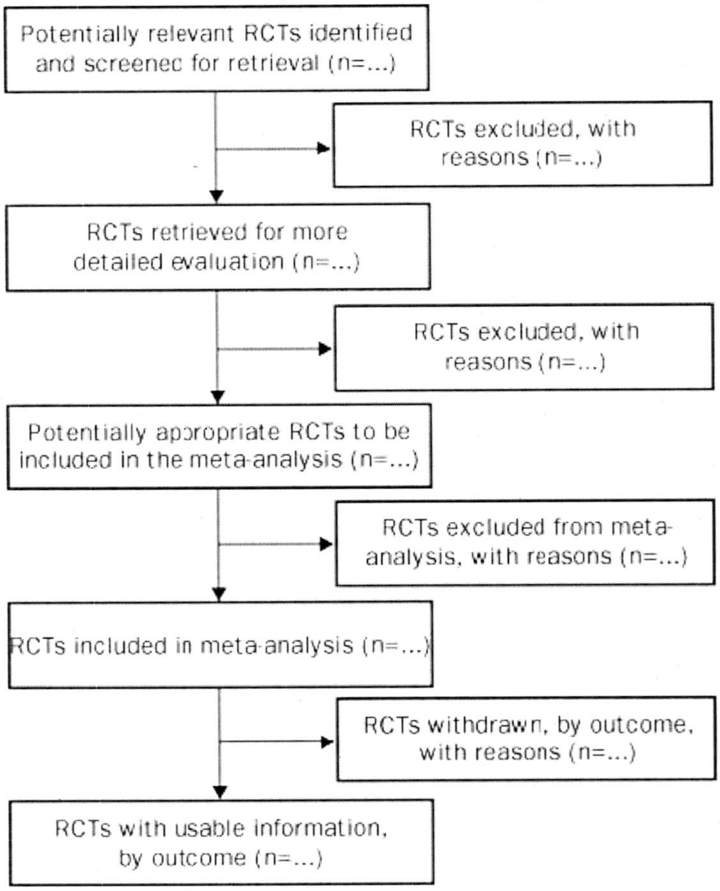

Figure 1 QUOROM diagram illustrating the sequential process used in a systematic review to identify and select articles for a meta-analyses. *Abbreviation*: RCTs, randomized controlled trials.

search and selection strategies and inclusion of post-hoc subgroup analyses of cancer patients in largely noncancer trials (28).

Primary Prophylaxis

Only three studies of a primary prophylaxis strategy in ambulatory cancer patients have had VTE as a primary outcome and no meta-analysis of this issue has been reported. On the other hand, a number of RCTs of anticoagulation treatment in cancer patients without a diagnosis of VTE have addressed overall or cancer-specific mortality as a primary outcome. No significant impact on one-year mortality of vitamin K antagonists (VKAs) administered in cancer patients without VTE was found in a meta-analysis including 1443 patients in nine disease groups from five separate studies (OR = 0.89; 95% CI: 0.70–1.13); however, this meta-analysis was not based on a comprehensive systematic review, allowed trials in the analysis with a combination of anticoagulants, and does not address the impact of bleeding complications (29). Another meta-analysis by the same authors explored the impact of unfractionated heparin (UFH) on survival in cancer patients (28). Only one study was identified as an RCT that studied UFH for more than seven days (21). Two other RCTs investigated UFH given intraportal continuously for seven days, which found a detrimental effect for UFH compared to control (OR = 1.66; 95% CI: 1.02–2.71) (30,31).

Secondary Prophylaxis

The comparative impact of low-molecular-weight heparin (LMWH) versus VKA on recurrence of VTE (secondary prophylaxis) specifically in cancer patients has been addressed in four RCTs, all of which have shown a trend toward a lower risk of recurrent VTE for LMWH (32–35). The comparative impact on cancer-specific mortality of different anticoagulants given for VTE has been studied in a number of RCTs that included post-hoc analyses of cancer subgroups in these trials (36). These investigators found no significant difference in cancer mortality in eight RCTs that compared LMWH and VKA for either all patients (OR = 0.95; 95% CI: 0.73–1.23) or limited to cancer patients (OR = 0.96; 95% CI: 0.73–1.25). It is important to note that none of these studies was specifically designed to study cancer-specific mortality. In another meta-analysis of RCTs of VTE patients comparing initial LMWH and UFH, Hettiarachchi et al. reported a significantly lower three-month mortality for the subgroup of 629 cancer patients treated with LMWH than those receiving UFH (OR = 0.61; 95% CI: 0.40–0.93) (37). Similar results were reported by an earlier meta-analysis also suggesting a reduction in VTE and major bleeding complications comparing LMWH to UFH for the initial treatment of VTE before starting oral VKA (38). However, it remains unclear how short courses (five to seven days) of LMWH improve survival whereas treatment LMWH courses for several months without increasing major bleeding events do not favorably impact survival in cancer patients.

Surgical Prophylaxis

A large number of RCTs of prophylactic anticoagulation have been performed in the perioperative and postoperative setting although few have addressed outcomes specifically in a cancer surgical population. Many methods for VTE prophylaxis have been studied, including compression stockings, intermittent compression devices, and various anticoagulants. Smorenburg et al. found that despite a significant reduction in three-year mortality in four retrospective studies of UFH given prophylactically to 1435 patients with resectable gastrointestinal cancer (OR = 0.65; 95% CI: 0.51–0.84), there was a significant increase in three-year mortality in two prospective RCTs in 418 similar patients (OR = 1.66; 95% CI: 1.02–2.71) (29). A recent review of deep venous thrombosis (DVT) prophylaxis including subgroup analysis of cancer patients undergoing nonorthopedic surgical procedures identified 26 studies involving 7639 patients (39). A significant reduction in DVT was observed in patients treated with high-dose LMWH found to be more effective than low dose. No significant difference was observed between LMWH and UFH treatment either in the low-dose setting or in the high-dose setting. A meta-analysis of RCTs of prolonged LMWH compared to standard postoperative prophylaxis in cancer patients undergoing abdominal surgery has been reported by Rasmussen et al. (40,41). The most recent of these studies identified four RCTs demonstrating that LMWH prophylaxis extended four to five weeks after surgery significantly reduced the risk of venographically detected DVT [relative risk (RR) = 0.44; 95% CI: 0.28–0.70; $P = 0.0005$] but not symptomatic VTE (RR = 0.35; 95% CI: 0.06–2.22; $P = 0.27$). An individual patient data meta-analysis of the two studies of the LMWH tinzaparin confirmed these findings (42).

Clinical Practice Guidelines of Prophylactic Anticoagulation in Cancer Patients

The Institute of Medicine has defined clinical practice guidelines as "systematically developed statements to assist practitioner and patient decisions about appropriate health care for specific clinical circumstances" (43). Clinical practice guidelines are developed to assist health-care providers to make rational and generally evidence-based decisions about the optimal delivery of medical care. Good guidelines should be reliable, valid, and reproducible as well as explicit, transparent, and clinically applicable. Guidelines should assist in the delivery of optimal care in a timely fashion while potentially reducing costs by improving outcomes, minimizing practice variation, educating clinicians and patients, assisting in self-evaluation, providing benchmarks for quality review, and ideally clarifying reimbursement and coverage issues among other potential benefits. Clearly, guidelines cannot fully address individual patient variation; they are not intended to replace clinical judgment as applied to specific clinical situations and cannot necessarily include all reasonable methods of care or treatment. In the end, guidelines should help align clinical practice with the available evidence and expert opinion. Guidelines should be considered as recommendations with their application to a specific patient's individual circumstances determined by the practicing clinician. Guidelines are intended to address interventions in clinical practice that may differ with those addressed in clinical trials of innovative approaches to patient care. However, clinical practice guideline may also help define gaps in our understanding, providing important questions for further research. A limited number of clinical practice guidelines have been developed to date that address VTE prophylaxis in cancer patients and include the following.

American College of Chest Physicians

The ACCP previously developed guidelines for VTE prevention (44). The ACCP guidelines consider a range of indications for the prevention and treatment of VTE under a variety of clinical situations. VTE prophylaxis is recommended for surgical patients as well as hospitalized medical patients considered acutely ill, including cancer patients. These guidelines focus on general medical patients with limited attention to the extensive information available on prophylaxis specifically in cancer patients.

National Comprehensive Cancer Network Guidelines on VTE

The National Comprehensive Cancer Network (NCCN) represents a consortium of some 20 National Cancer Institute (NCI)-designated cancer centers which develops and distributes clinical practice guidelines in oncology. Expert panels on a wide variety of clinical topics are assembled from the membership of the participating institutions. The panels develop clinical practice guidelines utilizing primarily a consensus process and then review and update the guidelines annually. The guideline panels rank recommendations based on the strength of the evidence and the degree of panel consensus as Level 1 (high level of evidence such as large randomized clinical trials or meta-analysis and full consensus); Level 2A (lower level evidence such as phase II studies but still consensus); Level 2B (incomplete consensus) and, Level 3 (strong disagreement). A Venous Thromboembolic Disease Panel was convened in 2005 and provided updated guidelines in 2006. The current version of the NCCN Venous Thromboembolic Disease Guideline (version 2.2006) can be found at http://nccn.org/professionals/physician_gls/PDF/vte.pdf (45). Clinical management pathways are presented as algorithms or diagrams defining decision pathways. The guidelines cover the diagnosis and evaluation of VTE in cancer patients, risks and contraindications of anticoagulation, available therapies for prophylaxis and treatment of VTE, and assessing response to treatment.

Italian Association of Medical Oncology Guidelines

The Italian Association of Medical Oncology published its recommendations for the management of VTE in cancer patients in 2004 and has periodically updated these guidelines (46). For each recommendation, levels of evidence are rated according to a five-point rating scale. The Italian guidelines focus on six areas including VTE and occult cancer;

prophylaxis in cancer surgery, prophylaxis during chemotherapy, or hormonal therapy; prophylaxis for central venous catheters; treatment of VTE in patients with cancer; and the impact of anticoagulation on cancer survival.

The Development of Clinical Practice Guidelines for the ASCO

ASCO has developed more than 20 clinical practice guidelines and technology assessments on a variety of important oncology issues. The development of guidelines is overseen by the Health Services Committee of ASCO, undergo extensive internal and external review and ultimately must be approved by the ASCO Board of Directors. ASCO guidelines are developed by panels of both content and methodology experts from both within and outside of the Health Services Committee and address widely recognized practice issues. The guidelines development process has recently been formally summarized in a Guideline Procedures Manual, which is available online at www.asco.org (47). Any ASCO member can propose a guideline topic by providing a written proposal including a brief overview highlighting relevant background information and addressing a number of specific questions. Issues that need to be addressed include the burden of the health-care problem, the importance of the intervention as well as the availability of sufficient high-quality scientific evidence, and the degree of uncertainty or controversy concerning the effectiveness of available strategies (Fig. 2). The proposed panel members must commit to the guidelines process and the ASCO confidentiality policy which requires disclosure of any financial or other interest that might be considered a conflict. Once approved and funded by the Board of Directors, the guideline process involves a series of actions orchestrated by the ASCO staff and nominated panel members (Table 2). The panel must also complete a guideline development protocol summarizing the proposed panel membership, define the overall purpose, target population and intervention and the specific clinical question(s) to be addressed by the guideline, and define the details of the systematic review of the topic required as a basis for all ASCO guidelines. Finally, a detailed timeline for achieving essential milestones in the guideline development process must be presented.

THE ASCO VTE GUIDELINE DEVELOPMENT PROCESS

Overview of the ASCO VTE Guideline Process

A proposal for development of ASCO guidelines for VTE prophylaxis in cancer patients was approved the Health Services Committee in 2005. In early 2006, a systematic review of the VTE literature related to prophylactic anticoagulation and cancer was commissioned. Shortly thereafter, the guideline panel was convened consisting of experts in clinical medicine and research relevant to VTE in cancer patients along with experts in the methodology related to systematic reviews and clinical practice guidelines. The entire panel met twice to discuss the results of the systematic review and resolve any differences in the interpretation of the results and the appropriate recommendations to be made. Writing assignments were made and a guidelines document is under review to be published in 2007.

Rationale and Primary Questions for the ASCO VTE Guidelines

The following rationale was provided in gaining approval for the development of the ASCO VTE Guidelines. Patients with cancer are clearly at increased risk of developing VTE. Nevertheless, the role of thromboprophylaxis in many common clinical settings in

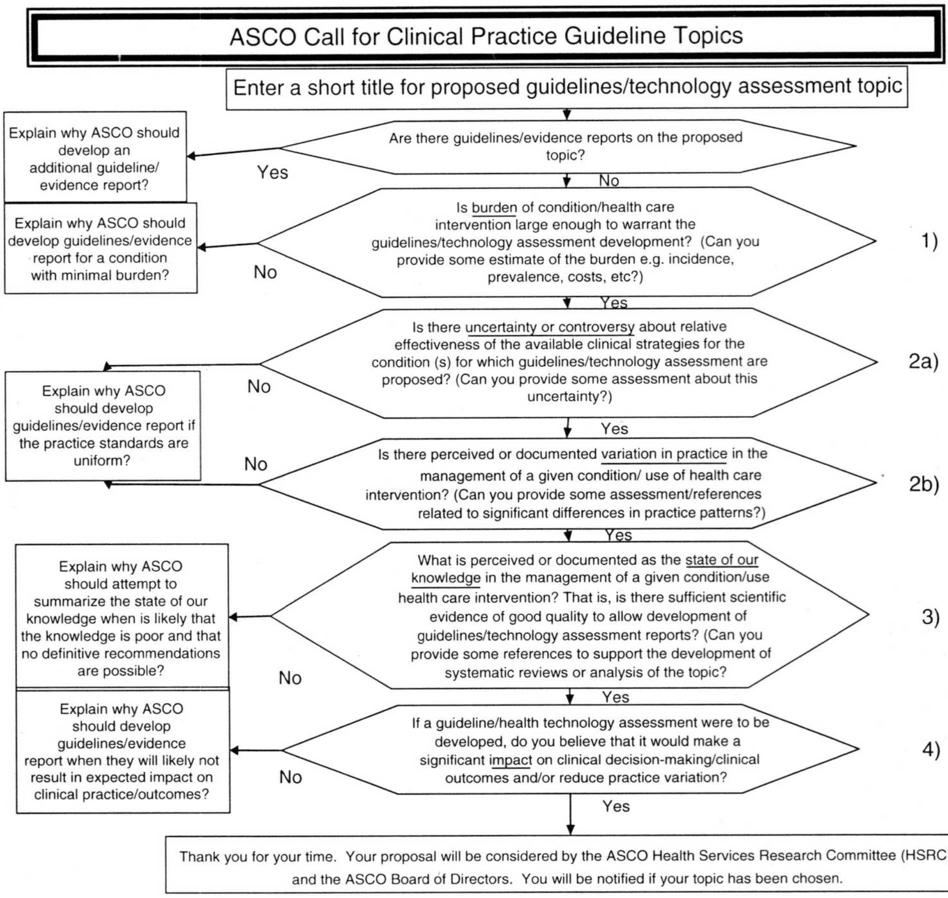

Figure 2 Schematic diagram of the series of question utilized in evaluating and selecting topics for guidelines by the American Society of Clinical Oncology (ASCO). *Abbreviations*: ASCO, American Society of Clinical Oncology; HSRC, Health Services Research Committee.

oncology remains unclear with considerable variation in practice in the application of VTE prophylaxis based on general medical guidelines. RCTs have been reported addressing many but not all of the areas of uncertainty. Primary questions to be addressed by the ASCO VTE Guidelines included the following:

1. Should hospitalized cancer patients receive anticoagulation for VTE prophylaxis?
2. Should ambulatory cancer patients receive anticoagulation for VTE prophylaxis during systemic chemotherapy? Specific issues involved with high-risk patients, e.g., multiple myeloma and thalidomide, were to be addressed
3. Should cancer patients undergoing surgery receive perioperative VTE prophylaxis? What is the best type of VTE prophylaxis in this setting? What is the role of mechanical devices, UFH, LMWH, and dual prophylaxis? What is the risk of hemorrhage with anticoagulation in postoperative patients? What is the optimal duration of prophylaxis following surgery? What is the optimal method for VTE prophylaxis in patients following gynecologic oncology surgery? What is the optimal method for VTE prophylaxis in patients following neurosurgical oncology operations?

Table 2 The ASCO Guideline Process

Subject of Guideline Proposed and Approved
Panel members Nominated and Approved
A Comprehensive Systematic Review Commissioned
Panel Convened to Review Evidence and Develop Preliminary Recommendations
Author Assignments Made to Panel Members
Draft Manuscript Assembled from Author Sections
Panel Reviews Draft Manuscript and Submits Comments and Modified Sections
Final Draft Approved and Sent for External Review
Manuscript Modified Based on Reviewer Comments
Panel Approves Final Manuscript
Guideline Manuscript Submitted to the Health Services Committee
Manuscript Revised Based on Health Services Committee Comments
Revised Manuscript Approved by Health Services Committee
Manuscript Forwarded to ASCO Board of Directors for Review
Manuscript Revised Based on Board Comments
Final Revised Manuscript Approved by the Board
Final Manuscript Sent to the *Journal of Clinical Oncology* for Publication
Guideline Published Online and in Print
Derivative Products Developed (Patient Guide, Executive Summary, Slide Set; Work Sheet) and Made Available Online
Executive Summary and Worksheet Published in the *Journal of Oncology Practice*

Abbreviation: ASCO, American Society of Clinical Oncology.

4. What is the best method for treatment of cancer patients with established VTE to prevent recurrence? How should treatment failures be managed? How should VTE be managed in patients with central nervous system (CNS) tumors and in the elderly?
5. Should cancer patients receive anticoagulants in the absence of established VTE to improve survival?

Systematic Review and Meta-Analysis in Support of the ASCO VTE Guidelines

Literature Search

A systematic and exhaustive review of the medical literature was performed through May of 2006 with weekly updates to December of 2006 of both published and unpublished randomized controlled clinical trials examining the efficacy of anticoagulation therapy in patients with cancer in both the medical and the surgical setting. Electronic databases included in the search were Medline, EMBASE, Cancerlit, Cochrane Database of Systematic Reviews, Cochrane Central Register of Controlled Trials (CENTRAL), Database of Abstracts of Reviews of Effect (DARE), and National Guidelines Clearing House and Conference Proceedings (International Society of Thrombosis and Hemostasis, ASCO, American Society of Hematology). Citations were hand-searched from identified articles, relevant excluded reports, and other meta-analyses and guidelines. In addition, expert panel members of the ASCO VTE guideline committee reviewed the list of identified articles to ensure completeness. Subject headings and keywords used in the search process included four major categories: (*i*) VTE; (*ii*) All types of malignancies; (*iii*) Type of anticoagulation including VKA, UFH, and LMWH, and (*iv*) RCT using the recommended search strategy from the Cochrane Collaboration (48). In the effort to minimize any potential publication bias, no language restrictions were imposed on the literature search (49).

Inclusion and Exclusion Criteria

Included studies represented controlled clinical trials of adult cancer patients randomized to anticoagulation drug therapy or to an appropriate control group. Anticoagulant therapy considered in the review included LMWH, UFH, or VKA. Anticoagulation had to be given on a continuous basis for more than four weeks without interruption unless clinically indicated, to allow for a reasonable therapeutic time period. Included studies had to report an a priori planned primary outcome such as objectively confirmed VTE or mortality and described an appropriate method of regular patient followup in both study arms that was identical. Nonrandomized reports, post-hoc subgroup analyses, or studies with noncancer patients and indwelling catheters were excluded. Trials were not allowed to study combinations of anticoagulation therapy or have treatment differences between study arms other than the assigned anticoagulation therapy under investigation. Only the most updated results among duplicate publications were included.

Meta-analysis

Data on basic study design, patient characteristics, study outcomes, and study quality were extracted by two independent reviewers. Discrepancies between reviewers were arbitrated by consensus and a third reviewer. Data abstracted from the published reports included (*i*) authors and citation; (*ii*) type and stage of malignancy; (*iii*) patient characteristics; (*iv*) drugs, doses, and schedule of anticoagulation therapy; (*v*) study design including the type of control group, description of randomization, blinding, treatment concealment, description of withdrawals or dropouts, sample size calculations, and intention to treat analysis; (*vi*) number of patients randomized, the number of evaluable patients, and the cumulative proportion experiencing primary or secondary outcomes. Study quality was evaluated by the validated method of Jadad et al. (50). Overall survival, VTE, and all bleeding complications represented the primary outcomes whereas major and fatal bleeding complications and fatal venous thromboembolic events were considered secondary outcomes. After assessment for significant heterogeneity, summary measures of RR were estimated by the method of Mantel and Haenszel. Forest plots were generated and potential publication bias was evaluated (49,51).

An Overview of the ASCO VTE Guidelines

Recommendations have been extensively discussed by the ASCO VTE Panel based on the results of the above systematic review and the cumulative background and knowledge of the panel members. The following clinical issues and the available supporting medical literature are presented.

Should hospitalized cancer patients receive anticoagulation for VTE prophylaxis? The reported frequency of VTE in hospitalized cancer patients varies widely (4,52–54). Although several multicenter studies of thromboprophylaxis with LMWH in acutely ill, hospitalized medical patients have been reported, none of these trials were designed specifically for cancer patients (55–59). The ACCP Conference on Antithrombotic and Thrombolytic Therapy guidelines strongly recommends pharmacologic prophylaxis with either low-dose UFH or LMWH for bedridden patients with active cancer. Although these recommendations are based on studies with a limited number of cancer patients, they appear to demonstrate both efficacy and reasonable safety of prophylactic anticoagulation in high-risk hospitalized cancer patients (44). Therefore, hospitalized cancer patients should be considered for VTE prophylaxis in the absence of contraindications to anticoagulation.

Should ambulatory cancer patients receive anticoagulation for VTE prophylaxis during systemic chemotherapy? The rate of thrombosis in ambulatory cancer patients appears to vary widely with the type of cancer, treatment, and comorbid conditions present. A single study has demonstrated the efficacy of low-dose warfarin in reducing the risk of thrombosis during systemic chemotherapy for breast cancer (60). Without more data, the apparent low risk of VTE in this setting and the possible risk for bleeding, anticoagulant prophylaxis has not been routinely recommended. However, a number of new cancer therapies and supportive care agents are associated with an increased risk of thrombosis, again raising the potential value of VTE prophylaxis in this setting (10,61–72).

Should cancer patients undergoing surgery receive perioperative VTE prophylaxis? VTE is a common complication in patients undergoing major surgical intervention for cancer (73–75). Cancer patients undergoing major surgical procedures consisting of laporscopy, labortory or thoracotory for more than 30 minutes are at increased risk for VTE as well as at greater risk of bleeding complications (76). Methods for the prevention of VTE in the perioperative period include mechanical devices such as graduated compression stockings or intermittent pneumatic calf compression devices as well as medical thromboprophylaxis with UFH, LMWH, or VKA (77–82). The optimal duration of anticoagulant prophylaxis in the postoperative setting continues under active investigation (83,84). Unless contraindicated, patients undergoing major surgical procedures for cancer should receive VTE prophylaxis with a consideration of combined mechanical prophylaxis and anticoagulation in high-risk patients (44).

What is the best treatment for cancer patients with established VTE to prevent recurrent VTE? Although the options for the appropriate treatment of a documented VTE are well recognized, the optimal method for preventing recurrent VTE (secondary prophylaxis) continue to be discussed (85). In the prevention of recurrent VTE, LMWH given for three to six months appears to be more effective than VKA with similar rates of bleeding complications (32,34,86). A number of special circumstances need to be considered in the treatment and prevention of VTE including patients with CNS malignancies (87–89). Likewise, patients undergoing neurosurgery for malignant disease are considered at high risk of VTE (1,90,91). Elderly patients with cancer are at a particularly high risk of death and disability of VTE-associated complications as well as the risk of serious bleeding (92–94). Nevertheless, the risk of recurrent VTE and possible fatal pulmonary embolism appear to outweigh the risk of serious bleeding (95).

Should cancer patients receive anticoagulants in the absence of established VTE to improve survival? The impact of anticoagulation on the survival of cancer patients has been studied in controlled clinical trials of anticoagulants for the treatment or prevention of VTE as well as cancer therapy. Meta-analyses of trials that compared initial therapy of VTE with UFH versus LMWH demonstrate a survival benefit in cancer patients randomized to LMWH (37,38,96,97). In addition, several RCTs have studied whether anticoagulants administered to cancer patients without VTE improve overall survival and reported mixed results (18–21) (98–101). Although overall these data do not justify the treatment of cancer patients with anticoagulation as antineoplastic therapy, the small study sizes and low power of these studies preclude a definitive conclusion on the efficacy of such treatment in the treatment of patients with nonmetastatic disease. Cancer patients should be encouraged to participate in clinical trials designed to evaluate anticoagulant therapy as an adjunct to standard anticancer therapies.

CONCLUSIONS

Patients with cancer, especially those hospitalized and those undergoing surgery or systemic treatment, are at significantly increased risk for VTE. The primary prevention of VTE in high risk settings as well as secondary prevention of recurrent VTE represent a continuing clinical problems for the practicing oncologist. Likewise, the possible adjunctive role of anticoagulants in improving survival represents an intriguing opportunity that will require further controlled clinical trials. All of these issues and others are being addressed in new guidelines for VTE prophylaxis in patients with cancer from the ASCO. These guidelines are based on an exhaustive and systematic review of the literature and a thorough deliberation by an international panel of thrombosis experts and methodologists. These guidelines provide oncologists with a balanced discussion of the benefits and risks associated with the use of anticoagulants in the specific management of patients with cancer.

REFERENCES

1. Heit JA, Silverstein MD, Mohr DN, et al. Risk factors for deep vein thrombosis and pulmonary embolism: a population-based case-control study. Arch Intern Med 2000; 160:809–815.
2. Chew HK, Wun T, Harvey D, et al. Incidence of venous thromboembolism and its effect on survival among patients with common cancers. Arch Intern Med 2006; 166:458–464.
3. Khorana AA, Francis CW, Culakova E, et al. Risk factors for chemotherapy-associated venous thromboembolism in a prospective observational study. Cancer 2005; 104:2822–2829.
4. Khorana AA, Francis CW, Culakova E, et al. Thromboembolism in hospitalized neutropenic cancer patients. J Clin Oncol 2006; 24:484–490.
5. Komrokji RS, Uppal NP, Khorana AA, et al. Venous thromboembolism in patients with diffuse large B-cell lymphoma. Leuk Lymphoma 2006; 47:1029–1033.
6. Gosselin MV, Rubin GD, Leung AN, et al. Unsuspected pulmonary embolism: prospective detection on routine helical CT scans. Radiology 1998; 208:209–215.
7. Storto ML, Di Credico A, Guido F, et al. Incidental detection of pulmonary emboli on routine MDCT of the chest. AJR Am J Roentgenol 2005; 184:264–267.
8. Sebastian AJ, Paddon AJ. Clinically unsuspected pulmonary embolism—an important secondary finding in oncology CT. Clin Radiol 2006; 61:81–85.
9. Cavo M, Zamagni E, Cellini C, et al. Deep-vein thrombosis in patients with multiple myeloma receiving first-line thalidomide-dexamethasone therapy. Blood 2002; 100:2272–2273.
10. Kabbinavar F, Hurwitz HI, Fehrenbacher L, et al. Phase II, randomized trial comparing bevacizumab plus fluorouracil (FU)/leucovorin (LV) with FU/LV alone in patients with metastatic colorectal cancer. J Clin Oncol 2003; 21:60–65.
11. Kuenen BC, Levi M, Meijers JC, et al. Potential role of platelets in endothelial damage observed during treatment with cisplatin, gemcitabine, and the angiogenesis inhibitor SU5416. J Clin Oncol 2003; 21:2192–2198.
12. Bohlius J, Wilson J, Seidenfeld J, et al. Recombinant human erythropoietins and cancer patients: updated meta-analysis of 57 studies including 9353 patients. J Natl Cancer Inst 2006; 98:708–714.
13. Ambrus JL, Ambrus CM, Mink IB, et al. Causes of death in cancer patients. J Med 1975; 6:61–64.
14. Khorana AA, Francis CW, Culakova E, et al. Thromboembolism is a leading cause of death in cancer patients receiving outpatient chemotherapy. J Thromb Haemost 2007. 5: 632–634.
15. Chew HK, Wun T, Harvey DJ, et al. Incidence of venous thromboembolism and the impact on survival in breast cancer patients. J Clin Oncol 2007; 25:70–76.
16. Prandoni P, Lensing AW, Piccioli A, et al. Recurrent venous thromboembolism and bleeding complications during anticoagulant treatment in patients with cancer and venous thrombosis. Blood 2002; 100:3484–3488.

17. Kucher N, Koo S, Quiroz R, et al. Electronic alerts to prevent venous thromboembolism among hospitalized patients. N Engl J Med 2005; 352:969–977.
18. Zacharski LR, Henderson WG, Rickles FR, et al. Effect of warfarin anticoagulation on survival in carcinoma of the lung, colon, head and neck, and prostate. Final report of VA Cooperative Study #75. Cancer 1984; 53:2046–2052.
19. Chahinian AP, Propert KJ, Ware JH, et al. A randomized trial of anticoagulation with warfarin and of alternating chemotherapy in extensive small-cell lung cancer by the Cancer and Leukemia Group B. J Clin Oncol 1989; 7:993–1002.
20. Maurer LH, Herndon JE II, Hollis DR, et al. Randomized trial of chemotherapy and radiation therapy with or without warfarin for limited-stage small-cell lung cancer: a Cancer and Leukemia Group B study. J Clin Oncol 1997; 15:3378–3387.
21. Lebeau B, Chastang C, Brechot JM, et al. Subcutaneous heparin treatment increases survival in small cell lung cancer. "Petites Cellules" Group. Cancer 1994; 74:38–45.
22. Elting LS, Escalante CP, Cooksley C, et al. Outcomes and cost of deep venous thrombosis among patients with cancer. Arch Intern Med 2004; 164:1653–1661.
23. Moher D, Cook DJ, Eastwood S, et al. Improving the quality of reports of meta-analyses of randomised controlled trials: the QUOROM statement. Quality of reporting of meta-analyses. Lancet 1999; 354:1896–1900.
24. Lyman GH, Kuderer NM: The strengths and limitations of meta-analyses based on aggregate data. BMC Med Res Methodol 2005; 5:14.
25. Vigna-Taglianti F, Vineis P, Liberati A, et al. Quality of systematic reviews used in guidelines for oncology practice. Ann Oncol 2006; 17:691–701.
26. Guyatt G, Schunemann HJ, Cook D, et al. Applying the grades of recommendation for antithrombotic and thrombolytic therapy: the Seventh ACCP Conference on Antithrombotic and Thrombolytic Therapy. Chest 2004; 126:179S–187S.
27. Atkins D, Best D, Briss PA, et al. Grading quality of evidence and strength of recommendations. BMJ 2004; 328:1490.
28. Smorenburg SM, Hettiarachchi RJ, Vink R, et al. The effects of unfractionated heparin on survival in patients with malignancy—a systematic review. Thromb Haemost 1999; 82:1600–1604.
29. Smorenburg SM, Vink R, Otten HM, et al. The effects of vitamin K-antagonists on survival of patients with malignancy: a systematic analysis. Thromb Haemost 2001; 86:1586–1587.
30. Fielding LP, Hittinger R, Grace RH, et al. Randomised controlled trial of adjuvant chemotherapy by portal-vein perfusion after curative resection for colorectal adenocarcinoma. Lancet 1992; 340:502–506.
31. Nitti D, Wils J, Sahmoud T, et al. Final results of a phase III clinical trial on adjuvant intraportal infusion with heparin and 5-fluorouracil (5-FU) in resectable colon cancer (EORTC GITCCG 1983–1987). European Organization for Research and Treatment of Cancer. Gastrointestinal Tract Cancer Cooperative Group. Eur J Cancer 1997; 33:1209–1215.
32. Meyer G, Marjanovic Z, Valcke J, et al. Comparison of low-molecular-weight heparin and warfarin for the secondary prevention of venous thromboembolism in patients with cancer: a randomized controlled study. Arch Intern Med 2002; 162:1729–1735.
33. Deitcher SR, Kessler CM, Merli G, et al. Secondary prevention of venous thromboembolic events (VTE) in patients with active malignancy: a randomized study of enoxaparin sodium alone vs. initial enoxaparin sodium followed by warfarin for a 180-day period. J Thromb Haemost 2003; 1, Abstract OC194.
34. Lee AY, Levine MN, Baker RI, et al. Low-molecular-weight heparin versus a coumarin for the prevention of recurrent venous thromboembolism in patients with cancer. N Engl J Med 2003; 349:146–153.
35. Hull RD, Pineo GF, Brant RF, et al. Self-managed long-term low-molecular-weight heparin therapy: the balance of benefits and harms. Am J Med 2007; 120:72–82.
36. Conti S, Guercini F, Iorio A. Low-molecular-weight heparin and cancer survival: review of the literature and pooled analysis of 1,726 patients treated for at least three months. Pathophysiol Haemost Thromb 2003; 33:197–201.
37. Hettiarachchi RJ, Smorenburg SM, Ginsberg J, et al. Do heparins do more than just treat thrombosis? The influence of heparins on cancer spread. Thromb Haemost 1999; 82:947–952.

38. Siragusa S, Cosmi B, Piovella F, et al. Low-molecular-weight heparins and unfractionated heparin in the treatment of patients with acute venous thromboembolism: results of a meta-analysis. Am J Med 1996; 100:269–277.
39. Leonardi MJ, McGory ML, Ko CY. A systematic review of deep venous thrombosis prophylaxis in cancer patients: implications for improving quality. Ann Surg Oncol 2006.
40. Rasmussen MS. Preventing thromboembolic complications in cancer patients after surgery: a role for prolonged thromboprophylaxis. Cancer Treat Rev 2002; 28:141–144.
41. Rasmussen E, Wille-Jorgensen P, Jorgensen LN. Extended out-of-hospital low-molecular-weight heparin prophylaxis against venous thromboembolism in patients after cancer operations: a meta-analysis [abstr]. ISTH 2005.
42. Jorgensen LN, Lausen I, Rasmussen MS, et al. Prolonged thromboprophylaxis with low molecular weight heparin (tinzaparin) following major general surgery primarily for, cancer: an individual patient data meta-analysis. J Thromb Haemost 2005; 1:abstract P1870.
43. Field MJ, Lohr KN. Clinical Practice Guidelines: Directions for a New Program. The National Academies Press, 1990.
44. Geerts WH, Pineo GF, Heit JA, et al. Prevention of venous thromboembolism: the Seventh ACCP Conference on Antithrombotic and Thrombolytic Therapy. Chest 2004; 126:338S–400S.
45. http://nccn.org/professionals/physician_gls/PDF/vte.pdf
46. Mandala M, Falanga A, Piccioli A, et al. Venous thromboembolism and cancer: guidelines of the Italian Association of Medical Oncology (AIOM). Crit Rev Oncol Hematol 2006; 59:194–204.
47. www.asco.org.
48. Dickersin K, Scherer R, Lefebvre C. Identifying relevant studies for systematic reviews. BMJ 1994; 309:1286–1291.
49. Egger M, Smith GD, Schneider M, et al. Bias in meta-analysis detected by a simple, graphical test. BMJ 1997; 315:629–634.
50. Moher D, Jadad AR, Nichol G, et al. Assessing the quality of randomized controlled trials: an annotated bibliography of scales and checklists. Control Clin Trials 1995; 16:62–73.
51. Begg CB, Mazumdar M. Operating characteristics of a rank correlation test for publication bias. Biometrics 1994; 50:1088–1101.
52. Sallah S, Wan JY, Nguyen NP. Venous thrombosis in patients with solid tumors: determination of frequency and characteristics. Thromb Haemost 2002; 87:575–579.
53. Stein PD, Beemath A, Meyers FA, et al. Incidence of venous thromboembolism in patients hospitalized with cancer. Am J Med 2006; 119:60–68.
54. Levitan N, Dowlati A, Remick SC, et al. Rates of initial and recurrent thromboembolic disease among patients with malignancy versus those without malignancy. Risk analysis using Medicare claims data. Medicine (Baltimore) 1999; 78:285–291.
55. Samama MM, Cohen AT, Darmon JY, et al. A comparison of enoxaparin with placebo for the prevention of venous thromboembolism in acutely ill medical patients. Prophylaxis in Medical Patients with Enoxaparin Study Group. N Engl J Med 1999; 341:793–800.
56. Leizorovicz A, Cohen AT, Turpie AG, et al. Randomized, placebo-controlled trial of dalteparin for the prevention of venous thromboembolism in acutely ill medical patients. Circulation 2004; 110:874–879.
57. Cohen AT, Davidson BL, Gallus AS, et al. Efficacy and safety of fondaparinux for the prevention of venous thromboembolism in older acute medical patients: randomised placebo controlled trial. BMJ 2006; 332:325–329.
58. Gardlund B. Randomised, controlled trial of low-dose heparin for prevention of fatal pulmonary embolism in patients with infectious diseases. The Heparin Prophylaxis Study Group. Lancet 1996; 347:1357–1361.
59. Mismetti P, Laporte-Simitsidis S, Tardy B, et al. Prevention of venous thromboembolism in internal medicine with unfractionated or low-molecular-weight heparins: a meta-analysis of randomised clinical trials. Thromb Haemost 2000; 83:14–19.
60. Levine M, Hirsh J, Gent M, et al. Double-blind randomised trial of a very-low-dose warfarin for prevention of thromboembolism in stage IV breast cancer. Lancet 1994; 343:886–889.

61. Wun T, Law L, Harvey D, et al. Increased incidence of symptomatic venous thrombosis in patients with cervical carcinoma treated with concurrent chemotherapy, radiation, and erythropoietin. Cancer 2003; 98:1514–1520.
62. Rosenzweig MQ, Bender CM, Lucke JP, et al. The decision to prematurely terminate a trial of R-HuEPO due to thrombotic events. J Pain Symptom Manage 2004; 27:185–190.
63. Barlogie B, Tricot G, Anaissie E, et al. Thalidomide and hematopoietic-cell transplantation for multiple myeloma. N Engl J Med 2006; 354:1021–1030.
64. Rajkumar SV, Blood E, Vesole D, et al. Phase III clinical trial of thalidomide plus dexamethasone compared with dexamethasone alone in newly diagnosed multiple myeloma: a clinical trial coordinated by the Eastern Cooperative Oncology Group. J Clin Oncol 2006; 24:431–436.
65. Zonder JA, Durie BGM, McCoy J, et al. High incidence of thrombotic events observed in patients receiving Lenalidomide (L) + Dexamethasone (D) (LD) as first-line therapy for multiple myeloma (MM) without Aspirin (ASA) prophylaxis. Blood 2005; 106:3455.
66. Zangari M, Anaissie E, Barlogie B, et al. Increased risk of deep-vein thrombosis in patients with multiple myeloma receiving thalidomide and chemotherapy. Blood 2001; 98:1614–1615.
67. Zangari M, Barlogie B, Anaissie E, et al. Deep vein thrombosis in patients with multiple myeloma treated with thalidomide and chemotherapy: effects of prophylactic and therapeutic anticoagulation. Br J Haematol 2004; 126:715–721.
68. Rus C, Bazzan M, Palumbo A, et al. Thalidomide in front line treatment in multiple myeloma: serious risk of venous thromboembolism and evidence for thromboprophylaxis. J Thromb Haemost 2004; 2:2063–2065.
69. Rajkumar SV, Hayman SR, Lacy MQ, et al. Combination therapy with lenalidomide plus dexamethasone (Rev/Dex) for newly diagnosed myeloma. Blood 2005; 106:4050–4053.
70. Barlogie B, Jagannath S, Desikan KR, et al. Total therapy with tandem transplants for newly diagnosed multiple myeloma. Blood 1999; 93:55–65.
71. Weber D, Rankin K, Gavino M, et al. Thalidomide alone or with dexamethasone for previously untreated multiple myeloma. J Clin Oncol 2003; 21:16–19.
72. Zangari M, Barlogie B, Thertulien R, et al. Thalidomide and deep vein thrombosis in multiple myeloma: risk factors and effect on survival. Clin Lymphoma 2003; 4:32–35.
73. Kakkar AK, Williamson RC. Thromboprophylaxis in malignant disease. Br J Surg 1995; 82:724–725.
74. Kakkar VV, Howe CT, Nicolaides AN, et al. Deep vein thrombosis of the leg. Is there a "high risk" group? Am J Surg 1970; 120:527–530.
75. Agnelli G, Bolis G, Capussotti L, et al. A clinical outcome-based prospective study on venous thromboembolism after cancer surgery: the @RISTOS project. Ann Surg 2006; 243:89–95.
76. Kakkar AK, Haas S, Wolf H, et al. Evaluation of perioperative fatal pulmonary embolism and death in cancer surgical patients: the MC-4 cancer substudy. Thromb Haemost 2005; 94:867–871.
77. Clarke-Pearson DL, Synan IS, Dodge R, et al. A randomized trial of low-dose heparin and intermittent pneumatic calf compression for the prevention of deep venous thrombosis after gynecologic oncology surgery. Am J Obstet Gynecol 168:1146–1153; discussion 1993:1153–1154.
78. Clarke-Pearson DL, Dodge RK, Synan I, et al. Venous thromboembolism prophylaxis: patients at high risk to fail intermittent pneumatic compression. Obstet Gynecol 2003; 101:157–163.
79. Roderick P, Fens G, Wilson K et al: towards evidence based guidelines for the prevention of venous thromboembolism; systematic reviews of mechanical methods, oral anticoagulation, dextran and regional anaesthesia as thromboprophylaxis. Health Technology Assessment 2005; 9.
80. Kakkar VV, Corrigan TP, Fossard DP prevention of fatal post operative pulmonary embolism by low doses of heparin. An international multi centre trial. Lancet 1975:2:45-51.
81. Bergqvist D, Burmark US, Flordal PA, et al. Low molecular weight heparin started before surgery as prophylaxis against deep vein thrombosis: 2500 versus 5000 XaI units in 2070 patients. Br J Surg 1995; 82:496–501.
82. Wille-Jorgensen P, Rasmussen MS, Andersen BR, et al. Heparins and mechanical methods for thromboprophylaxis in colorectal surgery. Cochrane Database Syst Rev 2003; CD001217.

83. Bergqvist D, Agnelli G, Cohen AT, et al. Duration of prophylaxis against venous thromboembolism with enoxaparin after surgery for cancer. N Engl J Med 2002; 346:975–980.
84. Rasmussen MS. Does prolonged thromboprophylaxis improve outcome in patients undergoing surgery? Cancer Treat Rev 2003; 29(suppl 2):15–17.
85. Buller HR, Agnelli G, Hull RD, et al. Antithrombotic therapy for venous thromboembolic disease: the Seventh ACCP Conference on Antithrombotic and Thrombolytic Therapy. Chest 2004; 126:401S–428S.
86. Deitcher SR, Kessler CM, Merli G, et al. Secondary prevention of venous thromboembolic events in patients with active cancer: enoxaparin alone versus initial enoxaparin followed by warfarin for a 180-day period. Clin Appl Thromb Hemost 2006; 12:389–396.
87. Levin JM, Schiff D, Loeffler JS, et al. Complications of therapy for venous thromboembolic disease in patients with brain tumors. Neurology 1993; 43:1111–1114.
88. Olin JW, Young JR, Graor RA, et al. Treatment of deep vein thrombosis and pulmonary emboli in patients with primary and metastatic brain Tumors. Anticoagulants or inferior vena cava filter? Arch INT Med 1987: 147:2177-2179.
89. Schiff D, DeAngelis LM. Therapy of venous thromboembolism in patients with brain metastases. Cancer 1994; 73:493–498.
90. Agnelli G, Piovella F, Buoncristiani P, et al. Enoxaparin plus compression stockings compared with compression stockings alone in the prevention of venous thromboembolism after elective neurosurgery. N Engl J Med 1998; 339:80–85.
91. Iorio A, Agnelli G: Low-molecular-weight and unfractionated heparin for prevention of venous thromboembolism in neurosurgery: a meta-analysis. Arch Intern Med 2000; 160:2327–2332.
92. Bates SM, Ginsberg JS. Clinical practice. Treatment of deep-vein thrombosis. N Engl J Med 2004; 351:268–277.
93. Lopez-Jimenez L, Montero M, Gonzalez-Fajardo JA, et al. Venous thromboembolism in very elderly patients: findings from a prospective registry (RIETE). Haematologica 2006; 91:1046–1051.
94. Garcia D, Regan S, Crowther M, et al. Warfarin maintenance dosing patterns in clinical practice: implications for safer anticoagulation in the elderly population. Chest 2005; 127:2049–2056.
95. Copland M, Walker ID, Tait RC. Oral anticoagulation and hemorrhagic complications in an elderly population with atrial fibrillation. Arch Intern Med 2001; 161:2125–2128.
96. Gould MK, Dembitzer AD, Doyle RL, et al. Low-molecular-weight heparins compared with unfractionated heparin for treatment of acute deep venous thrombosis. A meta-analysis of randomized, controlled trials. Ann Intern Med 1999; 130:800–809.
97. Dolovich LR, Ginsberg JS, Douketis JD, et al. A meta-analysis comparing low-molecular-weight heparins with unfractionated heparin in the treatment of venous thromboembolism: examining some unanswered questions regarding location of treatment, product type, and dosing frequency. Arch Intern Med 2000; 160:181–188.
98. Altinbas M, Coskun HS, Er O, et al. A randomized clinical trial of combination chemotherapy with and without low-molecular-weight heparin in small cell lung cancer. J Thromb Haemost 2004; 2:1266–1271.
99. Klerk CP, Smorenburg SM, Otten HM, et al. The effect of low molecular weight heparin on survival in patients with advanced malignancy. J Clin Oncol 2005; 23:2130–2135.
100. Sideras K, Schaefer PL, Okuno SH, et al. Low-molecular-weight heparin in patients with advanced cancer: a phase 3 clinical trial. Mayo Clin Proc 2006; 81:758–767.
101. Kuderer NM, Khorana AA, Gyman GH, Francis CW: A meta-analysis and systematic review of the efficacy and safety of anticoagulants as cancer treatment. Cancer, published online July 17, 2007.

Index

Cancer-Associated Thrombosis